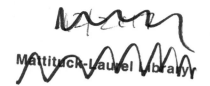
Nutritional Healing
with
Chinese Medicine

+175 Recipes for Optimal Health

Ellen Goldsmith, MSOM, LAc, DipCH
with **Maya Klein**, PhD

Robert
ROSE

For complete cataloguing information, see page 480.

Disclaimer
This book is a general guide only and should never be a substitute for the skill, knowledge and experience of a qualified medical professional dealing with the facts, circumstances and symptoms of a particular case.

The medical and health information presented in this book is based on the research, training and professional experience of the authors, and is true and complete to the best of their knowledge. However, this book is intended only as an informative guide for those wishing to know more about health and nutrition from the perspective of Traditional Chinese Medicine; it is not intended to replace or countermand the advice given by the reader's personal physician. Because each person and situation is unique, the authors and the publisher urge the reader to check with a qualified health-care professional before using any procedure where there is a question as to its appropriateness. The authors and the publisher are not responsible for any adverse effects or consequences resulting from the use of the information in this book. It is the responsibility of the reader to consult a physician or other qualified health-care professional regarding his or her personal care.

The recipes in this book have been carefully tested by our kitchen and our tasters. To the best of our knowledge, they are safe and nutritious for ordinary use and users. For those people with food or other allergies, or who have special food requirements or health issues, please read the suggested contents of each recipe carefully and determine whether or not they may create a problem for you. All recipes are used at the risk of the consumer. We cannot be responsible for any hazards, loss or damage that may occur as a result of any recipe use. For those with special needs, allergies, requirements or health problems, in the event of any doubt, please contact your medical adviser prior to the use of any recipe.

Design and production: Daniella Zanchetta/PageWave Graphics Inc.
Editor: Fina Scroppo
Recipe Editor: Tina Anson Mine
Copyeditor: Sheila Wawanash
Indexer: Belle Wong

Cover image: Gingerroot on wooden table © Villagemoon/iStock/Getty Images Plus
Back cover images: Bok choy © Elenathewise/iStock/Getty Images Plus; Superfoods in bowls
© Marilyna/iStock/Getty Images Plus
Interior images & illustrations: p.44 Balanced pebbles © VictorBurnside/iStock/Getty Images Plus;
pgs.35, 206, 210, 242, 286, 320, 366, 410 and 422 Seamless patterns © Ulimi/Gettyimages.ca/
DigitalVision Vectors

Published by Robert Rose Inc.
120 Eglinton Avenue East, Suite 800, Toronto, Ontario, Canada M4P 1E2
Tel: (416) 322-6552 Fax: (416) 322-6936
www.robertrose.ca

Printed and bound in Canada

1 2 3 4 5 6 7 8 9   MI   25 24 23 22 21 20 19 18 17

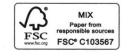

Contents

Introduction — Why This Book?

*"Those who take medicine and neglect their diet,
waste the skill of the physician."*

— *Chinese proverb*

If you struggle making the right food choices to improve your health, you're not alone. Many of us are confused about what to eat, driven by things other than common sense. But there is a solution, and it is rooted in the ancient wisdom of Chinese medicine. It's a system focused on accessing the therapeutic potency of food for healing that you can learn to adopt and integrate into everyday living — and its effectiveness is well documented over centuries of use.

So, why do so many us end up at the doctor's office with problems directly related to our diet? In these modern times, we have gotten lost on the path to eating well. We see the fallout in the rising rates of preventable chronic diseases, such as obesity, childhood diabetes and cardiovascular disease. Where do we turn? Do we source the latest research or hop on the latest diet craze?

There are lots of diets but there is also a treasure trove of wisdom about food and health right before us in nature that we can access. It's precisely what this book is about. The ancient Chinese were excellent observers of nature, cultivating and developing a system of health and healing that is embedded in their traditions in which food and its medicinal value are deeply intertwined.

As an acupuncturist and practitioner of Chinese medicine who has studied and taught food therapeutics over the last three decades, I see how confused people are about the link between what they eat and how they are feeling. They want help on how to create a daily diet that they enjoy and adapt without added stress. People come to me, as an acupuncturist, because they want relief from pain, from fatigue, from feeling out of balance; they want change, and they want it instantly. However, change is incremental — it took some time to not feel well and it will take some time to reverse the trend, but it is well worth it and its effects are enduring. Food is one of the best places to start. If you have ever tried to change your diet only to slip back to old habits, you know how tricky it is to maintain long-lasting change. I know because I was that person for many years. I started out as a vegetarian, became a lousy one at that, eating lots of cheese, nuts, fruit and essentially hardly eating meals. Then the macrobiotic diet —

a whole foods, mostly plant-based diet that includes a small amount of fish and whose energetic principles are similar to Chinese dietetics — helped steer me in the right direction. I learned about the energy of food as well as the cooking methods to optimize nutrients. I felt fantastic, for a couple of years, and then I hit a plateau. What I did not understand is that diet is dynamic and needs to change as we change, as our health changes, as the seasons change and as our activities change. Adopting the Chinese medicine approach to diet, whereby food and its inherent properties can support health, has made the biggest difference.

Studying Chinese medicine and its underlying principles of food as medicine has provided a solid understanding that I can apply to modern life. It has helped me learn to listen to my body and its needs, to be more patient, and to be attuned to how climate and the changing seasons affect my body, knowing what worked for me months ago or years ago may need to be adjusted at different stages of life. I have more energy than I did 30 years ago, my weight is stable and I know how to adapt food to support health and treat illness.

In *Nutritional Healing with Chinese Medicine*, you will learn about the wisdom of using food to heal the body. You will not find a prescribed diet, rather a guide to cultivating and increasing your innate power of observation and capacity to make and prepare vibrant food choices that support your health and well-being. Allow yourself to embark on a journey, albeit through a new land and language, with some familiar foods along the way. If you are not familiar with Chinese medicine, this book will serve as a guide to understanding how food and medicine are inseparable. For those with some knowledge of Chinese medicine and herbalism, you may discover strong healing parallels of herbs in everyday foods. As I tell my Chinese medicine students, "Your patients may come to you for a while for acupuncture, they may take the herbs you prescribe for a period of time, but they will eat every day for the rest of their lives."

The foundations and principles of Chinese medicine and food therapy traditions are applicable to you wherever you live, no matter your food culture and traditions, because Chinese medicine is rooted in nature and the order of change. Once you understand its principles, you will learn how to adapt eating to the seasons, the climate, your state of health and vitality. I have witnessed the role good food and eating habits play in improving and transforming people's health, energy and mood.

I hope this book helps you connect to food in a way that works for you, frees you from a fixed and static diet and helps you feel better in both mind and body. Use this book as you wish — you can start at the beginning, or in the kitchen by cooking up more than 175 recipes provided (see page 206 to start), or by learning about the nature and flavors of specific foods (Chapter 3, page 38). Let's go on a journey together to good health. When you sit down to eat, take a moment to take in the colors and aroma, and as the Chinese say, *Màn man chi* or "eat slowly and enjoy your food." Get ready to appreciate a new way of eating that helps build health and vitality for years to come.

Part 1

Foundations of Chinese Medicine

Chapter 1

Traditions of Food and Healing in China

"To the people, food is heaven."

— *Chinese proverb*

It goes without saying that, for most of us, eating is an enjoyable experience, filled with a variety of delightful tastes and textures. What you may *not* know is how that same food can help you heal, maintain good health and increase longevity. The ancient Chinese knew how to eat this way for centuries and developed traditions of food and healing that have endured to this day.

In modern Western culture, the enjoyment of "heavenly foods" is often equated with decadent, sensuous and often unhealthy fare that my daughter describes as "food that is usually sweet or salty and creamy or salty and crunchy — packed with intense flavor and texture that makes you want more!" To her, heavenly food includes pizza, cookies, brownies and ice cream. Why is it that she, like so many others, considers foods that are bad for our health, especially when we eat them in excess, heavenly fare? Why does the association with heavenly foods have to be a love-hate relationship? For most of us, it is difficult to stop eating these foods until we either feel full or reach the point of feeling sick. The aftermath is not pretty either. We feel guilty for giving in to temptation and have an intense desire to clean out our bodies with a nutritional cleanse or a special diet.

It's easy to understand the attachment we may have to these foods. When you take the intense flavor — often produced by high amounts of salt, sugar and fat — out of a diet, real whole food can seem dull and boring. But it doesn't have to be that way. There is a middle ground where food can be delicious and also be good for us, leave us feeling satisfied and act as our medicine ... quite a heavenly proposition.

Food as Medicine

In Chinese culture, people know that "food heals and medicine is food." Food and medicine are one and the same and part of everyday life. Many Chinese families still live by this maxim, knowing what and how to eat when, for example, they are sick or fatigued or a family member is recovering from childbirth. This ancient wisdom is embedded in the culture.

This cultural wisdom also introduces another way to think about food that we could adopt in the West, something I learned to do when studying the ancient traditions of Chinese medicine. For the Chinese, the relationship to food is grounded in the values of preventing harm and promoting longevity, which emerged out of the ancient traditions and practices of "nurturing life." Nurturing life (*yang sheng* — 杨生), which forms the core and foundation of Chinese medicine, was written about in the classic text of Chinese medicine, the *Huangdi Neijing Suwen* (*The Yellow Emperor's Classic of Medicine*), which emphasized that an individual's lifestyle and habits play a key role in maintaining and cultivating long-lasting health. Sun Simiao, the 7th century sage and "father" of Chinese medicine, also wrote about it in the classic text the *Bei Ji Qian Jin Yao Fang* (*Essential Formulas Worth a Thousand in Gold to Prepare for Emergencies*), written around 625 CE. He emphasized daily habits to nurture the body with food and herbs, regular exercise to promote internal strength and flow, adequate rest, and moderation in food, drink and work to nurture physical, mental and emotional health. At the root of nurturing life practices is the use of food as medicine.

Early Evidence

Nurturing life practices were adopted by Chinese herbalists, sages and physicians and written about in Chinese medical texts. After tasting and testing the effects of herbs and foods, they documented and codified their energetic and healing properties.

The importance of food and health was later evident in the Imperial Court of the Yuan dynasty in the 14th century, where the emperor employed Hu Sihui to serve his family as a court therapist and dietitian, recommending foods that would ensure long life and good health. Hu Sihui went on to write the *Yinshan Zhengyao* (*A Soup for the Qan Chinese Dietary Medicine of the Mongol Era*), one of the early pivotal texts in the development of Chinese dietary therapy. The book became a manual for eating for health, with guides on eating in moderation, variety in the diet and special diets for pregnant women and children.

"Medicine and food share the same origin."

— *Common expression in Chinese medical theory*

Did You Know?

The earliest texts where foods and herbs were classified according to certain properties can be found in three foundation books — the *Jin Gui Yao Lue* (*Essentials from the Golden Cabinet*), the *Shang Han Lun* (*Treatise on Cold Damage*) and the *Shen Nong Ben Cao Jing* (*The Divine Farmers' Materia Medica*) — written more than 2,000 years ago and still used today to guide the practice of Chinese medicine and nutritional healing.

It also recognized cross-cultural influences with the inclusion of Mongolian, Turkic and Islamic foods that had influences on Chinese food therapeutics. The kitchen became not just a place to make meals, but also a sort of alchemical laboratory where the preparation of specific foods were discovered to have heavenly attributes of health, vitality and longevity. And many of the foods, including adzuki beans, cardamom, goji berries, orange peel and lamb, are still considered important therapeutic ingredients in today's cooking.

The continued exchange of medicine and food traditions spread with migrating tribes, traders and explorers along the Silk Road through China into Eurasia, the Middle East and Southern Europe. At the same time, traditions of food as medicine were also alive and being practiced by the Romans, Greeks, Mayans, Egyptians and Indigenous people throughout the world, whose civilizations shared similar insight into the power of food for healing. Indeed, it was Hippocrates, the Greek father of modern medicine, who wrote, "Let food be thy medicine and medicine be thy food." These traditions continue, seeded by ancient wisdom and continuous practice by Ayurvedic doctors and practitioners in India, as well as Native American and Indigenous peoples throughout the world. We also see these practices passed down from one generation to another in Europe, Africa, Iran and Mexico and all throughout Central and South America.

Adopting Traditional Practices

We know that generations before us knew how to soothe an aching throat, nourish a mother after childbirth and calm tension with soups or teas. They knew how to cook and use foods, alone or combined with other foods and herbs, to restore health and harmony in each season and each stage of life. Our ancestors knew how to make food taste good by using the coveted herbs and spices they grew or procured. They understood that spices and herbs made certain flavors in food come to life in the distinct flavor palate of their culture. They were aware of the plants that activated and improved digestion, and increased and balanced energy.

While numerous cultures have healing traditions of dietary practices, the Chinese articulated their concepts well over thousands of years and wrote about them extensively. Their wisdom continues to play an important role in their medicine and culture to this day.

Food from the Earth: The Influences of Location and Climate

The Chinese have taught us that, to live in harmony with the forces of nature, location and climate can affect and determine what one eats. In ancient times, Chinese and other early civilizations learned through necessity how to balance natural forces through the foods they grew, prepared and ate — these populations were indeed the original locavores. There was no global food system, so people had to invest in raising and accessing the best food possible from the region in which they lived. Food and eating was really a regional matter. As crops were susceptible to fluctuations in weather and climate, people had to work with their geographic location, soil, climate and water sources, among other elements, to optimize food production, and they had to make their food last beyond the growing season. To nourish, maintain and protect their health, methods of extracting optimal nourishment in the preparation and preservation of food were developed.

Preserving Nourishment through Food Preservation

In the past, without refrigeration, eating fresh food throughout the year was not possible. With some chance discoveries, experimentation and invention, people found ways, such as fermenting and drying, to preserve foods to sustain themselves and their families through the colder months.

Fermentation

Fermentation brought us alcohol from fermented grains, herbs and fruits. In fact, the use of alcohol as a medicinal agent in ancient China dates back approximately 4,000 years. Fermentation is also the process used in the making of tamari, miso, tempeh, vinegar, kombucha, fish sauce and many types of pickled vegetables and fruits. Fermented foods are not only used to improve the flavor of dishes, but also to assist digestion by breaking down complex proteins and adding beneficial bacteria to the gut. Today, fermented foods like sauerkraut, pickles and yogurt are enjoyed around the world for their intense flavor as well as health benefits.

Did You Know?
Fermenting and drying foods are two of the oldest preservation methods.

Drying

Like fermentation, the drying of grains, herbs, spices, vegetables, fruits and animal products also assured food's longevity. Drying intensifies the flavor and potency of foods, rendering them usable throughout the seasons. Many of the same dried spices and herbs we find in today's pantry are a treasure trove of culinary flavors and medicinal benefits that have been used in Chinese and Western healing traditions for centuries.

While we now have refrigeration as an additional method of preservation, we can use both dried and fermented foods to support and maintain health in addition to enjoying their intense flavor.

Climate and Diet

The effects of climate play a key role in the foods recommended in Chinese nutrition. We know that each locale generates different types of foods. But how does climate play a role in what we eat at different times? Differing types of climates — such as damp and temperate, hot and humid, dry and hot, and dry and cold — can affect decisions about what to eat to support optimal health.

The ancient Chinese knew that, to preserve health, you need to create an internal environment that balances the external forces of climate. If it is constantly damp outside, for example, it's important to counter that dampness internally by eating foods that counter external dampness. If you live in a cold climate, you would need to consume foods that provide inner warmth without drying you out. Likewise, in warmer climates, it is recommended that you eat foods that keep you cool. So warming foods to keep you warm when it's cold outside, cooling foods to keep you cool when it's hot outside, and foods that counter dampness when it's damp outside. Many people instinctively eat to cool down or warm up, but there is a bit more to it when eating for balance. According to the foundations of Chinese nutritional healing, it is also essential to know which foods are considered warming or cooling, moistening or drying and best at different times of the year, as well as how the flavors of food act on the body.

Where you live matters. The climate you live in matters. Chinese nutritional healing advocates that not all people eat the same way. In later chapters, you will learn what specific foods to eat according to where you live and the state of your health.

The Seasons Go Round and Round

Our bodies are affected in many ways by the change of seasons. The ancient cultures recognized that as the weather changes, so too does the need to adapt and change activities, habits and nourishment to maintain health. Attuning to the activity of each season is one of the cornerstones of Chinese medicine and nutritional therapy. No matter where we live on the planet, there are variations in temperature, light, dryness and dampness, with each element impacting human health. Eating salads, some fresh local berries or ice cold watermelon during the summer may be a typical way to enjoy the foods and flavors of a hot season, but eating these same foods near the end of summer or during the winter is counter to what the ancient Chinese taught us about balance and "heavenly" eating. Why? Because those foods are cooling, and as the summer wanes, our body needs to protect its inner warmth as it adapts to the oncoming cooler weather.

Let's go back to the idea of location and climate and apply it to seasonal eating: eat locally as much as possible and eat the foods that protect and promote internal balance to the external forces. If it is windy, we need to protect ourselves from the wind; if it is hot, we need to maintain an even internal temperature to avoid becoming overheated; and when it is cold, we need to protect ourselves from the cold while generating internal warmth and hydration.

We do this by including the foods that are in season, by adjusting our cooking styles, and by understanding what the thermal nature and flavor of foods are and how they influence the body so we can make choices appropriate to the prevailing energy of the season.

Let's Start with Spring

Spring, for example, is a time when we emerge from of a long period of hibernation and of storing nourishment and warmth internally — a shift that requires energy and force. In spring, we move from indoors to outdoors and start to clear out and shed some of the winter "weight" in order to participate fully in the season. Our cooking becomes lighter and fresher; foods with pungent and sweet flavors — as well as a range of foods that are neutral, cooling and warming — are added to the diet to help us move up and out into spring. Foods that promote upward and outward movement are some of the first foods of spring — pungent and sweet flavors found in chives, arugula, radishes, sweet peas, fresh spring greens, baby carrots and beets. Balance is key. As much as eating shifts to lighter and fresher fare, the body

> "The *qi* of the body flows in accordance with the changes of heaven and earth (the seasons)."
>
> — *Huangdi Neijing Suwen, The Yellow Emperor's Classic of Medicine*

still needs to maintain internal warmth, a type of counterbalance, which can be found in the warming pungent and aromatic herbs and spices, such as ginger, garlic, dill, basil, rosemary, thyme, fennel, nutmeg and cardamom.

When Winter Arrives

Did You Know?

As we stay indoors physically and figuratively during winter, Chinese medicine also encourages us to make time to rest, protect ourselves from the elements and meditate to restore our deepest energy, reflecting the energy of winter, which goes underground to regenerate.

In contrast, winter eating needs to support inner warming and storage — with foods that generate warmth, such as certain soups, stews, tonic wines and beverages, herbs and spices. Foods with a cooling bitter flavor need to be added to the diet to counter and drain the buildup and storage of that internal heat. Some of those foods include bitter greens, grapefruit and black or green tea. Winter is a time to build inner resources and capacity through the foods we eat and the activities we participate in.

The ancient Chinese considered living in harmony with the seasons as fundamental to protecting vitality. As the *Huangdi Neijing* says, "Therefore the change of yin and yang through the four seasons is the root of life, growth, reproduction, aging and destruction. By respecting this natural law it is possible to be free from illness. The sages have followed this, and the foolish people have not." (See Chapter 5 and the recipes in this book to learn more about seasonal eating.)

The Basics: Thermal Nature, Flavor, Yin and Yang

In understanding what to eat, the teachings of the ancient Chinese tell us that it is impossible to separate food from life, nature, location, climate and the seasons. In essence, the key to understanding the Chinese medicine approach to diet is by learning about the foundational principles of the medicine as it applies to food; its thermal nature and flavor, together with the forces of yin and yang, and their combined action and potency on the body.

Thermal Nature

In the West, we have common-sense instincts about eating foods to warm us or cool us down. The ancient sages, Daoists and practitioners of nurturing life built upon those same instincts and added another dimension, creating distinct classifications for the warming and cooling actions that foods and herbs have on the body. Their documents termed the thermal nature of food as *xing* or *qi* (see Chapters 2 and 3 for more information). Together, the thermal nature (*qi*) and flavors of foods are considered to influence the internal balance of yin and yang balance within the body and can give people a dynamic way in which to adapt their diet.

Flavors

In Chinese medicine, flavors are not defined in the way we think about them in the West; that is, the sensory experience of tasting food. Flavor is therapeutic. To be sure, we taste foods and have flavor preferences, too, but in Chinese medicine, flavor is another key to understanding how to choose appropriate foods according to what action those flavors have on the body. A sweet flavor will nourish and balance; sour will contain and draw into the body; salty will descend, consolidate and soften; bitter will drain and purge; and the pungent flavor will lift and disperse. Flavor combinations make a meal "heavenly" and healthy.

Yin and Yang

Finally, flavor and thermal nature are woven into the foundational principles of yin and yang — the most complex concept of Chinese medicine — as a guide to creating balance. Simply put, yin and yang are the opposing and connecting forces of nature. Yang is the energy of the sun, warming, motivating, energizing and the embodiment of *qi* (vital force). Yin is the energy of the moon and night, cooling, moistening, nourishing, embedded in the substance of vital body fluids and blood, the anchor for our spirit (*shen*). All flavors and thermal natures are related to yin and yang — sweet and pungent are yang, while sour, bitter and salty are yin. The spectrum of food's capacity to warm or cool also falls on the spectrum of yin and yang — hot and warming are more yang, while cooling and cold are more yin, and neutral rests as the balancing point. Yin and yang can be difficult to grasp, but when you experience a sustained sense of flow and ease in your energy, the food you eat and your health, the yin and yang are considered to be in a dynamic state of balance.

> **Did You Know?**
>
> The foundations of Chinese medicine and the Chinese use of food for nutritional healing is classified according to yin and yang, the thermal nature (*qi*) and the classification of flavors in foods. The practice of Chinese medicine also includes herbal medicine, acupuncture, bodywork, qi gong and shamanism.

> **Note**
>
> Some of these concepts may seem confusing at this point, but they will become clearer as you read on. For now, it is helpful to understand that the ancient traditions of food and healing that emanated from China can be a vital component in your journey to health. We can learn from them — we simply have to learn a new language and apply it to the foods available to us in our own locale, climate and seasons. By adopting the traditions of food and healing developed by Chinese medicine and practiced by generations for thousands of years, we can bring that "heavenly" wisdom into our kitchens to enhance our long-term health.

Chapter 2

Chinese Medicine — Straight From Nature

"Look deep into nature, and then you will understand everything better."

— *Albert Einstein*

Albert Einstein was not a practitioner of Chinese medicine, but he fundamentally understood it. He understood that everything in nature and the universe are inherently connected. Many of his theories derived from his keen observation of natural phenomena in his environment as he noted patterns, causes and effects, ultimately developing theories about the cosmos and the universe.

Likewise, the underlying theories of Chinese medicine, and the practice of healing with food — the subject of this book — are also based on the observation of nature, change and transformation. Chinese medicine practitioners study the interaction of humans and nature in the natural world and are trained to identify patterns of change and recognize their interplay within the human body.

In Chinese medicine, everything is connected. All the parts make a whole; every symptom and lifestyle habit is part of an individual's total health picture. It's an integrative, holistic and individualized approach that can provide a powerful medicine in the high-tech 21st century. The tools and therapies of Chinese medicine offer an "energetic" intervention in the forms of nutritional therapy, acupuncture, herbal medicine, bodywork and movement and exercise (qi gong) to promote balance and activate healing.

What is Qi Gong?

Qi gong is the practice of gentle movement, breathing and meditation to strengthen and circulate *qi*. Many Chinese medicine practitioners will recommend that their patients practice qi gong.

Chinese Medicine: Its Origins

Dating back more than 3,000 years, Chinese medicine is one of the oldest holistic healing traditions and complete medical systems that has been practiced, continuously adapting and evolving through time. Ancient Chinese Daoists, sages and physicians worked with the only resource they had to help people stay healthy: foods, plants and herbs, as well as the power of the human body. They observed patterns in nature, tested foods and herbs, and noted their effects. They developed physical techniques and exercises to build and maintain vigor and vitality. Then they codified what they observed and discovered. The ancient texts, which date back to the Han dynasty in China in the 2nd century BC, are still used today. For example, the *Huangdi Neijing Suwen*, also known as *The Yellow Emperor's Classic of Medicine,* describes the philosophy, diagnostic and therapeutic concepts that practitioners use to diagnose and treat disease. Even though this important book was written more than 2,500 years ago, the following quote from Chapter 1 still holds true:

> *In the past ... they ate a balanced diet at regular times, arose and retired at regular hours, avoided overstressing bodies and minds, and refrained from overindulgence of all kinds. They maintained well-being of body and mind; thus, it is not surprising that they lived over 100 years. These days people have changed their way of life. ... They fail to regulate their lifestyle, diet and sleep properly. So it is not surprising that they look old at 50 and die soon after.*

Eastern and Western Medicine: What's the Difference?

Chinese medicine differs from Western medicine, yet they can both help relieve suffering. Western medicine looks at the mechanisms of disease, examines the parts of the body that are affected and treats the symptoms. Chinese medicine seeks to identify patterns of disharmony. Practitioners analyze the "part" in relation to the whole person, which is why so much attention is paid to the patterns and details of an individual's health history and lifestyle. Chinese medicine practitioners treat to relieve suffering while considering the pattern and relationship of these symptoms to possible underlying root causes and patterns, and offer energetic intervention to stimulate healing. While Western medicine can provide excellent care for acute and urgent emergency health problems, Chinese medicine can

> **Tip**
> If you're experiencing a serious health problem, consult your primary health-care provider, whether they are a medical doctor, naturopathic or osteopathic physician, physician assistant or nurse practitioner, to support your health. A Chinese medicine practitioner and acupuncturist can work with you at the same time as you see your medical doctor.

be effective in the treatment of many chronic lifestyle diseases. However, Chinese medicine also has a long history in resolving more acute problems, including relieving some types of acute and chronic pain, headaches, allergies, indigestion, viruses and common colds.

Another important distinction is that health is not considered separate from illness in Chinese medicine. Health and illness are connected, two sides of the same coin. Recognizing that disease does not come out of the blue but rather that many chronic illnesses develop from an underlying pattern of disharmony and conditions fed by a combination of poor lifestyle habits, genetics and environmental factors, Chinese medicine doctors first focus on *preventing* disease. And as first noted by the ancient doctors, what you eat and how you live have long been considered important factors in the prevention and subsequent treatment of disease. Among a number of therapies and lifestyle recommendations used to optimize health and prevent disease, practitioners offer guidance in nutritional recommendations, the focus of this book.

The Big Language of Chinese Medicine

"If you grasp the wisdom that is contained in the workings of the universe and expressed in the realm of philosophy, you will be able to safeguard your physical health."

— The Book of Songs: The Ancient Chinese Classic of Poetry (Shijing)

Chinese medicine developed a dynamic language, describing and representing the nature of phenomena as reflected through the theory of yin-yang and its manifestations in the body. There are patterns, rules — or, as we call them — laws of nature, which are seen outside every day, whether it is in the energy of the rising sun, the changing winds, the growth of spring or the barren, cold terrain of winter. Such patterns influence and, in some ways, dictate our level and type of activity throughout the changing seasons as well as the quality and length of our rest every night. Cycles in nature and life are constant, and how we interact with them affects health.

The constant interplay of opposites forms the foundation of Chinese medicine's fundamental understanding of change and transformation, known as yin and yang — dark and light, rest and activity, night and day — and is the basis for explaining all phenomena as it relates to life. It is the relationship of yin and yang in the body, along with other concepts known as *qi* (pronounced *chee*), blood, *jing* (constitution) and *shen* (spirit), that make up a Chinese medicine diagnosis, lifestyle recommendations and treatment.

In this chapter, the concepts of Chinese medicine are introduced. In Chapter 3, you will learn how these theories form the foundation of Chinese nutritional therapy. Once you learn the basics and some new language, it will be easier to understand nutritional healing with Chinese medicine.

The Basic Principles

If you can understand that the underlying principles of Chinese nutritional healing with Chinese medicine are all about balance, connectedness and wholeness, it will be easier to grasp presumably abstract concepts. The ideas discussed later in the chapter are easily and potently applied to food, from specific choices of foods and how they are cooked to how they are put together to create balanced meals during each season.

As noted earlier, the concepts that form the foundation of Chinese medicine and represent processes and substances in the body are yin and yang, *qi*, blood, body fluids, *jing* and *shen*, which are all part of a body-mind tapestry that interacts with external environmental influences, such as the changing seasons and the elements of climate (wind, heat, dampness, dryness and cold). In addition, the Five Phases of transformation, more commonly known as the Five Elements, a theory used more extensively in the West to better grasp the concept of yin and yang, will be explained later in this chapter. Understanding these basic concepts will help when we look at how food is used to promote healing with Chinese medicine. Let's begin.

> **Did You Know?**
>
> Chinese medicine is becoming more and more common in the West and is often offered to people in hospitals, as well as in pain and integrative medicine clinics, to supplement conventional medical treatment or in some cases as a standalone treatment option to resolve a wide variety of health issues.

Yin and Yang: A Dynamic Balance

Yin-yang may seem abstract as a concept, but these two seemingly opposing forces in nature are easily observed and are part of our daily experience. According to Chinese medicine, their dynamic state of balance is key to our health. Waking in the morning to start the day, the sun (warming yang energy) streams through the window, we begin to move and the day's activities begin. As evening descends, the cooling and moist (yin) energy begins to pervade; the moon rises as the day comes to a close and we slow down to stillness and rest. Day in and day out, season after season, cycles of activity and rest follow each other and the cycle is repeated. Seemingly opposite forces interact and function together within our bodies and in nature. The energetic effects of food, flavor, nature and how we use them to maintain and improve

> "The law of yin and yang is the natural order of the universe, the foundation of all things, mother of all changes."
>
> — *Huangdi Neijing Suwen, The Yellow Emperor's Classic of Medicine*

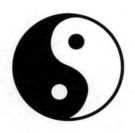

Yin and Yang symbol

health throughout the seasons all depend on balancing yin and yang, as we will see in the coming chapters.

Within each of us, yin and yang are constantly interacting and responding to changes in our environment, food and state of health (see table below). How can these opposite energies exist together? Think of a hillside, where we may only see one side of it and yet, there is another beyond our sight. Both the sunny side (the warming yang side) and the shady side (the cool yin side) of a hill comprise the whole hillside. The hill can't exist without these two terrains, together. The same analogy can be used with yin and yang to describe a day: the brightness of the day turns to night, comprising one cycle of a day. This brings to the fore another aspect of yin and yang — everything changes and can turn into its opposite; day becomes night, night becomes day. Yin and yang exist together and are inseparable. We cannot have day without night and vice versa. Thus, in Chinese medicine, yin and yang are always considered as relative to and in relation to each other in the body.

Qualities of Yin and Yang

Yin	Yang
Night, the moon	Day, the sun
Dark	Light
Winter, autumn	Summer, spring
Interior	Exterior
At rest	Active
Substance and storage	Function and activating
Cooling, moistening	Warming, drying
Blood and body fluids (moisture)	*Qi*
Contracting, consolidating, astringent	Expanding, dispersing
Flavors: sour, salty, bitter	Flavors: pungent (aromatic), sweet (not added sugar)
Descending	Rising
Turbid	Clear

There are times, however, when yin and yang are out of balance. Perhaps yin becomes predominant, in which case we can feel weaker, lethargic, colder and "damp" (more on this later in the chapter). If yang, the more active and warming force in the body, becomes predominant, it is easier to feel agitated, hot, impatient, prone to fever or even outbursts of frustration, irritability or anger. As much as the yin-yang balance can be disrupted, there is a lot we can do to bring it back into balance. Adjusting the food we eat to tip the scale back to center to counter an excess of yin or yang will become clearer in the following chapters.

Cycles of Yin-Yang

Before we examine how yin and yang are expressed through food, let's look at some of the principles that explain the fundamental concept of yin and yang.

Yin and yang are opposites, yet they coexist and are indivisible at all times.

Even though we can distinguish the qualities of activity and rest, hot and cold, day and night, front and back; yin and yang, nothing in life exists without its opposite. Yin and yang are opposites, yet relative, and inseparable. Day and night are not separate; rather, they are part of the cycle of one full day. They exist in relation to each other. Imagine endless days without night, activity with no rest, or endless winters with no summer.

Yin and yang exist within each other and are interdependent.

Think of our bodies, for example, when applying this concept. The back of our body — the bony spine and ribs (more yang) — protects our soft internal vital organs (more yin). We are active (yang) only to need rest (yin) to come back into activity. Nothing is purely yang or yin; they coexist. Outwardly, we express ourselves through our words, activities and movement. This outward manifestation is more yang, more active. Internally, we experience emotions and body processes happening without our conscious knowledge: our heart beats, we breathe, we digest and we feel. We do not see what happens inside, yet these internal activities (yin) generate our blood (our nourishment) and is the foundation for our yang, our warmth, our outward vitality and activity. Without the deep internal yin, our outward yang expression and activity would be compromised. One cannot exist without the other.

"Humankind has not woven the web of life. We are but one thread within it. Whatever we do to the web, we do to ourselves. All things are bound together. All things connect."

— *Chief Seattle*

Yin and yang transform each other and turn into its opposite.

"We call them laws of nature. If I throw a stick up in the air, it always falls down. If the sun sets in the west, it always rises again the next morning in the east. And so it becomes possible to figure things out."

— *Carl Sagan*

As the yang energy of the day emerges and progresses from sunrise, it reaches its pinnacle of yang at high noon. From here, the sun begins its slow descent and eventually brings sunset and the yin energy of the night, which reaches its pinnacle at midnight when it begins its movement toward the yang energy of sunrise. Yin and yang are in a constant dynamic state of change. Think of a hot summer day. As heat rises, it can cause water to condense and form into a possible tempestuous thunderstorm, causing the earth to cool (yang gives rise to yin). The extreme cold of winter eventually makes way for spring (the yin of winter submerges the yang of regeneration deep underground, which later gives rise to the yang of spring). Everything turns into its opposite. Thus yang gives rise to yin and conversely yin gives rise to yang.

Yin and yang counterbalance each other.

Just as any change in weight affects the balance of a seesaw, a shift in the balance of yin (cooling, moistening and calming) or yang (warming, drying and activating) will create a new proportional relationship. For instance, a high fever with sweating (yang excess) will deplete our body's fluids, weakening our yin (moistening and cooling capacity). An excess of yin (moisture, dampness) tampers with and obscures the body's yang.

Balance is key. To understand that yin and yang are indivisible, interdependent, turn into its opposite, and balance each other presents the building blocks for understanding change in the body and how to treat it. But what happens when the internal balance is off, when the seesaw tilts one way or the other and our equilibrium is off? We don't feel right. There can be too much (an excess of) yin or yang, drawing resources away from the other resulting in its lack (deficiency).

Think of a seesaw where a small child is sitting at either end. The seesaw rocks back and forth easily and pleasurably. But then, suddenly, one of the children jumps off. Because there is no weight at the other end to create balance, boom, the child left on the seesaw slams to the ground, with no force to lift her back up. Then a big kid, heavier and stronger than the first one, jumps on and the small child flies up. The difference in weight creates a lack on one end — a deficiency. The big kid is too heavy for the weight at the other end; the heavy kid creates excess weight.

Excess and deficiency are important concepts to understand and treat, and this book will help you understand about how foods affect our yin-yang balance. Now let's look at some of the imbalances of excess and deficiency when it comes to yin and yang.

Yin-Yang Imbalance

We continually experience all the elements of yin and yang within us, which is a normal process. Chinese medicine practitioners look for the "too much, too hot," or excesses, and the "too little, too cold" those lacks or deficiencies that show up as yin-yang disharmony in the body. Treating the patterns of these imbalances and disharmony can relieve external manifestations — your symptoms — while working on the underlying sources or root of the problem.

Here are five distinct yin and yang disharmonies that can occur, along with accompanying symptoms.

1. Yang Excess, Yin Deficiency

Excessive yang causes a buildup of heat sensations in the body. This buildup is often due to emotional stress and strain, which can impede the free flow of *qi*. Symptoms can include the body feeling hot, a red face, irritability, a feeling of thirst, excessive perspiration, a tendency to headaches, pent-up frustration, anger and outbursts of anger. A good example of how yang excess creates yin deficiency is fevers with sweating (yang excess). Once fluids are lost, the moistening and cooling aspect, the yin, becomes deficient. In cases of yang excess, it is important to disperse excessive yang (heat) to protect the yin.

2. Empty Heat (Yang)

Empty heat (yang), is the sudden rising feeling of heat that can occur as a result of yin deficiency, as in the case of menopause and perimenopause. In this case, because of hormonal changes, the underlying yin (cooling and moistening) deficiency allows the yang (warming) to flourish without any counterweight. The result is experienced most commonly as hot flashes or night sweats. Remember the seesaw. There has to be a balance of cooling and warming — here, the lack of yin causes heat to proliferate.

Did You Know?

One thing is certain for health to exist: the dynamic balance that happens at the fulcrum is where one can experience ease, interaction and movement.

3. Yin Excess

Yin is important to our functioning. It is the body's moisture, the cooling and lubricating part of the body (blood and body fluids are considered yin); yin is the substance of our fluids, including blood. An excess of yin, however, means that fluid is stagnating in the body, and this is considered to be dampness. (Dampness occurs outside in nature, but it can also accumulate in the body.) For example, if there is yin excess, you may be lethargic, lack drive, feel a sense of heaviness, experience bloating, have a tendency toward diarrhea, snore at night, lack a sensation of thirst, retain water and weight, feel worse in damp weather and experience melancholy or depression. Because dampness indicates some sort of stagnation, it is considered a yin pathogen.

4. Yin Deficiency

Yin deficiency can result after a long acute illness and recovery or chronic illness, long-term use of drugs, medications or excessive alcohol intake, long-term stress or overwork, aging, long-term sleep deprivation due to night work, and poor diet. With the loss of yin, hair, skin and lips can lose their shine and feel continually dry and you may experience constipation. Symptoms can also include all the signs of empty heat (due to yin deficiency): hot flashes, night sweats, sensations of heat in the palms of the hands and feet, nervousness and restlessness, feeling anxious and easily stressed and having trouble sleeping.

5. Yang Deficiency

Yang is warming and activating; it fuels the digestive processes and metabolism. Yang deficiency is the body's inability to generate warmth. People experiencing yang deficiency can feel cold, especially in the hands and feet, feel overall weakness, lack of strength and motivation, and experience edema, poor digestion and an inability to lose weight.

VITAL CONCEPTS
Qi 氣

Qi (pronounced *chee*) has no literal translation in the West, even though it is often referred to as "energy" or "vital force." *Qi* is the force of life itself, derived from breathing and eating once we are born. *Qi* may be invisible, but it is potent and affects all life. The Chinese character for *qi* illustrates the steam rising from a pot of rice. Inherent in this steam is the energy that cooks the food in the pot. This energy, or *qi*, is the invisible force that animates the rising steam in the cooking pot and everything in nature. *Qi* is the "invisible steam" behind our energy, the force behind the wind, the emanation of warmth of the sun, the refreshment of a rushing stream. It can be felt and sensed. *Qi* is the potential we can feel when we're inspired; it is the motivator that activates movement and propels us into action. We can experience *qi* as vibration, pulsing, flowing and tingling energy in the body. *Qi* is also in the land where our food grows. It imbues vitality in the food we eat and is in the cook who prepares the food. The quality and strength of our *qi* enables us to digest the food we eat, turning it into vital energy, blood and nourishment. *Qi* is not finite, but it is mutable: we can build our *qi* or deplete it. The quality of *qi* influences everything in life and is the progenitor of all material substance.

Qi *and Its Functions*

Just as the planet Earth has a magnetic field that extends from beneath its crust out into space, Chinese medicine attributes the magnetic flow of *qi* as a vibration that has an energetic function moving and flowing through every organ system and every pore of the body.

Qi has a number of core functions in the body. It transforms, transports and holds. When *qi* is abundant, flowing and circulating harmoniously through our bodies, we feel at ease, "in the flow" and full of energy. We *can* feel resourceful, impervious to the elements.

Let's look at the five main functions of *qi* in the body.

Transforms

Qi is the motivator that transforms the air we breathe and the food we eat into vital substances that nourish the body: the *qi* itself, the blood and body fluids. Without *qi*, what is eaten has little value. *Qi* and yang are considered part of each other — the act of transforming needs yang and *qi*.

Moves and Transports

The power and potency of *qi* generates movement throughout the body. If the *qi* is deficient, a person feels tired and nourishment cannot be transported to the tissues and cells.

Warms

Qi motivates, activates and warms the body by helping it maintain normal body temperature. As yin is related to blood and cooling, *qi* is related to yang and warming.

Protects

When the *qi* is strong, it serves as a force shield protecting the body from external climactic influences like cold, wind, damp, heat and dryness. *Qi* warms and protects the body via an aspect of itself known as defensive (*wei*, pronounced *way*) *qi*, which can be equated with the Western concept of the immune system.

Contains and Lifts

Qi moves in all directions throughout the body, up and down, in and out. Vibrant *qi* holds things in place, including the organs, and blood in the vessels. It also holds, or contains, the pores' capacity to remain closed to prevent sweat from pouring out.

Qi *Disharmony*

To ensure optimal health, we need to tend to our *qi* with good food, exercise and rest. When we experience variations in our energy levels, an illness or persistent and unresolved body or emotional tension, the free and abundant flow of *qi* is affected; disrupting the harmonious flow of *qi*. In this instance, *qi* is in disharmony.

Qi *Stagnation*

Stagnation of *qi* can be likened to a bad traffic jam in the body. With *qi* stagnation, tension is the overriding experience: tense muscles, headaches, feeling "uptight," irritable, short-fused and stressed out, and shallow breathing are all signs that the *qi* is stagnant and stuck. *Qi* needs to be free and easy in order to transport nourishment to every pore in the body.

So what causes *qi* stagnation? Modern life; being on 24-7; constant stimulation; overwork; hormonal imbalances; stress, stress and more stress; and too much alcohol consumption, poor-quality foods, overeating and too many stimulants like coffee and spicy foods. When *qi* is stagnant, it aggravates premenstrual syndrome symptoms, including headaches, digestive disturbances (such as irritable bowel syndrome) and constipation.

Reduce or avoid: foods that are greasy, fatty or too spicy and tend to overheat the body; excessive alcohol and coffee consumption; all processed foods.

Add foods that ease and move qi: pungent vegetables such as arugula, mustard greens, radish, leeks and ginger; herbs and spices: basil, dill, fennel and rose.

Qi *Deficiency*

Qi deficiency is marked by the pervasive feeling of not having enough energy to get going in the morning or get through the day. The condition is prevalent when, in the dead of winter, you are the one who keeps catching everyone else's cold. It is also marked by low appetite, a general feeling of weakness, looking pale and not having the energy to project your voice and energy. Stress, prolonged illness or lack of adequate rest and nourishment, compounded by overwork and a feeling of burnout, can lead to *qi* deficiency. We need to tend and replenish *qi* every day with good food, exercise and rest. The good news is that in most cases, a change of lifestyle habits, such as food, rest, exercise and stress management, can do just that.

Avoid foods that do not build qi: foods straight from the fridge, which are cold, and cold juices; excessive raw food; dairy products; tofu; cooling beverages, such as black or green tea and beer; fruit; refined sugar; hot spices such as chiles, cayenne and hot peppers, as they are too dispersing.

Add foods that build qi: foods that are sweet and slightly pungent in flavor, and include whole grains such as brown rice and oats; nuts and seeds; some animal meat (lamb, chicken, beef); some organic eggs; sweet vegetables such as winter squash and pumpkin; tonic herbs such as astragalus or cordyceps.

Rebellious Qi

Rebellious *qi* can exist in different forms. When we eat food, it naturally moves down to the stomach and through the digestive system, but in some cases, the stomach rebels and food moves upward, causing symptoms of nausea, hiccups, belching and possibly vomiting. Coughing is another example of rebellious *qi* and also the body's natural response to expel phlegm and mucus. Other symptoms include mental restlessness, headaches, dizziness and irritability.

Avoid foods that aggravate qi *rebellion:* stimulants, such as caffeine and alcohol; greasy, fatty foods; heating or spicy foods such as garlic or hot chile peppers.

Did You Know?

A more extreme level of *qi* deficiency is sometimes referred to as sinking *qi* when there are cases of organ prolapse and incontinence.

Add foods that calm rebellious qi: cooked carrots and celery; foods that are light and easy to digest, such as light vegetable soups, congee, miso soups and ginger (which helps to calm and harmonize digestion).

Blood 点

"Qi is the commander of blood and blood is the mother of qi."

— Common expression in Chinese medicine

In Chinese medicine, "blood" has a different meaning than in the West, even though both know it is a life-giving substance. As a substance, blood is also considered a form of *qi* — a dense fluid inseparable from *qi*. Qi infuses life force into the blood, generating movement, activating circulation through all the organs, bathing, moistening and nourishing all the cells and tissues of the body. As *qi* is to yang and warming, blood is to yin — cooling, lubricating and moistening.

What makes the blood? Food. What we eat matters because when we eat, the *qi* of the spleen transforms the food into blood (more on this in Chapter 7). The spleen extracts nourishment from the food, and that nourishment (nutritive *qi*) moves throughout the body via the pumping of the heart. Blood circulates throughout all the tissues and vessels of the entire body and is stored in the bone marrow.

Blood and Its Functions
Blood Nourishes the Body

Wherever *qi* goes, blood will follow, and they cannot be separated in function. As *qi* moves blood, blood nourishes and promotes *qi*. It is said that the nourishing *qi* circulates with the blood in the blood vessels; blood nourishes the organ systems, muscles and tendons. The quality of blood, derived from the quality of the foods we eat and the body's capacity to transform that food into nourishment, is mutable and is enhanced by proper nourishment.

Blood Moistens the Body

The blood is a fluid that bathes all the tissues of the body, ensuring that they are resilient and do not dry out. Blood nourishes the muscles and tendons to enable a level of flexibility. Blood also moistens the eyes, skin, hair and tongue. If you have dry hair, skin and eyes, there may be a "blood" deficiency.

Blood Supports the Mind and Spirit

The brain needs good blood circulation for clarity of thought. Just think about how hard it is to think when you are tired or hungry. The blood is seen as helping to stabilize and "ground" the mind and spirit (known as *shen*) to ensure that we have clear thoughts, a good memory, restful sleep and a calm mind.

Blood Disharmony

When blood disharmonies come to the forefront, nourishment, vitality and ease are compromised. Where nourishment is compromised, there is blood deficiency; where there is pain, there can be blood stasis; and where there is heat, there can be irregular bleeding and dryness.

Blood Deficiency

You wouldn't instantly recognize a blood deficiency, as it doesn't imply that there is not enough blood in the system. It *does* mean that the body is not receiving enough nourishment via the blood. The tissues and organs are not being enveloped in nourishing blood to ensure flexibility and vibrancy of the muscles, skin, hair and eyes. Blood deficiency can occur when there is poor nourishment, poor absorption (it can be a digestive and metabolism issue), excessive bleeding (as in excessive menstrual flow), or chronic disease.

The symptoms of a blood deficiency are: the skin and lips are pale and listless; the skin and hair are dry without sheen; and memory is poor, the mind is restless and you may suffer from depression, fatigue and insomnia. The good news is that blood deficiency can be easily improved with diet.

Avoid or reduce foods that have a warming or hot thermal nature (drying): drinks such as coffee, chocolate and black tea; too many spicy foods; alcohol; and processed salty foods like chips, canned or processed soups (which are very high in sodium) and pretzels.

Add nourishing foods that are neutral and mildly warming in nature: foods with a sweet flavor, such as squid, mussels, chicken soup and broth, red cabbage, red beets, carrots and spinach. Also include sea vegetables; bone broths; adzuki beans; organic meats such as chicken, lamb and liver; oysters and mussels; red fruits such as cherries, strawberries and red grapes; dates; longan fruit; goji berries; figs; nettles; and watercress.

Did You Know?

For women, blood is their fundamental essence. Women lose and rebuild blood monthly and blood is the vehicle for nurturing the life of a fetus. It is easier for women to experience symptoms of blood deficiency because they lose blood every month. Women should include foods that nourish the blood right after their menses. See Blood Tonic Recipes, page 410, for more information.

Tip

For vegans, add blood-nourishing herbs to your cooking (see Qi Tonic Vegetable Broth, page 417).

Blood Stagnation and Stasis

If the *qi* is weak or stagnant, it cannot move blood effectively and blood stagnation can occur. Blood stagnation can lead to blood stasis. If you have a physical injury, the trauma itself can cause swelling and black and blue markings (a sign of blood and fluid stagnation), which can typically include pain that is sharp and fixed in one place. Other signs of blood stagnation or stasis are premenstrual pain, menstrual cramps with blood clots or purplish lips.

Avoid foods that congest and stagnate: greasy, fatty, fried foods; baked goods; crackers; chips; and excess salt and sugar. (No matter the health problem, eliminating processed, overly salty, sugary, fatty, artificial foods and flavors from your diet will ensure better overall health.)

Add foods that are more activating and can help break up stasis: vinegar (poultices soaked in vinegar can be applied to areas of black and blue to disperse and heal it) and medicinal wines with herbs such as salvia, dang gui and thyme. Other additions can include eggplant, peach, crab, onion, mustard greens and Chinese leeks.

Blood Heat

Symptoms related to blood heat can be more serious and warrant seeing your health-care provider. They can include feeling hot, a dry mouth, skin eruptions that are itchy, red and inflamed, bright red menstrual bleeding, excessive menstrual bleeding and breakthrough bleeding between periods.

Reduce or avoid foods that cool blood: foods that are greasy, fatty or too spicy.

Add foods that are cooling and clear heat: bitter greens such as dandelion, chicory and escarole; artichokes; eggplant; asparagus; celery; spinach; mung beans; sea vegetables; and rabbit.

Body Fluids (*Jin Ye*) 金叶

The body needs hydration, moisture and lubrication to function. How else would we sweat, cry, urinate or digest our food? In Chinese medicine, "body fluids" (*jin ye*) refers to the two types of physiological fluids that circulate throughout the body: *jin* fluids lubricate the skin and muscles, are clear, and include sweat, tears, saliva and mucus. *Ye* liquids include synovial fluids, which bathe

the joints, and fluids that circulate in the brain, bone marrow, eyes, ears, nose and mouth. Body fluids are extracted from the food we eat and are circulated throughout the entire body, from the deepest level of the bone marrow to the most superficial layer of the skin and hair.

Body Fluid and Its Functions

The prime function of fluids is to moisten and lubricate the body, and contribute to a healthy blood consistency. We see fluids in the joints that are covered in synovial fluid, the digestive juices that facilitate the breakdown and digestion of food, and the sweat and tears that help the body release heat or emotion.

Disruption of Body Fluids

Healthy production of body fluids can be disrupted in two ways: there can be an accumulation of fluids, experienced as water retention or excess phlegm and mucus, or there can be a deficiency in body fluids, which causes a cascade of dryness symptoms, from dry cough to constipation to joint inflammation to dry skin, hair and eyes.

Avoid foods that dry body fluids: crackers, hot and spicy foods, too many baked foods and excessive caffeine.

Add foods that moisten: pears; apples; tofu; wheat (if tolerated); coconut milk; almonds; peanuts, spinach; chia, flax and hemp seeds; honey; lotus roots; persimmon; and lily bulbs.

The Three Treasures:
Jing, Qi and Shen

The ancient Chinese recognized that as human beings — *ren in Mandarin,* 人 — we hold within us three treasures that connect us to our genetics (*jing*), physical characteristics nourished by air and food after we are born (*qi*), and mind and spirit (*shen*). Each of us is born with unique characteristics that we inherit, and they dictate our growth and development (*jing*). When we are born, the food we eat, the environment we live in (both physical and mental/emotional) and every breath we take nourishes our *qi*, and *qi* supports healthy movement, continued growth and development. Finally, the most subtle of the three treasures — the mind and spirit — is built upon the physical foundation of vitality (*qi*). A healthy body vibrant with *qi* manifests in our *shen* with clear thinking and calmness of mind.

"*Qi* is the forefather of spirit and essence is the child of *qi*. When *qi* accumulates, it produces essence. When essence accumulates, it renders spirit wholesome."

— Li Dong Yuan,
Pi Wei Lun

A proper diet can nourish the three treasures: *jing*, *qi* and *shen*. Think of someone you know who has a Type A personality — hard-driving, strong and on a fast track to burn out. This person was probably born with an incredibly strong constitution (*jing*) but used it all up and depleted all its resources. It is not what we are born with that dictates the health of our body and mind in the future; it is how we nurture it and what we do with it that counts.

Foundational Treasure: Jing 景

Jing is what we inherit from our ancestors — our genetic makeup, our essence, our constitution, the foundation responsible for healthy development. It is stored in the bones and bone marrow, and revealed through the health of the teeth and hair. *Jing* determines inherent constitutional strength and vitality and is a precursor of *qi*. Each individual is born with a fixed amount of *jing*, yet as soon as we are born, *jing* can be protected and nourished by the food we eat. *Jing* is weakened by the potential excesses of modern life — work, stimulants, prolonged physical exertion, drug use and excessive sexual activity — and this weakening can lead to premature or rapid aging.

Did You Know?

Protecting the *jing* requires a healthy and well-balanced diet as well as lifestyle habits that ensure rest and rejuvenation.

Add foods that protect and support the jing: seaweed and
    sea vegetables, bee pollen, nettles, almonds, bone marrow,
    black beans, ghee (clarified butter), black sesame seeds,
    raspberries, wheat and barley grass.

Physical Treasure: Qi 氣

The interaction of *jing* and *qi* are like yin-yang: inseparable. Following our first breath, our postnatal *qi* serves to protect and enhance the *jing* as well as the day-to-day rhythms of vitality and activity. (See the section on *qi* earlier in this chapter for more information). *Qi* is mutable and can be supplemented as well as protected.

Subtle Treasure: Shen 神

We are not a body and mind, we are one body-mind. Whatever affects the body affects the mind and spirit. *Shen* is an all-encompassing concept of the spirit and consciousness of an individual. Our spirit, or mental state, is extremely important to our overall health. In Chinese medicine, a person's mental health is inextricably dependent on sound *jing* and *qi*. *Shen* is the subtlest energy in the body and manifests through our emotions, thinking and natural spiritual development. It makes sense, then, that the organ associated with *shen* is the heart. Where *jing* represents our inherent constitution and *qi* our physical state, *shen* represents the combination of these two treasures. If our *shen* is disturbed, we can experience insomnia, depression or restlessness and unstable emotions. The saying "You are what you eat" has a deeper connotation when it comes to feeling calm and clear in the mind.

Add foods that nourish the shen: dates, longan fruit, lily bulbs, mussels and lotus seeds. Fragrant flowers open the heart and are calming — include violets, jasmine, rose and orange flowers.

The Five Phase Theory

The ancient Chinese took the natural chaos of nature and found a sense of dynamic order that is explained by the Five Phase Theory of change and transformation, more commonly known in the West as the Five Element Theory. The Five Phases emerged from Daoist thought in the 4th century BCE as a rational, orderly and self-sufficient system that expanded the foundation of yin-yang theory to explain how the elements interact and influence one another. The cycle and movement of natural change was applied to human beings centuries later by the Confucian school. It notes the perpetual cycle of change in nature and human beings through the seasons, and their continuous interaction with each other. It includes the *five elements* (wood, fire, earth, metal and water) correlating with the concept of *five seasons* (spring, summer, late summer/seasonal transition, autumn and winter), the *five climates* (wind, heat, dampness, dryness and cold), the *five organ pairs* (liver/gallbladder, heart/small intestine, spleen/stomach, lung/large intestine and kidney/bladder), the *five flavors* (sour, bitter, sweet, pungent and salty), *five colors* (green, red, yellow, white and black), the *five imbalances of emotions* (anger, joy, pensiveness, grief and fear),

"*Wuxing* has been translated into English as 'five elements,' but when we actually watch the work that *xing* does in the Chinese language, it is used to describe movement (e.g., walking), alteration, changing states of being, permutations or metamorphoses."

— *Ronnie Littlejohn, Wuxing (Wu-hsing)*

the *five tissues* (tendons, blood vessels, flesh, skin and bones) and the *five sensory organs* (eyes, tongue, mouth, nose and ears).

The Five Phase Theory is a complex and nuanced system that takes into account the phenomenon of change through physiology, pathology, diagnosis and treatment, and is used in classifying foods and Chinese medicinal herbs. As in yin-yang theory, no phase is isolated from any other. Cycles of generation and control are considered in various schools of acupuncture (Five Element acupuncture), while aspects of nutritional and herbal therapy are partly based upon the Five Phase Theory when it comes to flavor and the association of flavor with organ systems and the seasons. Even though this system is invaluable in the practice of Chinese medicine, its complexity is beyond the scope of this book. While we introduce it here to highlight its influence on the principles and concepts of Chinese nutritional healing, it will not be covered in depth.

The Five Phases

The chart below represents the Five Phase Theory — the relationship of seasons to organ systems, directions, climates, movements, emotions, flavors, sense organs and parts of the body. It can be useful as a point of reference when making food choices in light of what you will learn in the upcoming chapters.

The Five Phase Theory					
	Wood	**Fire**	**Earth**	**Metal**	**Water**
Season	Spring	Summer	Late summer and seasonal transition	Autumn	Winter
Organ system	Liver, gallbladder	Heart, small intestine	Stomach, spleen	Lung, large intestine	Kidney, bladder
Direction	East	South	Center	West	North
Climate	Wind	Heat	Dampness	Dryness	Cold
Movement	Upward growth and renewal	Expansive and abundant	Harmonizing, nourishing and stabilizing	Contracting and containing	Downward and inward
Emotion	Anger	Joy	Pensiveness	Grief	Fear
Flavor	Sour	Bitter	Sweet	Pungent	Salty
Sense organ	Eyes	Tongue	Mouth	Nose	Ears
Part(s) of the body	Sinews, muscles and tendons	Blood vessels	Muscles, flesh and limbs	Skin	Bones

Wuxing: The Five Phases

FIRE
Summer
BITTER

Heart / Small Intestine

Heat • South • Expansion/
Abundance • Red • Joy •
Blood vessels •
Tongue

EARTH
Late Summer /
Seasonal Transition
SWEET

Spleen / Stomach

Dampness • Center •
Harmony/Stability • Yellow •
Pensiveness • Flesh
• Mouth

WOOD
Spring
SOUR

Liver / Gallbladder

Wind • East • Upward/
Growth • Green • Anger
• Tendons • Eyes

METAL
Autumn
PUNGENT

Lung / Large Intestine

Dryness • West • Contraction/
Containment • White •
Grief • Skin • Nose

WATER
Winter
SALTY

Kidney / Bladder

Cold • North • Downward/
Inward • Black • Fear
• Bones • Ears

The Five Phases with corresponding elements, seasons,
flavors, organ systems, climates, directions, movements,
colors, emotions, parts of the body and sense organs.

External Environmental Influences

Did You Know?

If you live in a temperate climate, you are most often exposed to the first five conditions, but if you live in a hot climate, it is easier to be exposed to the high and intense heat known as summer heat.

In Chinese medicine, the ill effects of the external environment and fluctuations in climate are known as external pathogenic factors that can adversely affect the body's equilibrium. When we are strong and resilient, it is easy to deal with a climate's fluctuations. When a person is run-down, however, the body is more susceptible to the external forces of climatic changes. External weather conditions are known as the "six pernicious influences or pathogens" and they include heat, dryness, cold, wind, dampness and summer heat. Each climatic influence has a unique effect, and food is used to help strengthen the body's resiliency against them, as well as to help clear its ill effects.

Wind

Winds are quick, forceful and changeable and move through the body. Wind is most predominant in spring, when the weather can abruptly change. In Chinese medicine, protecting the body from "wind invasion" is key to preventing the invasion of other climatic effects. Wind symptoms are most often seen as manifestations that come on and progress quickly. Wind invasions most always carry cold, heat or dampness with them. Think of the times you may be well one moment and suddenly you are experiencing fever or chills, body aches or a burning sore throat. That is wind. Wind is countered with pungent herbs, which are either warming or cooling.

Heat

The Chinese consider a "heat invasion" something that also comes on quickly and is usually associated with wind. Heat exposure can cause inflammations, strong allergic reactions, skin eruptions, fevers, sudden irritability, headaches or drying out of the body, causing excessive thirst or hunger. Heat is countered with either cooling yin or pungent and cooling foods and herbs.

Dampness

Fog, humidity, gray skies and cloud cover (like we have in the U.S. Pacific Northwest for months on end) are all signs of external dampness. But when there is internal dampness, the following symptoms are prominent: lethargy, bloating, indigestion, diarrhea, a feeling of heaviness, foggy thinking, slowness of thought and movement, pain along with aching in the joints. Dampness is countered by foods that nourish the stomach and spleen, such as whole grains and beans, aromatic herbs and spices such as basil, dill, parsley and coriander, and small amounts of bitter foods.

Dryness

Dryness most always occurs with cold or heat symptoms and can lead to feelings of dryness, dehydration; excessive thirst; dry skin, lips or nostrils; or a dry cough that won't go away. Dryness is countered with moistening yin foods.

Cold

The invasion of cold winds and cold weather, usually in winter and colder months, causes us to contract physically to protect and conserve inner warmth. Catching a cold wind can cause chills, headaches and body aches and can aggravate joint pain. Cold is countered with warming yang foods.

Summer Heat

Summer can bring with it debilitating heat. Every summer, we hear about people falling ill or dying from heat exposure or heat stroke. Just as you need to protect yourself against the fierce cold winds of winter, you need to protect yourself from the drying, dehydrating effects of summer heat. Such extreme weather can cause heat stroke, exhaustion, fever, heavy sweating, a dry mouth and excessive thirst. Summer heat is countered with hydration and cooling yin foods.

Bring the Concepts Together

What do all these concepts have to do with food and nutritional healing? Everything. We eat every single day and the quality of what we eat can make or break our health. Food has energy (*qi*), which can cool (*yin*) or warm (*yang*). Food nourishes *jing*, *qi* and *shen*, connecting our body-mind so that we feel at ease, energetic and resilient. Everyone in the world experiences weather patterns and can feel when heat, cold, dampness or dryness effects a sense of well-being. Chinese medicine is the language of nature. Learn the language, look "deep into nature," observe it all around you in its dynamic dance of change and you may understand things in a new way. Once you learn the language, you can attune to yourself and the food you eat in a more holistic way to promote balance and vitality.

Part 2

Foundations of Chinese Dietary Therapy

Chapter 3

The Foundations: Thermal Nature and Flavor

"Dietary therapy should be the first step when one treats disease. Only when this is unsuccessful should one try medicines."

— *Sun Simiao*

Now that you've been introduced to a distinct system of nutritional healing that has its roots in Chinese medicine, you might be curious, willing and eager to learn more about how food can be a delicious and foundational medicine that helps build and maintain health and vitality for years to come.

The system uses the properties inherent in foods — in particular, the thermal nature (*qi*), flavor, and their actions and effects on the body — to guide what to eat to support the internal balance of the body. The dynamic classifications of food emerged out of observation, trial and error, and meticulous recordings that have endured over millennia.

In comparing Chinese dietary therapy to the Western approach to eating for health, we see similarities — both stress the elimination of poor-quality, processed foods with excesses of refined flour, sugar and fat, and both encourage an abundance of fresh whole foods in the diet. Both systems advocate the role and value of healthy eating for the prevention of disease.

This, however, is where the two approaches diverge: Western nutritional and dietary therapy looks at food's potency through its parts — micro- and macronutrients, vitamins, amino acids, proteins and calories, to name a few. Unlike the ancient classifications used by Chinese medicine, foods are recommended in the West as new research brings the role of specific nutrients to light.

So how can we adopt a system that was created thousands of years ago to our way of eating in modern-day life? In this chapter, we dive a little deeper to better understand the effects of thermal nature and flavor and how to apply these when choosing what to eat. We start first by learning about the dynamics of food and healing from the vantage point of thermal nature (*qi*) and flavor.

Thermal Nature, or *Qi*, of Food

Simply put, the thermal nature or *qi* of foods is the categorization of foods according to their capacity to warm or cool the body. If we tend to run hot or cold, it would be important to eat foods that counterbalance those tendencies to create internal balance. Earlier, we learned that yang is warming and yin is cooling. Applied to food, yang foods warm the body while yin foods will counter heat and cool it down. By attuning to our body temperature, we can choose and incorporate foods with warming or cooling effects to help support inner balance.

When you consider the effect of the thermal nature of foods on health, consider your inner thermostat. If you're someone who tends to be cold and has sluggish digestion, drinking cold protein smoothies may not be the best approach for your long-term digestive health. Cold begets cold. If you're someone who often feels hot and is easily agitated, spicy and warming foods may aggravate an already hot and inflammatory condition. Heat begets heat. Therefore, it will be important to consider your warming and cooling tendencies, as well as the current season, when making food choices. Follow this simple rule when choosing foods based on their thermal nature: if you tend to run cold, dispel it by choosing warming foods. If you run hot, clear the heat by choosing more neutral or cooling foods.

> "If something is cold, heat it. If something is hot, cool it. Supplementing the opposite polarity restores balance."
>
> — *Huangdi Neijing Suwen, The Yellow Emperor's Classic of Medicine*

Flavor and Its Effects on the Body

The second distinguishing component of food in Chinese dietary therapy is flavor of which there are five. The five flavors — sweet, sour, salty, pungent and bitter — have specific movement, actions and effects on the body. Flavor is distinguished in Chinese medicine from the sensory experience of taste in the mouth by its specific action on the body (disperse, nourish and harmonize, drain and purge, astringe or consolidate) and the movement it promotes (upward and out, inwards, down, down and out). Here's an example of a dish that incorporates the five flavors and varying

Did You Know?

Some of the five flavors have sub-divisions of flavors, such as sweet (*full, bland* and *empty*) and pungent (*pungent and warming,* and *pungent and cooling*). Aromatic, a subdivision of pungent, denotes the warming and activating action of many culinary spices and some Chinese herbs. See more information later in chapter.

thermal natures: a fresh salad made with arugula (pungent — cooling), grapefruit slices (sour, bitter and sweet — cooling), olive oil (bitter and sweet — cooling), vinegar (sour and bitter — cooling), salt (salty — cooling) and black pepper (pungent — warming). The combination of flavors in this salad has all the five flavors categorized in Chinese dietary therapy; each of them is a catalyst of action within the body. Meanwhile, the thermal nature, or *qi*, of the foods in the salad is supporting or adjusting the body's internal thermostat. This salad will ultimately cool you down, due to the heat-clearing actions of certain foods, and counter any buildup of internal heat. So if you run hot and have a strong digestive system (more about that later), this salad is a good choice. Why? The thermal nature, or *qi*, of the foods in this salad are mostly cooling with a bit of warming pungent black pepper to add a counterbalance to the cooling aspect of the dish. The combination of the five flavors is deliciously acting upon the body to move *qi*, stimulate digestion, clear excess heat, nourish, calm and hydrate.

Flavor and Culture

Every culture has its distinct flavor palate — from preferences in grains and produce to spice selection to cooking styles. Of course, each of us has developed food preferences and tastes based on our upbringing, cultural traditions and exposure to foods. In fact, many cultures have similar traditions and connections to food and healing that can correlate to the foundational principles of Chinese medicine as it has been applied to food. Those principles are entrenched in nature and can be adapted to any cuisine in any culture.

Cultural variations in tastes, flavor profiles and preparation methods are distinct and grounding for people and are imbued with a sense of home and heritage. China's flavor palate includes green onions, ginger, garlic and soy sauce. Mexican cuisine emphasizes the use of peppers, tomatoes, onions and chiles, while India's culinary preferences lean toward the addition of spices like cumin, coriander and turmeric to dishes. Italian cooking is known for its use of olive oil, fresh vegetables, basil, oregano and tomatoes. The flavor palate of Iran, influenced by the interaction of Chinese traders along the Silk Road, includes pungent green herbs such as basil, parsley and mint, dried limes, rose petals and rose water, and saffron. In the United States, according to Sarah Lohm, author of *Eight Flavors: The Untold Story of American Cuisine*, flavors include a veritable melting pot of the cultures that make up the country and include black pepper, vanilla, curry powder, chili powder, soy sauce, garlic, monosodium glutamate (MSG) and Sriracha (a hot pepper sauce).

Over the past few decades, the United States has been known internationally as an exporter of fast and manufactured foods infused with man-made combinations of salty and sweet flavors and varied textures that make us want more: a veritably manufactured food palate. A diet of this type makes it difficult for people to enjoy simpler foods with flavors created under the sun — sweetness, sour, pungency, saltiness and bitterness; each flavor, potentially satisfying and nourishing. Mark Schatzker, in his book *The Dorito Effect: The Surprising New Truth about Food and Flavor*, illustrates how flavor can function in a species: "If goats had a word for delicious, it would have two meanings. The first would be: I like this. The second would be: This is what my body needs. For goats, they are the same thing." If we are continually eating foods that have been designed to make us "crave" them, stimulating the addictive centers of our brain, it can be difficult to like simple and fresh flavors, but it can be done. If we remove the obstacles that eating mostly manufactured foods and flavors has and replace them with real, fresh foods, we can regain our intuitive sense of what flavors we *need* at any given time. Our bodies are designed to seek out foods and nourishment that meet our physical needs, and yet we are often pulled in another direction by other food preferences and desires. Building a new foundation for healthy eating can start with first eliminating manufactured foods and understanding the dynamic concepts of Chinese dietary therapy — food's thermal nature and flavor — along with how they affect our bodies.

Types of Food

A whole-foods diet consisting of fresh fruits and vegetables,* whole grains,* nuts and seeds,* beans, pulses and other legumes, sustainably and pasture-raised meat and eggs, sustainably fished seafood, and culinary herbs and spices are foods mostly neutral, slightly warming or cooling in thermal nature (see image on page 44). If you eat a large quantity of raw foods or a diet heavy in meat and potatoes, you're likely sitting way out on the edge of the thermal seesaw.

Raw food = cooling and cold.

Heavy meat and potatoes = warming or even hot, depending on your food combinations and methods of cooking.

* Organic when possible

Thermal Nature = *Qi* = Warming and Cooling

Our health is a continuous balancing act that includes our body's self-regulating inner thermostat. Much like sitting on a seesaw, we move in one direction or another to achieve a dynamic state of balance. Expanding on the analogy we used in Chapter 2, if you have ever had the experience of sitting on a seesaw with a much bigger kid on the other end of it, you know how much effort (sometimes futile) it takes to raise yourself up to hover at equilibrium. It's much easier when the person on the opposite end is equal in weight or both parties stick closer to the fulcrum (center) of the seesaw to achieve balance. How we eat is much like that. It's much easier to maintain and adjust our eating to support health than it is to make those BIG changes to get back to health. The path is longer and the effort more vigorous and concentrated. So you have to choose: do you want optimal health and to learn how to choose the right foods for your needs? Or do you prefer to go with the flow without discretion, teetering back and forth with great effort?

Take Inventory

Understanding your body's nature, or your body temperature tendencies toward being too cold or too warm, is a good place to start. It's relatively easy to gauge where you are and how to balance our internal thermostat: if you feel cold much of the time, you would eat foods that are neutral, warming or mildly cooling — to help maintain internal warmth and balance. We want to stay close to the center on foods, however, and want to avoid foods that build an excess of heat (grilled meats, alcohol, spicy and hot foods and fried foods). Why? Because *too* much heat in the body can cause us to feel dried out or thirsty, driving us to crave cooler or cold foods to balance the buildup of this excess heat. If that happens, then we're back on the seesaw, trying to move from one end to the other and using a lot of internal energy in the process to bring us to balance.

Where are you eating on the seesaw? Take a look.

Warming to hot: shrimp, mussels, chicken, lamb, beef, cinnamon, thyme, rosemary, garlic, black pepper, chile peppers, alcohol, fatty foods, greasy foods.

Neutral: most whole grains, legumes and beans, soybeans, almonds, peanuts, winter squash, sweet potatoes, carrots, catfish, salmon, pork, dairy, honey, grapes.

Cooling to cold: clams, tofu, cucumbers, apples, pears, dandelion greens, spinach, watermelon, bananas, grapefruit, mint, cold juices, ice cream, foods from the fridge.

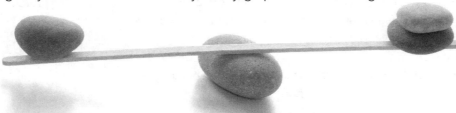

Hot or Cold: What to Drink

Drinking something hot makes us feel warm. This is pretty straightforward. In Chinese medicine, however, we are not *only* considering the external temperature of a food, rather the resulting internal effect.

Take iced drinks, for example. Drinking an icy drink makes us feel cold. Yes, ice *is* cold in its thermal nature, or *qi*. Here is where the logic shifts. Remember, in the theory of yin-yang, everything turns into its opposite at its extreme. Extreme cold, therefore, can create extreme heat. How? Its iciness demands more internal heat from the body to make it digestible. Inversely, iciness and cold in winter make us feel cold, so we drink a cup of hot tea, which initially warms the body. It's common sense that when you are cold, you drink something hot, yet there is a twist to drinking hot tea in winter. The temperature of the water (hot) warms us up, so the hot tea initially warms, but the inherent thermal nature of tea is cooling, which can be balanced by adding warming spices or ginger to render it less so.

Being able to distinguish and identify the thermal nature of foods in relationship to our condition, what season we are in and what our tendencies are can help guide our choices in foods and cooking styles (more on this later).

Yin-Yang in Foods

As we learned earlier, all foods that are characterized as having a warming and/or hot nature have yang characteristics and can be helpful for those who cannot generate enough internal warmth. If we cannot generate inner warmth (yang), it is difficult to thrive in the cold. Conversely, we can easily become overheated if we are unable to activate internal cooling (yin) and ventilation during the hot and dry or hot and humid months of summer.

Yang is the energy of the sun. Foods that are inherently warm and activating have yang characteristics. Foods that are characterized as having a cooling and/or cold nature have yin characteristics. Yin is the energy of the night, the moon, cool rivers and streams. Finally, foods that are neutral in nature have an harmonizing influence on our internal thermostat, helping to manage the dynamics of staying in the center and supporting the body's responsiveness to the changes and movement of the day, the season and the stages of life.

Did You Know?

The cooling thermal nature of tea will protect us from becoming overheated. Coffee, on the other hand, whose beans are roasted, is warming, so a hot coffee creates more internal warmth and is drying.

The Five Thermal Natures of Food

Thermal Natures of Food

1. Neutral
2. Warming
3. Cooling
4. Hot
5. Cold

Let's take a look at the five thermal natures (*qi*) of food and their actions to help us better understand their effects. What action do these varying thermal natures have on the body and where do we find them?

NEUTRAL: The neutral thermal nature supports harmony and balance in the body. It is found mostly in whole grains, beans, pulses and other legumes, some nuts and seeds, sweet vegetables, some fish and meats (such as pork).

WARMING: The warming thermal nature of foods is activating. It warms our innards, reinforces our vitality, stimulates digestion and increases circulation. Taken in excess, warming foods also have the tendency to build internal heat and dry us out. Warming foods include many common aromatic cooking spices, such as cinnamon, nutmeg and rosemary; many meats; nuts such as walnuts and chestnuts; some fruits, such as peaches and raspberries; wine; coffee; and alliums, including garlic, shallots, chives, leeks and onions.

COOLING: The cooling thermal nature of foods reduces internal heat, activates hydration in the body and calms the liver. An excess of cooling foods can tax the digestive network, slowing down the breakdown, digestion, absorption and transformation capacities of the digestive system. Many fruits and vegetables are quite cooling, including lettuce, cucumbers, tomatoes, tangerines, apples and pears. Green tea is cooling.

HOT: The hot thermal nature of foods is used sparingly and therapeutically to forcefully dispel internal cold, somewhat like activating your internal fireplace. Its movement is ascending. Hot foods are used in the treatment of cold conditions, as in the case of some pain syndromes. An excess of hot foods can aggravate irritability and impatience, as well as cause internal drying. Foods that have a hot nature include hot peppers (such as habanero, jalapeño, ghost peppers and chiles), Sichuan peppercorns, fried and greasy foods, alcohol and dried ginger.

COLD: The cold thermal nature of foods is also used sparingly and is most useful in very hot and humid climates or when someone suffers from hot conditions such as fevers caused by viruses. Cold puts out fire, as in the case of fever. It can be used to detoxify and is said to tranquilize. Its movement is descending. Many people in the West are accustomed to eating foods straight from the refrigerator and adding ice to drinks, but too much cold food can weaken digestion. Foods that have a cold thermal nature include grapefruit, bananas, watermelon, bamboo shoots, crabs, lettuce and sea vegetables, as well as ice cream and all foods eaten directly from the refrigerator.

Flavor

How do you consider flavor and taste when you choose what to eat? Are your senses fully engaged as you taste, sense, feel and experience the impact that flavor has on the entire body? Or does it stop at the mouth?

You actually can connect to flavor in a deeper and more visceral way. When you experience the simple, true flavors provided by nature, you can begin to *feel* the potency, the "destination" and impact of flavor on your body. Only then does flavor begin to have a new meaning.

In the traditional Chinese culture of food and its traditions of food as medicine, the use of flavor is key and vital in the foods and herbal formulas that Chinese medicine practitioners have been using for thousands of years. Flavors are chosen and put together to create harmonious dishes and herbal formulas to prevent illness, promote longevity and support treatment of acute and chronic health issues.

From the Chinese point of view, flavor is potent and has a clear destination and action in the body. It not only pleases our senses, but it also serves to activate bodily functions (such as digestion, sweating, moistening and excreting) and catalyzes actions within the body to transform and balance.

Just as with the thermal nature of foods, flavor is also categorized according to its yin and yang properties.

"The five flavors (五味 wǔ wèi) enter through the mouth. Each has a destination where it proceeds to, and each has a disease associated with it."

— *Huangdi Neijing Suwen, The Yellow Emperor's Classic of Medicine*

Flavors of Yin and Yang	
Yin	**Yang**
Sour — cooling	Sweet — neutral or warming
Bitter — cold	Pungent — warming and cooling; aromatic and warming
Salty — cooling	

Did You Know?

If you crave one flavor over another, your body may be out of balance. Each flavor is associated with a specific thermal nature and action on the body, which can help to resolve imbalances.

Appreciating the specific actions of these flavors, we can approach the organization of our plate, our meal and our way of eating differently. A balanced plate offers us a meal replete in the five flavors: sweet, sour, salty, pungent and bitter. We can fine-tune the predominance of any flavor depending on what the intention is for the meal, the season, and how we sense, as author Mark Schatzker says, "this is what my body needs." By adjusting flavors in cooking, we can direct the healing power of food, much like a Chinese herbalist who considers flavor and thermal nature when creating an herbal formula.

Each of us develops our flavor palate, some of which is based on our cultural upbringing and exposure to certain flavors and types of foods. Added to that is our exposure to and regular eating of manufactured or processed foods whose flavor is predetermined by food scientists in food laboratories. If your preferences include foods that have a strong and rich taste, foods that are high in sugar or salt or fatty foods, you'll have to start with staying clear of those manufactured foods and flavors, which obscure the capacity to truly taste and experience the vibrant simplicity of a food. If you're not currently optimizing the full spectrum of flavors noted by Chinese medicine, it may be time to add in whole fresh foods that reflect the spectrum of the five flavors, simply cooked, to reconnect with their potency and pleasure.

Reflection: What are Your Food Choices?

For the next week, or even the next few days, note your food choices based on flavor. It can be helpful to simply write down what you eat. Do not change any food choices; simply note what you eat and drink. Once you've taken stock, turn to the food chart starting on page 184 to analyze what flavors and thermal natures predominate in your diet. Now look at your notes:

- *Are you including all the five flavors in your meals?*
- *Do you tend to prefer one or two or only three flavors?*
- *Do you have an aversion to any flavors?*

The Five Flavors of Food

In Chinese medicine, each flavor is identified as having a taste (which may differ from its therapeutic actions) but is also associated with a particular thermal nature, and distinct effect and action on a specific body system. Let's look at the five flavors more closely.

Sweet

Thermal nature: Neutral to warming

Action: Yang — harmonizing, nourishing, supplementing, calming, nourishes body fluids

Meridian network: Stomach and spleen

Excess consumption damages: spleen *qi* (which is responsible for digestion) impedes breakdown and transformation of food, which can cause poor digestion, accumulation of dampness and weight gain due to the body's inability to transform and metabolize effectively

For a brief explanation of the meridian network, see box, below.

Sweet is the most universal flavor in our diet and important to our physical development. The *Neijing Suwen* says, "Sweet flavor adds flesh." Whole grains, most legumes and beans and nuts are sweet. So is meat. Even onions, with their pungent bite, are wonderfully sweet when cooked. Of course, maple syrup, sugar and dates are enormously sweet and delightful when used in baking. The addition of sweet helps to soothe the bitter flavor in food. It is the key flavor in a mother's milk, nourishing and fostering growth and development in infants.

What is a Meridian Network?

The meridian network is the system of channels that run through the body, associated with each of the organ systems as well as an ancillary organ system (pericardium and triple warmer) and utilized as a guide for treatment by acupuncturists, Chinese herbalists and practitioners of Asian bodywork. The 12 primary meridians connect the head to the foot, the front to the back and the surface of the body to each of the internal organs (lung and large intestine, stomach and spleen, heart and small intestine, bladder and kidney, triple warmer and pericardium, liver and gallbladder). There are six yang meridians (large intestine, stomach, small intestine, bladder, triple warmer and gallbladder) and six yin meridians (lung, spleen, heart, kidney, pericardium and liver). They are not related to nerves, blood vessels or lymph, rather they are the pathways through which *qi* and blood flow. In Chinese herbalism and dietary therapy, all herbs and foods are thought to have a correspondence and impact upon organs and their corresponding meridian.

In Chinese medicine, we consider "sweet" as the natural sweetness inherent in foods, *not* the added sweet found in most processed foods, from breads to ketchup to pasta sauces.

Neutral and warming in nature, the sweet flavor is considered to have a tonic effect — activating and supporting growth and development. This flavor is associated with the stomach and spleen, the center of the digestive network, where we transform the food we eat into nourishment for the body, in particular the yin aspects of the body — the tissues, blood and flesh. The sweet flavor is also calming, softening and harmonizing in the body.

Categories of Sweet

The sweet flavor is associated with the Earth element, late summer and the seasonal transitions at the end of each season.

The sweetness and neutral thermal nature of grains and beans, which are mostly neutral in their thermal nature, are quite different from the sweet flavor in meat, which is warming. Thus, there are several categories of sweet flavor:

Full sweet: This is the sweet flavor found in meats, dairy and nuts. It nourishes and warms.

Bland sweet: This flavor is prominent in grains and beans. It balances nourishment and elimination through its spleen tonifying and mild diuretic actions. The bland sweet flavor will not make us too warm or cool. It promotes growth and development.

Empty sweet: This flavor is found in fruits, which are cooling and hydrating and beneficial. Refined sugars are also considered empty sweet; they are warming and add no nutritional value to the diet.

Sour

Thermal nature: Cooling

Action: Yin — moistening, astringent; movement is inward; supplements yin; can ease muscle contractions

Meridian network: Liver and gallbladder

Excess consumption damages: muscles, in particular, it causes soreness and muscle contractions. Avoid sour if you come down with a cold from exposure to cold wind — the sour flavor pulls the cold deeper into the body (use pungent instead).

Bite into a lemon and you know what happens: your lips pucker up, you feel a cool burst of flavor and you start to salivate.

Sour is a flavor that stimulates digestive juices, activating the fluids that bathe our tissues and our whole body. The sour flavor is found in combination with other flavors in fruits, some vegetables, some lightly fermented black and green teas and fermented foods, including sauerkraut and plain yogurt. Because of its astringent properties, sour helps contain and reabsorb fluids and protects *qi*, the vital energy that runs through our body (see Chapter 2, page 25). It is a flavor that is beneficial in summer and autumn due to its hydrating and moistening actions on body tissues and mucous membranes.

Salty

Thermal nature: Cooling
Action: Yin — softens, loosens, moistens dryness and removes moisture as it moves *qi* downward to benefit the kidney function
Meridian network: Bladder and kidney
Excess consumption damages: Dries out fluids (through dehydration), can contribute to hypertension, hardens muscles and weakens bones

In the West, the *salty* flavor is associated with added salt. In Chinese dietary therapy, the salty flavor is found in various foods; in addition, actual salt is used as a condiment to enhance the flavors of other foods as well as to increase their palatability, absorption and digestion. While it may seem obvious that seafood and sea vegetables are inherently salty, even millet and buckwheat are considered to have a salty flavor. These foods can moderate the sourness and bitterness of foods. Salty is yin, due to its cooling thermal nature and moistening action. Salty moves the *qi* downward to benefit the kidneys. Too much salt can aggravate obesity and high blood pressure. It can also exert the opposite effect of its main action (moistening and softening) and become too drying.

> **Tip**
> All flavors need to be used in concert with each other to create an appealing, well-constructed, well-balanced dish or meal.

Pungent

Thermal nature: Warming or cooling
Action: Yang — uplifting, dispersing; breaks up stagnation, invigorates circulation, opens the pores, encourages perspiration, is useful in the beginning stages of a cold
Meridian network: Lung and large intestine
Excess consumption damages: pungent/warming can overheat the body and cause agitation, sleep and mood disturbances, dryness in the skin and inhibited bowel movements

Categories of Pungent

Did You Know?

A cooling pungent food, such as daikon radish or mint, can help to cool the heat of an acute fever or the burning heat of a sore throat. As we say in Chinese medicine, it releases the exterior.

"Variety is the spice of life," goes the old saying. The use of herbs and spices (whether they be *pungent and warming*, as in chile or hot peppers; *pungent and aromatic*, as in basil, rosemary, thyme, sage, cinnamon, nutmeg, cumin or cloves; or *pungent and cooling*, as in peppermint, spearmint, marjoram, lavender or lemon balm) transforms dishes and brings delight to the senses. Pungent foods and spices activate circulation, can clear heat or dissipate cold, dispersing and moving energy up and out to the surface of the body. Pungent can warm or cool. Aromatic spices and herbs serve mostly to activate *qi*, dissolve damp, and warm and strengthen digestion. The pungent flavor can help to clear built-up phlegm and mucus and activate circulation. Pungent warming flavors are also found in mustard greens, onions, Chinese spring onions, chives, leeks, shallots, arugula, garlic and ginger. Cooling pungent foods include radishes and broccoli. Alcohol, which is pungent and warm, is used therapeutically when infused with herbs or foods to increase circulation to the extremities and warm the body.

Did You Know?

Aromatic and warming: The aromatic quality of foods, certain herbs and spices assist the action of pungency through warming, activating digestion and dispelling dampness.

In Chinese medicine, the pungent flavor is a yang, active flavor with subtle yet powerful impact. Think of how you feel after eating a spicy pepper — it makes you sweat, activates circulation and helps to open the pores of the skin to promote sweating but then cools you down. Pungent foods disperse heat or activate circulation to promote warmth.

The pungent flavor is also used in culinary traditions to support the digestibility of fatty foods and animal meat.

Bitter

Thermal nature: Cooling and cold

Action: Yin — detoxifies, clears heat, dries dampness and phlegm, supports draining through urination and excretion; can have a calming effect through clearing heat and can dry the body fluids

Meridian network: Heart and small intestine

Excess consumption damages: bowel function and can cause diarrhea; can dry body fluids and the skin (dehydration)

Bitter is generally not one of the most preferred flavors. It has a strong taste to which many people react negatively. This is normal, as many bitter wild plants and herbs may have a certain level of toxicity in large doses. When it comes to the foods we eat, toxicity is generally not a big concern, but it does let us know just how potent the bitter flavor can be.

While the bitter flavor is something most of us will avoid in whole fresh foods, we regularly experience it in the form of stimulating foods such as coffee, chocolate or beer (which are not necessarily beneficial). The potency of the bitter flavor, with its strong healing impact on the body, means that a little goes a long way — small doses and additions to meals are enough to make a difference.

Human beings have gathered bitter greens and herbs in the wild for centuries and have eaten and drunk them (in the form of herbal teas and liquors) judiciously for health. In Chinese medicine, the bitter flavor is cold and is used to clear out toxicity. Bitter herbs are used to resolve viruses and dysentery, kill intestinal parasites and treat malaria and hepatitis C. They reduce blood sugar, cholesterol and any condition that involves heat buildup in the body. Using bitter foods adds balance to the daily diet and helps clear excessive damp conditions, which can lead to obesity and difficulty in losing weight, water retention and candida or other types of yeast overgrowth.

The bitter flavor is cooling, and therefore yin in nature. Its action is to move the energy in the body downward (think of how digestive bitters, whose movement is downward, help to stimulate digestion). The strength of the bitter flavor varies with the type of food and its preparation. Most foods considered to have a bitter flavor are not purely bitter but either bitter and sweet, as in amaranth, papaya, quinoa and celery; bitter and pungent, as in green onions, white pepper and arugula; or bitter and sour, such as vinegar. Other bitter foods include bitter melons, romaine lettuce hearts, artichokes, white grapefruit, rutabaga, tea (green and black), dandelion greens and dandelion root.

Explore and Enjoy

While the five flavors and five thermal natures of food have an effect on the body, we cannot simply choose foods for their therapeutic thermal nature and flavor. Eating is not a clinical experience but one that is sensuous, communal and nourishing in ways that make us feel satisfied and vibrant.

Initiating changes in how we eat is a bit of an adventure. Trying new foods and flavors can lead to new and satisfying discoveries. Planning meals, of course, can require some forethought and preparation, but once you get familiar with the food groups according to the principles of Chinese medicine and start expanding your food repertoire, it will become easier, more enjoyable and more gratifying.

Did You Know?

Many famous aperitifs of today — such as Cynar, Fernet-Branca and Campari, gentian liqueur, Aperol, Chartreuse, vermouth and many more — were formulations of healing herbs with bitter foods and herbs to stimulate digestion.

Chapter 4

Food Groups and Their Properties

"Medicine and food share the same origin."

— Chinese saying

Food is a gift from nature, coming to us in various forms that we grow, gather, harvest (and raise) to prepare, cook and eat. These simple actions are our way of interacting directly with nature each and every day. What and how we eat nourishes our body. It is the foundation for a sound mind and spirit. Eating fresh whole foods grown and raised under the heat of the sun are, indeed, our strongest health insurance. If we are what we eat, consuming such food infuses every cell of our body with vitality.

In the West, we evaluate and quantify food's health by breaking it down into nutrients — vitamins, minerals, amino acids — and calories. In Chinese dietetics, the evaluation of a food is based on its function, flavor and thermal nature. A food's health benefit is also considered in relation to the context of a person's life — their physical condition, physical activities and stage of life, as well as the season and the climate they live in.

Food Groups In Chinese Dietary Therapy

The functions of food — to nourish, fortify, fulfill, assist (as in, assist other bodily functions) and supplement — are crucial to understanding the food groups in Chinese dietary therapy. They form the basis of how foods are grouped and categorized. Some of these groupings will be familiar, overlapping with some of the Western food groups, while others are different, having been observed to add functional and nutritional value.

As our physical, mental and emotional needs change, so too can our food choices and how we use food to help us function. What was beneficial to us earlier in life may not apply as we age. For example, I was a vegan and vegetarian for at least a decade, but my needs started changing and I felt I needed to add a minimal amount of animal food to my diet to supplement my energy. At first, I had felt strongly and believed that eating a vegetarian and later a vegan diet would be best for my health, but then I started to experience less-than-optimal energy and motivation. I had reached a stagnant plateau with my eating and it felt more like a chore than a pleasure. It was clear that I needed to make adjustments. I realized that the foods I was choosing to eat were not fortifying enough for my active lifestyle, so over time, I added fish, small amounts of eggs, sustainably raised meat and small amounts of fermented goat's milk products into my diet, along with the mounds of vegetables I was already eating every day. It has made a big difference. In making the change, I needed to learn to prepare and integrate animal food into my diet in a way that was palatable to someone who loves a plant-based diet, creating meals that were not only fortifying but easy to digest and delicious. My eating repertoire has modified and expanded as I have matured, and I presume it will continue to change as I do.

The food groups in Chinese dietary and nutritional therapy are categorized in the following way:

- Whole Grains; beans, pulses and other legumes; nuts and seeds
- Animal foods, including meats, seafood, eggs and dairy
- Vegetables, including land vegetables, alliums (the onion and garlic family), fungi, wild vegetables and sea vegetables (seaweeds).
- Fruits
- Condiments, including salt, sweeteners, tea, alcohol, vinegar, herbs and spices, and fragrant flowers

Tip

Review the food groups discussed in this chapter to make the most of your diet and better understand their energetic effect on the body according to their thermal nature, flavor and action. Then, use the chart at the end of this chapter to track what you eat in each category and note your current preferences and eating habits. Do not make any changes now. Later on, once you've built an awareness of how and what you eat, review the recipes section, starting on page 206, and start to experiment with new recipes that are focused on achieving balance.

Food Groups in Chinese Dietary Therapy

Food Group	Includes	Flavor and Thermal Nature	Major Functions
Whole Grains, beans, pulses and other legumes, nuts and seeds	All whole grains All beans, pulses and other legumes All nuts and seeds	Mostly bland and sweet, neutral	Nourishing Tonifies spleen and *qi* Removes dampness Stops diarrhea Moistens
Animal foods	Land animals Fish and shellfish Eggs Dairy	Mostly sweet Neutral to warming, although some fish and shellfish are cooling or cold	Nourishes *qi* and blood Reinforces stomach and spleen, liver and kidney
Vegetables	Land vegetables Alliums Fungi Wild vegetables Sea vegetables	All flavors All thermal natures Alliums are warming	Cleanses the body Detoxifies Clears heat Promotes regular bowel movements Nourishes
Fruits	All land and tree fruit	Sweet and sour Cool to cold	Clears heat Hydrates Dissolves phlegm Detoxifies
Condiments	Salt Sweeteners Tea Alcohol Vinegar Herbs and spices Fragrant flowers	Varied	Improves palatability and absorption of food Flavors foods Can harmonize, activate, moisten, and reinforce stomach and spleen Activates circulation and digestion Relieves muscle spasms Promotes moistening and body fluids

Note: See the food property table in Chapter 10, page 184, for further information on the specific thermal nature, flavor, action and therapeutic indications for foods and herbs, as well as descriptions of distinct and uncommon foods and herbs used in this book.

FOOD GROUP 1
Whole Grains, Beans, Pulses and other Legumes, Nuts and Seeds

The multitudes of golden, earth-toned kernels of grains and multicolored beans and legumes, nuts and seeds have served at the center of traditional diets throughout human history. They are easily dried, stored, prepared and cooked, and offer vital nourishment throughout all the seasons.

This grouping of foods "nourishes" and "fulfills," according to the classic text *The Yellow Emperor's Classic of Medicine* (the *Neijing Suwen*), providing the stomach and spleen substance for the transformation of food into vital energy for the body. In Chinese medicine, the stomach and spleen network is considered the center of the body, the "earth," the foundation of *qi* and blood from which all nourishment flows. With a healthy stomach–spleen network, the body is able to absorb, transform, transport, nourish and create energy from the food we eat. If the stomach and spleen are out of balance or deficient in their functioning, however, the body holds onto excess, called dampness in Chinese pathology, possibly causing digestive disturbances, such as bloating, indigestion, a feeling of lethargy or sometimes an inability to lose weight.

"The five grains are used to nourish."

~ Huangdi Neijing Suwen, The Yellow Emperor's Classic of Medicine

Whole Grains

Whole grains and cereals are essential staples in every pantry. There is a wide range of whole grains and cereals that are typically grown and eaten in every culture. This category of food is most nourishing when eaten whole rather than as a refined and ground product or milled and processed into a refined flour in which the beneficial components of the grain, including the germ, are removed. Most grains are cooked on their own to accompany other main dishes, as in steamed rice, or cooked into a porridge, as in congee (rice porridge) or oat porridge. Grains are also added to soups and stews or cooked together with other ingredients, as in a pilaf or fried rice. Grains need to be cooked and chewed well to enhance their digestion. Expand your meal repertoire with the inclusion of different varieties of whole brown rice, such as short-grain and long-grain varieties, fragrant basmati and jasmine or sweet (glutinous) brown rice. After you've tried one group of grains (rice, for example), move on to another bunch, such as earthy buckwheat groats (which are technically an herb,

Did You Know?

Cereals are often interchanged with whole grains. Technically, cereals are the grains that are in the grass family, which includes wheat, rice, corn, millet, oats, barley, hato mugi (Job's tears) and wild rice.

not a grain), fragrant quinoa, silky amaranth or versatile millet (all technically seeds but cooked and utilized as grains), as well as stone-ground corn grits or polenta. Grains can be stored well in a closed jar in a dark, cool area for up to 1 year.

Thermal nature: neutral with minor variations of cooling to warming
Flavor: bland and sweet
Action: nourishes, strengthens and builds the body, tonifies spleen *qi*, mildly diuretic, relieves diarrhea
Cooking/preparation methods: boil, steam, slow cook, roast, bake

For deficient conditions, include: whole-grain brown rice, sweet (glutinous) brown rice, oats, buckwheat groats, millet, corn, quinoa
For excess conditions, include: a moderate grain intake, including hato mugi, barley (a gluten grain, which we do not use in this book's recipes along with other gluten grains), millet, basmati rice, whole-grain ancient organic wheat (a gluten grain; use only if tolerated, and only whole-grain berries)
To clear heat, include: millet, amaranth, barley and, if tolerated, whole-grain ancient organic wheat
To add warmth, include: sweet rice, oats, buckwheat groats
For those who have a difficult time losing weight: moderate your intake of grain and include grains that dry dampness to increase the diuretic effect, such as amaranth, wild rice, millet, rye, barley, hato mugi

Beans, Pulses and Other Legumes

Legumes such as beans, lentils and chickpeas and soybeans have been incorporated into many cuisines from around the world. For thousands of years, pulses and beans have been cultivated and eaten. While these plants enriched the soil without the use of synthetic fertilizers when they were planted centuries ago, today's farming practices are once again planting them to replenish soils with much-needed nitrogen. Pods and seeds from bean plants are eaten either fresh or their seeds are dried (pulses) and offer essential plant protein. Beans can be difficult to digest, however, so knowing how to prepare and cook them are essential. Beans and pulses can be eaten in soups, on their own or cooked with other vegetables or meats. Foods in this category are an excellent source for people who are transitioning from a high-meat diet or vegetarians seeking more forms of plant protein. In some cases, however, eating beans may not be as beneficial. If you find it

Cooking Tip
Soak beans for at least 8 hours. Drain the soaking water and rinse. Add a 1-inch (2.5 cm) piece of kombu (a seaweed) to the cooking water to increase digestibility. Alternatively, you can add the Mexican herb epazote to aid digestibility.

difficult to gain weight and have a yin-deficient condition, eating beans regularly may not be recommended, as beans can have a stronger diuretic and drying effect than whole grains.

Thermal nature: neutral with minor variations of cooling to warming

Flavor: bland sweet, some salty

Action: tonifies spleen *qi*, removes dampness, relieves diarrhea, acts as a diuretic through urination, helps reduce cholesterol, lowers blood pressure

Cooking/preparation methods: boil, steam, slow cook, roast or bake after beans have been cooked through boiling or slow cooking

For deficient conditions, include: fava beans, chickpeas, red beans, lentils, soybeans

For excess conditions, include: adzuki beans

To clear heat, include: mung beans

To add warmth: season with alliums (such as shallots, leeks, onions or garlic) or spices

Nuts and Seeds

Crunchy in texture and rich in essential fatty acids, nuts and seeds add warmth and energizing nourishment to any meal or snack. This category covers a range of plant parts and types, from fruit (almonds and pistachios) to legumes (peanuts) to seeds (sesame, sunflower, pumpkin, flax, chia, hemp) to Brazil nuts. They add a delicious and satisfying flavor and texture, enriching vegetables dishes and salads, dressings, spreads and desserts.

Nuts and seeds, rich in oils, should be eaten in moderation. An excess of nut consumption can contribute to a buildup of dampness in the body, as well as contribute to liver *qi* congestion due to its fat content. Of course, if you are allergic or have a high sensitivity to nuts or seeds, avoid them entirely.

Thermal nature: neutral with minor variations of cooling to warming

Flavor: bland sweet

Action: lubricates, moistens lungs and large intestine, eases constipation, tonifies spleen *qi*, nourishes energy, is restorative

Cooking/preparation methods: roast, toast, bake, eat raw, grind, soak, decoct as a tea or infuse in liquor

For deficient conditions, include: walnuts, peanuts, pine nuts, chestnuts, peanuts, sesame seeds

Did You Know?

To *decoct* is a method of extracting the essence of a food, either by heating or boiling in water as a tea. To *steep* is to place dry ingredients (such as herbs, tea leaves, spices, etc.) to soak in hot liquid until the flavor is infused into the liquid. To *infuse* is to allow dry ingredients to sit in a liquid, such as alcohol or vinegar until such time that the flavor and aroma has been absorbed.

Cooking Tip

To improve the digestibility of nuts, soak them overnight, then place them on a baking sheet and bake them in a preheated oven at a low temperature, about 200°F (100°C), for 30 minutes to 1 hour. To bring out the flavor of nuts and seeds, toast them in a dry skillet over low heat, stirring or shaking often, for 3 to 5 minutes or until golden and fragrant.

For excess conditions, include: white sesame, sunflower and
  pumpkin seeds

To clear heat: avoid nuts, as they build yang and can contribute to
  warming. You can substitute seeds, such as sesame, sunflower,
  flax, chia, hemp or pumpkin.

To add warmth, include: walnuts, chestnuts

FOOD GROUP 2
Animals: Land and Sea

"The five animals are
used to fortify."

— *Huangdi Neijing Suwen,*
The Yellow Emperor's
Classic of Medicine

While animal foods are known to fortify our bodies, it is
recommended they be eaten in moderation and always with plenty
of vegetables. Organic, grass-fed (for land animals), sustainably
raised or fished and fresh-to-market should be the criteria for
eating animal foods.

Land Animals

This category of foods is the most intensely nourishing, supplementing
your body's *qi*, blood, yin and yang. It is most useful when recovering
from childbirth or intense physical activity and in the cooler months
of the year to build blood and *qi*. On the other hand, much of
modern-day illness and life-threatening disease are exacerbated by
an excess consumption of meats, especially poor-quality meats. In
Asia, even though meat is ubiquitous, it is almost always used in
small amounts and in combination with many vegetables.

Meat can be dried, frozen or preserved using salt. Be sure to
always wash your hands and keep your preparation area clean
before cooking with meat. Follow appropriate cooking times and
methods (so that animal food is cooked thoroughly). If you prefer
not to eat meat and other animal foods regularly, learn how to use
them to support your health. For some individuals, drinking meat
and/or seafood broths is a preferred way to extract nourishment
from animal foods.

Thermal nature: neutral to warming; seafood tends to be more
  cooling

Flavor: sweet, salty

Action: tonifies *qi*, yang, nourishes blood and yin, fortifies the body

Cooking/preparation methods: boil, steam, slow cook, braise,
  sauté, roast, bake, grill

For deficient conditions, include: beef, chicken, lamb, venison

For excess conditions: consider removing meat from your diet
  for a period of 8 to 12 weeks. You can include seafood, which

is generally more cooling. Increase your intake of vegetables, especially dark leafy greens.

To clear heat: eliminate meat from your diet for 8 to 12 weeks while increasing vegetables, whole grains and fruit. Include sea vegetables. You may include fish broth and stock.

To add warmth, include: lamb, beef, chicken, beef

To treat dryness, include: pork

Fish and Shellfish

Fish and shellfish taken from both fresh and seawater offer light and refreshing sustenance. When eaten fresh, the sweetness, moisture and richness of fish come together to provide a lighter form of animal protein. It is important to choose the freshest fish and seafood possible. If you regularly visit a fish store or fish department in your local grocery store, ask the fishmonger when shipments are generally expected to arrive and how the fish has been caught or raised. I will never forget ordering a fish dish in a restaurant when I was in China and the waiter bringing over a bucket of live fish for me to approve and select — that is fresh!

Every region around the world that has access to fresh streams and rivers or seas also has distinct types of seafood or freshwater fish offering a particular flavor and texture. Although fish generally have a cooling thermal nature, freshwater fish are generally sweeter in flavor with a neutral to warming nature that nourishes the stomach and spleen. Saltwater fish are typically more cooling or cold and salty in flavor, nourishing the yin while reinforcing the liver and kidneys.

Thermal nature: freshwater fish, neutral to warming; saltwater fish, neutral to cooling to cold

Flavor: freshwater, sweet; ocean fish, salty

Action: supplements the stomach and spleen, reinforces the kidneys and liver, builds *qi*, nourishes blood and yin

Cooking/preparation methods: boil, steam, grill, sauté, smoke, poach, slow cook in soups

For deficient conditions, include: catfish, trout, mussels, sardines, oysters

For excess conditions, include: clams, crab

To clear heat, include: crab, clams

To add warmth, include: shrimp (do not eat if you have a cold or you are prone to hives, have eczema, psoriasis or red skin rashes; its warming nature can aggravate skin conditions), mussels, salmon, trout

To treat dryness, include: cuttlefish

Eggs and Dairy

Did You Know?

Many people can have a sensitivity or intolerance to eggs and dairy products, so it is best to consume them in moderation.

Much like animal foods, these foods offer concentrated and fortifying nourishment that is immensely satisfying for some while being difficult to break down and digest for others. Be attentive to the ubiquitous inclusion of dairy products in many dishes.

Eggs and dairy products (from milk and cream to butter and yogurt) are fortifying, moistening and yin-enriching; however, they can contribute to excessive damp conditions, with symptoms ranging from indigestion, allergies, chronic ear infections, excessive phlegm production, headaches with dull pressure or sinus and lung congestion. These foods are best used in moderation.

Many peoples around the world do not digest and metabolize cow's milk well. Reducing cow's milk consumption is recommended if you are prone to recurrent ear infections, colds and sinus congestion, allergies or experience digestive issues. Dairy is best used in small amounts and is beneficial when experiencing qi and blood deficiencies, but only if it can be tolerated. Organic, omega-3-rich eggs are more easily tolerated and contain both yang and yin respectively in the yolk and albumen.

From a Chinese medicine perspective, an excess of dairy products congests the spleen and causes an accumulation of dampness, which obstructs digestion (the body's ability to transform food into nourishment and elimination). This is especially true for young children, whose digestive systems are developing and not yet stable. If your child has a tendency to digestive distress or recurrent ear infections, colds or runny noses, consider eliminating dairy products from their diet for a minimum of 8 to 12 weeks. Any concern about calcium can be addressed by eating sufficient dark leafy greens, fish and nuts.

Thermal nature: neutral to warming (goat's milk and sheep's milk is more warming)

Flavor: sweet

Action: nourishes, reinforces the stomach and spleen, replenishes energy, moistens mucous membranes, tonifies qi

Cooking/preparation methods: for dairy: fresh or fermented, boil, poach. For ghee and butter: eaten alone or used to sauté, stir-fry or added to sauces. Eggs can be poached, boiled, steamed, fried, baked or preserved.

For deficient conditions, include: ghee, butter, fermented whole milk products (including kefir or yogurt), omega-3-rich organic eggs

For excess conditions: consider replacing cow's milk with goat's or sheep's milk fermented products — the fat molecules in goat's and sheep's milk are smaller and easier to metabolize

To clear heat: avoid all dairy products as they contribute to dampness, phlegm and stagnation in these conditions

To add warmth, include: ghee, omega-3-rich organic eggs

To treat dryness, include: ghee, butter, eggs

FOOD GROUP 3
Vegetables

Wherever you live, during whatever season, the vibrancy of vegetables is always available. Walk into any farmers' market, grocery store or ethnic food market and you'll see a rainbow of colorful vegetables, depending on the season. The hardy roots, the delicate green or red or mottled leaves of lettuce and the deep, earthy colors of eggplant, carrots, beets, radishes, winter squash, broccoli and beans are truly a visual feast. The wide range of flavors and textures can thrill anyone who loves to eat — all that is needed is clear guidance on how to prepare this assortment, from roots and tubers to leafy greens to the spicy alliums to wild vegetables to mushrooms to the marvels of sea vegetables. You will never be at a loss with vegetables in your fridge or on your table. They embrace all thermal natures, all flavors and all actions that contribute to inner renewal, vibrancy and health.

> "The five vegetables are used to fulfill."
>
> — *Huangdi Neijing Suwen,*
> *The Yellow Emperor's*
> *Classic of Medicine*

Land Vegetables

Land vegetables include root vegetables, tubers, winter and summer squashes, and leafy greens.

Thermal nature: cooling to neutral to warming

Flavor: varied — bitter, sweet, sour, salty, pungent

Action: varying dependent upon the vegetable, but in general detoxifies, clears heat, aids bowel movements, eases constipation

Cooking/preparation methods: boil, steam, slow cook, roast, bake, grill, sauté, braise, pickle, ferment

For deficient conditions, include: pumpkin, winter squash, leeks, fennel, cabbage, taro root, sweet potato, mushrooms

For excess conditions, include: dark leafy greens, seaweeds, celery

To clear heat, include: dandelion greens, mustard greens, bitter melon, spinach, seaweeds, celery, shepherd's purse, lotus root, cucumber

To add warmth, include: pumpkin, alliums, Chinese spring
onions (also known as green onions, scallions), chile pepper

To treat dryness, include: spinach, okra, sweet potato, eggplant

Alliums

The allium family includes onions, leeks, chives, Chinese spring
onions (also known as green onions, scallions), shallots and garlic.
Alliums bring sweet pungency and a warming thermal nature
to many dishes. They are best for people who tend to feel cold
often. If you run hot, avoid using alliums altogether or use them
in moderation.

Thermal nature: warming

Flavor: pungent, sweet, bitter

Actions: warms the interior and expels cold, aids digestion,
moves and activates *qi* and digestion

Cooking/preparation methods: boil, steam, slow cook, roast,
bake, grill, sauté, dry, braise, eat raw, pickle, ferment, decoct
as teas

Mushrooms

Mushrooms, or fungi, add deep flavor or umami to many
dishes. The ancient Egyptians believed they were the "plants of
immortality," and the Chinese have used them for thousands
of years as *qi* tonics and longevity foods. The mycelium, the
organisms that produce mushrooms, are powerful antimicrobial
and antiviral agents. Mushrooms offer powerful protection to
support and boost the immune system.

Mushroom varieties include shiitake, maitake, cremini, oyster,
chanterelles, morels, reishi, oyster, button, tremella, chicken
in the woods, lion's mane, reishi and cordyceps, among others.
Reishi, cordyceps, turkey tail, maitake and shiitake are just some
of the varieties known for their potent *qi*-building, blood sugar–
regulating and anticancer properties. The fragrant, earthy taste
of mushrooms also adds depth and richness to dishes.

Thermal nature: neutral to slightly warming or cooling

Flavor: sweet, fragrant

Actions: Reinforces the spleen; builds *qi*; strengthens immune
system; resolves phlegm; reduces cholesterol

Cooking/preparation methods: boil, steam, slow cook, roast,
bake, grill, sauté, dry, braise, pickle, ferment, decoct

For deficient conditions, include: shiitake, reishi, cordyceps,
maitake

For excess conditions: consider eliminating or reducing meat for 8 to 12 weeks while introducing mushrooms known for their heartiness, such as shiitake, morel and button

To clear heat, include: tremella, oyster mushrooms

To add warmth, include: mushrooms with ginger or warming spices

To treat dryness, include: button mushrooms, tremella

Seaweeds, or Sea Vegetables

Throughout history, coastal peoples have eaten and used the primordial vegetables of the sea. Sea vegetables bring minerals back into our bodies and link us to the primal vitality of the oceans and seas. The malleable seaweed and its mineral abundance can enrich many dishes. Sea vegetables are delicious eaten on their own, fresh, or in salads, stir-fries, stews, soups or bouillon. As a powerful category of vegetables with a high iodine content, seaweeds can be eaten daily in moderation. They are also high in calcium, magnesium, iron, phosphorus and other micro-minerals, and are effective in balancing hormones. If you have a thyroid disorder, consult with your physician or health-care provider about recommended amounts.

Sea vegetable (seaweed) varieties include agar-agar, kombu, wakame, dulse, nori, arame and hijiki. Bring these vegetables into your diet as a small daily side dish.

Thermal nature: cooling to cold

Flavor: salty

Action: dissolves phlegm, clears heat, softens accumulations, detoxifies, nourishes yin and blood, benefits the lymphatic system, benefits the thyroid

Cooking/preparation methods: eat fresh, smoke, boil, roast, stir-fry

For deficient conditions, include: hijiki, dulse

For excess conditions, include: kombu, nori, arame, wakame

To clear heat, include: nori, wakame, kombu, nori

To add warmth, include: sea vegetables in warming dishes — their salty and cooling nature will moderate warming dishes

To treat dryness, include: all sea vegetables — they are yin tonics and benefit the kidney network, therefore supporting the dissemination of fluids throughout the body.

> **Tip**
> Due to the high pollution levels in the world's oceans, it is important to know the sources for the sea vegetables you eat. This book recommends suppliers of sea vegetables who know their sources and may test for heavy metals. For more information, see Resources, page 466.

Wild Vegetables

Wild vegetables are plentiful underfoot. I have a ritual with my daughter in early spring, when we head to the hills in a local forest to pluck the sprouts of stinging nettle to add vibrant sweetness to a wild spring soup or risotto. In Veneto, Italy, I saw locals pulling wild dandelion from pastures to cook in a boiling pot of water along with a whole garlic clove, a pinch of salt and topping it with fresh olive oil after being cooked. These are both examples of how we can forage in our own backyards for wild vegetables. Take note of what grows in the fields near you and even in the big city — nutritious, delicious vegetables are everywhere, offering plenty of omega-3s, essential fatty acids and strong, unique flavors and actions. Their flavors may take some getting used to, but their potent health benefits are a perk. So venture beyond your normal vegetable consumption and try some foraged vegetables, but be sure to find out what you're picking by consulting a wild food guide, and pick only where you are sure there is no residue from pesticides or automobile pollution.

Wild vegetables include shepherd's purse, stinging nettles, lamb's-quarter, purslane, dandelion greens and chickweed (see page 192). Learn how to add them into your diet and you will not be disappointed.

> **Cooking Tip**
> Add wild greens to your soups, salads, stir-fries or risottos as you would any other green vegetable.

Thermal nature: neutral to cold
Flavor: bitter, bland, pungent, sweet
Action: clears heat, calms the liver, detoxifies, cools blood, diuretic, improves digestion
Cooking/preparation methods: eat raw, juice, steam, boil, pickle or ferment, sauté

For deficient conditions, include: wild nettles, purslane, shepherd's purse
For excess conditions, include: all wild vegetables
To clear heat, include: all wild vegetables
To add warmth: since wild greens are mostly cooling or cold in nature, they are not recommended to add warmth
To treat dryness, include: stinging nettles

FOOD GROUP 4
Fruits

Succulent, juicy, fragrant, sweet, tart and refreshing, the bounty of fruit delights our senses. Their sweet and sour flavor, as well as their juicy flesh, keep us hydrated and cool during the warmer months of the year. Eating fruits in season, and buying them locally when possible, ensures freshness and optimal flavor. Canning, drying and freezing ripe seasonal fruit seals in their freshness, preserves their nutritional value and guarantees a taste of spring or summer even when it's not.

Besides their refreshing taste, many fruits have a distinct therapeutic value to help clear excess heat, moisten internal dryness and, in some cases (such as with pears and papaya), dissolve phlegm.

Thermal nature: cold to warming

Flavor: sweet and sour, occasionally combined with minor bitter flavor (as in grapefruit)

Actions: cools heat, hydrates, stimulates appetite, dissolves phlegm, acts as a diuretic, eases thirst and dry mouth, laxative

Cooking/preparation methods: eat raw, juice, bake, dry, poach

For deficient conditions, include: figs, cherries and grapes, raspberries, red dates, longan fruit, peaches

For excess conditions, include: kiwifruit, pineapple, grapefruit, apples, persimmons, tangerines, pears, papaya

To clear heat, include: watermelon, grapefruit, banana, kiwifruit, tomatoes (technically a fruit), rose hips, tamarind, lemons, blueberries, cranberries

To add warmth, include: cherries, raspberries

To treat dryness, include: bananas, apricots, apples, mandarins, oranges, peaches, plums, lemons, kiwifruit, grapefruit, figs

"The five fruits are used to assist."

— Huangdi Neijing Suwen, The Yellow Emperor's Classic of Medicine

Did You Know?

Too much fruit can spike blood sugar and increase internal dampness, hindering the warming and yang action of the spleen, impeding digestion and causing an accumulation of mucus or phlegm. Fruit facilitates hydration, but too much sweetness can dam up the body's capacity to circulate and eliminate that excess.

FOOD GROUP 5
Condiments

Eating is a sensory experience. We smell aromas, we see colors, we feel the texture and taste the flavors of foods we eat, amplifying the joys eating can bring. Without the senses, eating does not satisfy or even hold our interest. This is where condiments come in.

In the Chinese materia medica of foods, condiments have a distinct purpose: to amplify and enhance the flavor of foods, heighten palatability and absorption, and energize digestion and circulation, as well as infuse our eating with pleasure. Preparing food for a group of people and satisfying all their tastes can be difficult, so supplementing a meal with a variety of condiments — from salt and sweeteners to alcohol and vinegars to herbs and spices to teas and flowers — transforms a meal, adding a customized "magic" to suit the eaters' preferences.

The range of condiments listed in this book is broader than the conventional thinking of what we call condiments used in North American cooking. Condiments incorporate all the five flavors (salt, sour, sweet, pungent and bitter), which can layer therapeutic actions and enhance culinary delight. They can heat up a meal or cool it down.

Salt

Many foods have some degree of naturally occurring saltiness, so adding salt at the table is not recommended. However, using condiments that include saltiness as part of their makeup can bring a rounder and more satisfying flavor or "saltiness" to a meal while countering strong bitter flavors. Salty condiments include miso, tamari, soy sauce, anchovies, katsuobushi (bonito flakes) or condiments that contain umeboshi or sea vegetables. (See Condiment Recipes, starting on page 422 for more ideas.)

Thermal nature: neutral
Flavor: salty
Action: adds flavor to foods, harmonizes digestion, clears heat, moistens dryness, supports kidneys, dissolves phlegm
Cooking/preparation methods: Salt and salty foods and seasonings, including tamari, miso, salt, seaweeds, katsuobushi and brined anchovies, are added to cooking to moderate and bring out the flavor of foods. Dissolve salt in water when cooking other foods or soups and stews.

Tip

See Condiment Recipes (starting on page 422) for a long list of condiments. These recipes are intended to add a dimension to even the simplest of meals and provide variety at a shared table of eating. Remember: a little will go a long way.

Health Tip

Pay attention to your consumption of salted foods, which is abundant in processed foods. Moderate your intake if you suffer from hypertension, kidney disease or edema.

Sweeteners

Sweet is the ubiquitous flavor that delights all ages, but we often overeat and overindulge in it. Used judiciously in dishes, sweeteners can moderate the bitter or sour flavor of a dish while enhancing its taste. Sweeteners can also warm and deepen the natural sweetness found in so many foods.

When added to dishes with a specific intention and action in mind, a sweetener's therapeutic effect is evident: people relax, tensions melt, a steady calm pervades any meal. However, too much sugar has the opposite effect — it creates a spike, or "sugar" high, only to cause the body to crash in energy or mood soon afterwards.

Many of the recipes in this book have no or little sugar added, yet when there is, the sweetener is from natural, less processed sources such as the fruit itself, coconut sugar, date sugar, honey and maple syrup. (See Condiment Recipes, starting on page 422, as well as the beverages and desserts recipes, for more inspiration.)

Thermal nature: neutral to warming; in excess, sweetness creates
   warmth and dampness
Flavor: sweet
Action: supports the middle burner (the digestive system),
   stomach and spleen, calms, relaxes muscle tension and spasm
Cooking/preparation methods: add as a condiment to flavor
   foods, stir into warm drinks, add to alcohol to aid in the
   decoction of herbs, use as a topping on foods

Tea

Legend has it that a legendary ruler in ancient China, Shennong, whose name translates as the "divine farmer," is credited with discovering tea. Shennong, who preferred his drinking water boiled, was sitting under a tree with his cup of boiled water when leaves from the *Camellia sinensis* (tea plant) blew into his cup and infused the hot water with fragrance and flavor. The legend goes on to say that he was intrigued by the fragrance, took a sip and felt its effects throughout his body, and thus tea was discovered more than 5,000 years ago.

In Chinese culture, as in many others, a meal is often finished with a cup of tea. Tea quenches the thirst and promotes hydration. Tea was also one of the first medicines drunk to dispel heat and clear the mind. To this day, many Chinese herbal remedies are taken as a tea. In Chinese medicine, we may add herbs to green tea to dispel a headache or to treat the first signs of a head cold. In this book, green tea leaves are lightly fermented as a condiment and used as a cooking liquid in a few dishes.

> **Did You Know?**
>
> In the Chinese culture, as in many others, a tea finishes off a meal to help refresh and relax.

Health Tip

Whether you prefer a black tea (which has the most amount of caffeine) or green tea (also rich in caffeine), teas are sure to stimulate your senses. If you are sensitive to caffeine, however, avoid drinking tea late in the day so you can get to sleep more easily.

In the beginning, all tea was green, but as tea drinking evolved, experimentation with drying, roasting, aging and adding flowers and herbs to tea leaves accelerated the evolution of tea. Today, teas include black tea, green tea, oolong tea, white tea and pu-erh tea, and the ritual of drinking them takes place in various cultures around the world, from China and Japan to India and Russia to the Middle East and England to South America and Australia, as well as in North America, where we see a revival and development of tea drinking. The ritual of tea is a high art, yet the simple act of taking time for tea kindles the slowing of time in our relationship with ourselves or another as we sit with the fragrance and flavor of a warm cup of tea.

Thermal nature: green, oolong and white tea are more cooling; black and pu-erh tea are more warming

Flavor: slightly bitter and sweet

Action: relieves thirst, energizes and refreshes the mind, acts as a diuretic, aids in digestion if drunk separately from a meal. Excessive tea drinking can be too drying, due to its slightly bitter flavor

Cooking/preparation methods: infuse, brew, steep, decoct

Alcohol

A bit of spirits can be powerfully therapeutic, as seen in Chinese medicine's medicinal and tonic wines. Alcohol is a potent carrier, enriching a dish or soup when it's added in the cooking process or infused with herbs or added to an herbal formula to vitalize and activate circulation to our extremities. *A bit of spirits* is the key, as taken in moderation, spirits open the mind, move *qi* and blood, and warm the body and extremities while lifting the spirit. Consumed in excess, alcohol is one of the great destroyers of the body and mind while wreaking havoc on personal lives and families. Alcohol should be used in moderation for the purpose of improving and invigorating our health.

The medicinal use in Chinese medicine usually refers to alcohol, such as rice wine (or sake), red wine or distilled liquor (such as vodka or brandy), that is used as a vehicle for soaking foods or herbs to create a medicinal wine or elixir. Medicinal wines are most often consumed during the winter in small amounts as a tonic to ward off cold and to build yang and *qi* while activating circulation. (See tonic wine recipes in each season for more inspiration.)

Young people (below the age of 18 and depending on your jurisdiction), who are rich in *qi* and blood should avoid alcohol (they can equally benefit from teas, water and other non-alcoholic beverages), as well as those with cardiac conditions, diabetes mellitus, autoimmune disorders, inflammatory bowel disease or any other chronic illness that is being monitored by a health-care provider.

Many food-grade liquors and wines, such as red date and walnut wine, are mild enough that they can be enjoyed just for their flavor while the user could still benefit from the *qi*-building therapeutics. For medicinal use, alcohol and wines can be taken in small amounts, 2 tablespoons (30 mL) twice a day. Many of the herbal alcohol and wines can be added to tea. It is also not uncommon for a Chinese medicine practitioner to prescribe an herbal formula that is added to a small dose of brandy to augment the reach of the formula throughout the body.

Thermal nature: warm to hot

Flavor: pungent, sweet, bitter

Actions: scatters the cold while warming the body and extremities, invigorates *qi* and blood circulation, augments the effects of herbs, aids digestion

Cooking/preparation methods: None. Herbs and food can be left to soak and decoct in alcohol for 10 days to up to 2 months. All of the recommendations below are to soak in alcohol, either vodka, brandy or dry rice wine, for 10 days to up to 2 months.

For deficient conditions, include: ginseng, walnut, astragalus, goji berries, red dates

For excess conditions: avoid alcohol altogether

To clear heat: mostly for those who have a combination of heat and damp, include: chrysanthemum flower tonic wine

To add warmth, include: cinnamon, cardamom, walnut, astragalus, dang gui

To treat dryness, include: honey

Vinegar

In Chinese folk medicine, vinegar is a medicinal food used to stop bleeding, relieve toxicity, increase blood circulation and improve digestion. In the ancient Chinese medicine text the *Shang Han Lun*, the *Treatise on Cold Damage*, vinegar is referred to as *ku jiu*, or "bitter liquor." Vinegar is used in Chinese medicine to dry-fry herbs (see Did You Know? at right), changing the potency and action of these specific herbs. It is also documented to be a simple remedy for common health problems such as hangovers, headaches, gingivitis, nausea and skin issues. In the West, a

Did You Know?

Dry-frying herbs, or *pao zhi*, is an ancient method of altering the tastes and potency of herbs through processing them in a pan with either honey, vinegar or salt. Doing this enhances and changes the direction and therapeutic action of herbs.

teaspoon (5 mL) of vinegar mixed in hot or warm water with some honey is commonly believed to jump-start digestion and increase stomach acid when taken before a meal.

Traditionally, in China, vinegar is made from rice, sorghum, millet or wheat. In the West, vinegars are also made from grapes or apples and added to salad dressings — the sour and bitter flavors awaken the digestive processes.

Thermal nature: varied, including warming
Flavor: sour and bitter (the *Neijing Suwen* states that when sour and bitter come together it serves to drain stagnation)
Action: moves *qi* and blood, stops bleeding, relieves toxicity, activates and assists digestion, eases pain, reduces food stagnation from overeating,
Cooking/preparation methods: Add to stews, beans, salads, teas

Herbs and Spices

Culinary herbs and spices brighten up any dish, activate the senses and digestion, and warm the body while elevating the intensity of flavor in dishes and evoking sensuous pleasure in eating. What's more, simple culinary spices and herbs are strong therapeutic and medicinal agents that add dimension to the inherent flavor of foods and enhance the therapeutic action of a dish. Every cultural tradition has a flavor palate that it values and is often known for in its cooking. If you embrace cooking as a way to affect your health, spices can play a key role — they can create balance in a dish, cooling down a warming dish (so it doesn't overheat you) or warming up cooling foods.

Spices have been traded and highly valued for thousands of years, and for good reason. Spices are defined as the seeds, fruits, roots or barks of a plant, whereas herbs (in the West) are considered the leafy parts of an herbaceous plant. Spices are usually dried and sometimes ground. Herbs are easy to grow and are most flavorful fresh, but can also be dried.

> "Sanctioned by the wisdom of the ancients — if wisdom it was — spices were believed to heal, mitigate, and rectify as much as they delighted.
>
> — *Jack Turner, Spice: The History of a Temptation*

Thermal nature: varied, including warming to cooling
Flavor: pungent, sweet, aromatic
Action: scatters the cold while warming and activating digestion, warms the center. Pungent and warming as well as cooling herbs and spices can disperse *qi*, hot or cold.
Cooking/preparation methods: decoct as teas or in wines, add to foods in all cooking methods

For deficient conditions, include: warming aromatic spices, such as rosemary, thyme, cinnamon, cardamom, fennel, garlic (if no heat symptoms), ginger

For excess conditions: avoid all hot warming spices, such as garlic, cayenne, chile peppers and galangal, which add to and exacerbate stagnation. You can use small amounts of ginger and culinary herbs.

To clear heat: avoid all spicy foods, including any type of pepper, chile peppers, cayenne and galangal. Instead, use cooling herbs, such as mint, lemon balm, lemongrass, lavender or turmeric.

To add warmth, include: ginger, cardamom, fennel seeds, mustard seeds

To treat dryness, include: lubricating and hydrating foods, such as spinach, fruit, almonds. Eliminate warming and hot spices from your cooking and diet.

Did You Know?

In Chinese medicine, herbs are considered to include a plant's or tree's roots, rhizomes, stems, bark, leaves, flowers, berries or fruits.

Fragrant Flowers

Flowers are said to open our hearts and lift our spirits. Their fragrance is evocative, their flavor subtle and their history on our plates ancient. There is a long tradition of including flowers in the diet, whether in salads, teas, spice mixes, honeys or wines. If you are feeling stuck or low, adding edible flowers to your meals, in a side dish, an herb and spice mixture, a tea or medicinal wine, will certainly move qi and affect your state of mind. In Chinese medicine, we say that fragrance, "opens the orifices," that is, the senses. (See the food table in Chapter 10, pages 199 and 200, to learn about the thermal nature and actions of edible flowers.)

Edible flowers include jasmine, gardenia, rose, violets, gardenia, chrysanthemum and lavender, but before adding flowers to any meal, ensure that they are indeed edible and organic.

Thermal nature: cooling, neutral or warming

Flavor: pungent, sweet, slightly bitter

Actions: dissolves dampness, assists in regulating digestion, activates blood circulation and qi, lifts the spirit

Cooking/preparation methods: raw, decoct, infuse or decoct in alcohol or wines, infuse in water, made into an electuary

Note: For more information on specific foods, see Chapter 10 (page 162) for food descriptions and food property tables. For more information on stocking a healthy kitchen, see Chapter 9 (page 144) for shopping lists for recommended foods.

Introducing New Foods

Note: Use the food tables in Chapter 10, starting on page 183, for specific information on flavor, thermal nature and actions.

When expanding your eating repertoire, approach it with the spirit of curiosity and inquiry. Try new foods and explore their flavors and textures. If you decide to drastically change the way you eat, it may take some time to acclimate to these new flavors and textures. Maybe you start with a couple of new foods, while eliminating those foods that create obstacles for your health, such as processed foods, fast foods, greasy and fatty foods, poor-quality meats, refined carbohydrates, sugar and artificial sweeteners. I often tell my patients to start with adding one new vegetable a week to their diet, and look for ways to prepare it.

As you approach a new diet, use the food groups to guide you. Experiment with different foods and learn to cook them or discover new ways to cook a familiar food to bring out more flavor and delight in what you eat. Take the time to sit down and enjoy it alone or in community with others. As you eat these new foods, chew, savor and enjoy the nourishment you are receiving. Food has energy and *how* we eat it is just as important as *what* we eat.

Reflection: The Food Groups and Your Diet

If you would like to better understand your patterns of eating, use the guide, opposite page, to record what you eat for a few days or a week. Tracking the foods you eat will help you become more aware of your patterns: the variety of foods you may or may not eat in relation to the food groups, flavor and thermal nature. Don't worry about analyzing the information you list. You might notice that you tend to lean toward one or two flavors or food groups and are missing out on others. If you find you're missing out on important food groups, use the chart as a guide to begin your exploration of new foods and flavors.

Food Groups and Your Diet

Food Groups	List foods you have eaten according to the food groups	Predominant Thermal Nature	Predominant Flavors
Whole grains Beans, pulses and other legumes Nuts and seeds			
Animal foods: Land and sea Eggs Dairy			
Vegetables: Land vegetables Alliums Fungi Wild vegetables Sea vegetables			
Fruits			
Condiments: Salt Sugar and sweeteners Tea Alcohol Vinegar Herbs and spices Fragrant flowers			

What patterns of eating do you notice?

What is the predominant flavor or nature (warming or cooling) of the foods you eat?

What patterns do you notice about yourself?

- Do you eat regular meals or snack?
- Do you eat on the go or sit down?
- Do you cook meals or eat take-out?
- Do you eat when stressed or tired?
- Do you have food cravings? If so, what are they?

Chapter 5

The Cycle of Change: The Seasons

"From ancient times it has been recognized that there is an intimate relationship between the activity and life of human beings and their natural environment."

— *Huangdi Neijing Suwen, The Yellow Emperor's Classic of Medicine*

The ancients understood the importance of attuning ourselves to and living in harmony with nature through the seasons in order to improve and maintain good health. We naturally acclimate to changes in temperature, light and weather. In these transitions, the availability of certain foods also changes and we can fine-tune our alignment with the season at hand by choosing more locally grown and seasonal foods, adjusting how we cook and becoming more aware of what and how we eat throughout the year. In Chinese medicine, eating according to the seasonal cycles is one of the key foundations in building and protecting health.

No matter where we live, whether it is a temperate four-season climate or a cold or warm region with more muted alterations, we are affected by the subtle and profound changes that occur over the course of a year — externally and internally. Our capacity to adjust internally to these changes and balance yin and yang is crucial to maintaining health and aided greatly by our dietary choices, cooking methods as well as our regular physical activities.

Eating in Tune with the Seasons

Each seasonal change has a direct impact on us. We may not be overtly aware, but we change, feel different and *make* changes. As spring ripens into summer, we may feel more inclined to be active and outdoors, extending our vitality out into the world. Or perhaps when autumn begins to descend, we feel the urge to move inside and contain our energy, seeking to organize, store and rest.

We may crave meals that are cooked more slowly over a longer period of time and richer types of food in winter to warm us, while we eat more fresh uncooked and cooling foods in summer to create an inner, cool lightness in contrast to the blazing summer sun.

Attuning to the energy of each season serves a deeper function: to nourish and protect the vital, subtle *qi* that animates energy and vital body functions and to balance our internal yin and yang with the surrounding environment.

You probably already know that eating *with* the seasons is good for you. Indeed, foods that are in season are fresh and vibrant and have peak flavor. Peak flavor equals peak nutrition — all the more so in that flavor heightens our eating pleasure. Eating seasonally means we are eating what nature provides at a given time, putting us in synch with our surroundings. It is also one of the primary ways we can participate in and enjoy the rhythm of the season at hand. It is fundamentally common-sense eating. To obtain the best flavor, nutrition and eating pleasure from where we live, doesn't it make sense to eat what grows where we live? Therefore, learning how to utilize foods' intrinsic flavor and how to prepare and cook each of them in each season for optimal health will enhance the eating experience and help integrate the vitality and rhythm of the season directly into our body.

In this modern, interconnected world, especially in the West, we have the world's foods available all year long. We can eat the world, at times forsaking the beauty and vitality of our distinct locale and its unique growing conditions. There is much to be gained from eating seasonally.

How Do We Eat in Harmony?

Eating in harmony starts with choosing locally grown seasonal foods, but there's more to it than that. At times we crave the opposite of what is actually good for us. Take summer, for instance. Even though you want to grab foods that cool you down quickly — foods like ice cream and cold drinks — they do not actually serve you best. Why? When we eat ice cold ice cream, our body needs to generate internal heat to warm the food to digest and absorb it. That is vital energy that our digestive system could be using to transform what we've eaten to build and nourish our vitality. It also means that we are generating heat in response to something cold — the exact opposite of what we want in summer.

The solution in this instance may seem counterintuitive, but if we eat or drink food in summer that is warmed or at room temperature, our body can adapt more easily. We also consider a food's thermal nature. Take tea, for example. Tea, even though

"If you truly get in touch with a piece of carrot, you get in touch with the soil, the rain and sunshine. You get in touch with Mother Earth and you feel in touch with true life."

— *Thich Nhat Hanh*

Did You Know?

In Chinese medicine, overindulging in cold foods contracts our stomach, slows our digestion, digestive capacity and weakens what is called our *digestive fire.*

we usually enjoy it warm or hot, is bitter in flavor and has a cold thermal nature that helps to cool internal heat, a necessary action in summer. Cooling pungent spices, such as peppermint, lemon balm, chamomile, coriander, lavender and dandelion, also keep us cool internally in hot weather. Warming spices, on the other hand, are important to help maintain an inner fire and warmth. The use of basil, rosemary, thyme, sage, dill, cumin, paprika, pepper, cardamom and chile peppers, can help to keep our inner heat active so that, when autumn comes around, we haven't weakened our internal furnace.

The Cycle of the Seasons

"To everything —
turn, turn, turn.
There is a season —
turn, turn, turn.
And a time to every
purpose under
heaven."

— *Pete Seeger, adapted from Ecclesiastes*

The seasons change, we change and our eating changes. What benefits us in spring may not be right for us in the middle of a dark, cold winter.

The energy of spring rises and pushes upward as new life is born. The full yang, the warmth and fire of summer, is the fuel for rapid growth and exuberant abundance in the natural world. As Earth pivots, the shorter days and cool air of autumn descends and the harvest comes to fruition. As the days shorten and the plants begin to dry and shed their leaves, we begin to harness our energy to begin moving inward. Finally, during winter, in the darkest time of the year, we come indoors both physically and spiritually to maintain internal warmth, protect our vitality and restore and renew ourselves. The energy of plants also moves down, deep into the earth — to consolidate, regenerate and prepare for the inevitable spring. So even though winter on the surface appears barren, it is one of the most important and active seasons as we too become more interior, preserving our energy for the inevitable upward force of spring.

Seasonal cycles have their ebbs and flows affecting each one of us differently. If we pay attention and learn how to adjust our food and activities appropriately, we will learn how to promote our inner balance in harmony with the seasons.

Spring: Renewal and Growth

Spring is that wondrous time of year when the earth reawakens and the energy that has been deeply stored in the earth begins to push itself vigorously upward and outward, as seen in the first emerging shoots of plants and leaves. This is the initiation of yang *qi* in nature. It is a time of new beginnings and internal movements, when we can generate inner renewal and emerge from the darkness of winter to the light outdoors. We often feel stirred to clear out the old and do a bit of spring cleaning, both in our homes and our bodies. We want to shed the buildup and accumulation of winter — but not so fast. Spring is a highly changeable time. In Chinese medicine, spring is a time of "wind" — quick and unpredictable changes. One moment it is warm, then it is cold, then the winds and rain come. My grandmother always told me, "Don't be fooled. Wear your jacket and keep it buttoned." Internally, we need to do the same: "button up" our outer layer (our defensive *qi*), keeping it strong to promote and protect our emerging yang *qi*.

> "The months of the spring season bring about the revitalization of all things in nature. It is the time of birth."
>
> — *Huangdi Neijing Suwen, The Yellow Emperor's Classic of Medicine*

Organ System

Spring is the liver's time of year. The liver, in Chinese medicine, is responsible for promoting harmonious *qi* flow in all directions and throughout our body and organs. The liver stores and supports the regeneration of the blood, which nourishes our muscles and tendons. As yang *qi* emerges, the body needs to dispel and disperse the excessive buildup that occurs in winter; coming out of winter, we need to mimic this movement internally and physiologically as well as externally in our physical activities to renew and stimulate revitalization throughout our being.

Spring is powerful and fragile, asking us to soften and become more receptive and relaxed. We need to cultivate our inner spring of growth and renewal. In Chinese herbal medicine, we often use an herbal formula, Xiao Yao Wan (Free and Easy Wanderer) — typically made up of eight Chinese herbs, including dang gui (aka dong quai), mint and fresh ginger — to help relieve internal muscle tension and ease the liver *qi*, which is responsible for promoting internal flow and harmony. The free and unobstructed movement of liver *qi* through the body contributes to a feeling of inner connection, ease, flow and capacity for increased mental clarity.

Did You Know?

In Chinese medicine, wind (*feng* 风) is one of the external influences that can cause an intense sore throat and cold to come on quickly.

Physical Activities

Spring invites us to walk in the woods, relax and spend more time outdoors — walking leisurely, breathing in the fresh spring air and absorbing the newness and energy of spring. Remember that we are coming out of the winter hibernation and it is not yet the time for full-on activity. Exercise should include stretching as well as movement to open up the muscles and loosen the tendons. It is still important that we protect ourselves from the changeable weather; the hard shell of winter is just beginning to crack open.

Flavors and Foods

The first leafy green vegetables of spring are rich in chlorophyll, which give plants their green color while offering nourishment and cleansing capacity. Eating these green vegetables helps us take in the revitalizing energy of spring. Here are the two flavors that are beneficial in spring:

Sweet and pungent: During this season, it is best to favor flavors that are sweet and pungent. The sweet and slightly pungent flavor of baby turnips is a perfect example as are snow peas, spinach, baby carrots and beets, whole grains, legumes and seeds, which help bring nourishment that is calming and support the digestive process. The spicy and pungent flavors found in many spring herbs — such as mint, lemon balm, rosemary, thyme, chives, Chinese green onions (aka scallions), garlic, ginger, watercress and arugula — awaken our senses.

The sweet flavor encourages the softening and relaxing of the body. The pungent flavor's action on the body is upward and outward, dispersing the buildup of the winter and mimicking the renewal of spring. To include Chinese herbs in cooking, add in food-grade herbs such as Chinese yam (*Dioscorea*, or *shan yao*), white peony (*bai shao*), goji berries, chrysanthemum flowers and honeysuckle (*Lonicera*) buds.

Cooking Methods

Note: For more information about cooking methods, see Chapter 6.

To help us soften and begin to expand upward and outward as we shed the constraints of winter and transition from a richer way of cooking, we use lighter cooking methods — steam, quick boil, quick sauté, light braise, stir-fry, spring soups — to help preserve the freshness of food. Adding lightly fermented foods, such as pickles and sauerkraut, stimulate digestion. Finally, if our digestion permits, we may eat more raw foods.

Foods to Avoid

Health cannot be built upon the addition of good foods without the elimination of certain foods that get in the way. In spring, as our bodies eliminate heavier and richer foods, we need good-quality fats and oils, such as those found in fish, nuts and seeds and avocados, to maintain our health. There is no reason to fear healthy fats, which are necessary for the production of cholesterol. Cholesterol is, in fact, a type of fat produced by the liver and is necessary for a healthy nervous and endocrine system, as well as optimal daily brain functioning. However, many processed foods are created with poor-quality oils, which oxidize in the body and create free radicals, contributing to cell damage, early aging and the onset of many modern-day chronic diseases.

These manufactured foods may have also been created by food scientists to give us a "taste" we may find hard to resist. Avoid the following:

- Processed and manufactured foods. Many are made with poor-quality oils and include too much sodium and sweeteners. Even the "healthy" and "natural" processed foods are usually higher in sugars and sodium.
- Greasy, creamy and fatty foods, in particular deep-fried fast foods.
- Processed meats, such as luncheon meats, bacon and sausages (the overconsumption of red meat is also attributed to many chronic diseases).
- Alcohol and stimulants like caffeine, which includes coffee, black tea, cola or caffeinated sodas and drinks or chocolate.
- Refined carbohydrates and refined sugars are a big factor in the development of fatty liver disease, chronic digestive disturbances, insulin resistance and diabetes.
- Hot and spicy foods, which can cause internal heat, irritate and cause inflammation, especially when used in excess.
- Overly salty foods.

Did You Know?

The liver is responsible for the free flow of *qi* throughout the body. It is important to avoid foods that congest the liver's capacity to detoxify and therefore impede its physiological function.

Lifestyle Habits

Besides the elimination of certain foods, particular lifestyle practices can "weigh" us down. Eating heavy meals late at night obstructs digestion. Using recreational drugs drain *qi* and *jing* (essence) and exert a strain on one's health and vitality.

Summer: Exuberance and Abundance

Summer is the most yang, exuberant and vigorous time of year, when *qi* and blood are most active throughout the body. We are open to the light of the sun and the abundance the earth produces in its harvest. This season invites our active participation, whether by simply being outdoors more, rising earlier in the morning or taking in the starry summer nights. The most yang time of the year is the brightest, the warmest and the most expansive time of growth and abundance.

Summer offers us an abundant variety of fruits and vegetables. We participate in summer by expanding our activity levels and eating a wide selection of fresh, vibrant and nourishing foods. Summer might, however, be the trickiest time of year to create balance. Our environment and climate invite us to participate in a non-stop party of light, warmth, activity and delightful food. During the warmest, brightest and most yang time of year, the challenge is to balance expansion and containment — staying cool while maintaining internal warmth.

Organ System

Summer is the time of the heart. In Chinese medicine, the heart is considered the emperor of the body, in charge of all the internal organs, responsible for pumping and circulating blood to all the tissues and organs throughout the body. The heart, the center of our being and hub of circulation is, in Chinese medicine, considered the home of the *shen* (or spirit) and houses the mind, the seat of consciousness. The *shen* corresponds to the mind, which is housed in the heart and signifies the entire sphere of mental, emotional and spirit. The state of and health of the heart will effect mental activities and balanced emotions.

Our heart energy, as big and expansive as it can be in the expression of joy, affection and love, still needs to be contained and balanced during the hot summer season. The balance to expansion is containment. Too much expansion can weaken our internal boundaries and make us feel scattered, tired and anxious. In the West, there are a number of risk factors that impact heart health and our state of mind, including chronic long-term stress, excessive intake of alcohol or stimulants, refined salt and sugar, fatty foods and high meat consumption.

Did You Know?

In Chinese medicine, there is no differentiation between the body and mind. The brain is considered an extraordinary organ dependent upon the heart for healthy functioning. On a physical level, the pumping of our blood throughout the body oxygenates every cell. This oxygenation nourishes the brain, promoting an harmonious state of mind.

Physical Activities

Staying physically active is most important. Our bodies want to participate in the sensuous pleasures of summer, and we do this by jumping into water, hiking, bicycling, spending time in nature and going on a new adventure, even if it is in our own town or city. We want to encourage free-flowing communication with our physical environment. It is a great time to be with loved ones and family in social activities outdoors.

Flavors and Foods

Summer requires a delicate balancing of the heat outside in relation to our own internal thermostat. We need to stay cool but not cold. We need to maintain an internal warmth and yang that will serve us as we move forward toward autumn. We therefore need flavors that clear excess heat, activate and maintain internal warmth, and promote and support the hydration sorely required during the hot summer months. Here are some of the flavors favored in summer:

Pungent; cooling and warming: In the intense heat of summer, we feel best when we are able to maintain a cooler body temperature. It is well known that hot tropical countries use pungent and warming spices to promote perspiration, bringing the inner heat to the surface and opening the pores so that we can perspire and cool the body down. Warming and, less often, fiery spices can be used sparingly to bring heat to the surface of the body while promoting internal warming. As much as we may love summer, we will need to be ready for the eventual autumn and cooler weather.

Bitter: Bitter is a much maligned flavor in Western cultures, except when it comes to coffee, chocolate and beer! But bitter is a flavor to befriend because of its tremendous benefits. The flavor stimulates digestion and excretion; it is calming (through its heat-clearing actions) and can dry excess internal dampness (plaque in the form of high cholesterol). Bitter is very cooling (the exception is bitter liquors, which are more warming) — the flavor descends and purges heat from the body through urination and is most useful to counter any internal heat buildup in summer. Include small amounts of bitter foods (remember, coffee beans are roasted, which warms up the food and is not recommended). Bitter foods such as endive, escarole, romaine lettuce, radicchio, asparagus, dandelion, bitter melon, cardoons and tea are wonderful additions to the summer diet.

> ## Tip
> *Cooling pungent foods and spices* include peppermint, spearmint, lemon balm, lavender, gardenia, zucchini blossoms, lily buds, hops flower used as a tea, arugula, endive, chicory, radishes and young mustard greens.

Sour: The sour flavor is found in most of the delicious fruits and berries of summer. The sour flavor produces internal hydration. Think of what happens to our mouth when we eat a lemon. First we pucker, and then we salivate. These fluids are crucial to our hydration to counter the heat of summer. Berries, peaches, apricots, plums and rhubarb are all partly sour in their flavor makeup. We can include lightly fermented foods as well to bring this flavor into summer.

Other foods to also include: Mung beans are very cooling and useful in clearing summer heat. Melons, cucumbers, tofu, tomatoes, corn, zucchini, radishes, celery, berries, hato mugi (Job's tears), basmati rice, corn, wheat (if you can tolerate wheat and gluten), fish and all vegetables, which grow abundantly in the summer months.

Tip

Add some moderately warming herbs or spices to raw foods to help add warmth to foods. Additions could include Chinese spring onions (scallions), black, white or red pepper, small amounts of garlic, fresh ginger or its juice, sage, rosemary, thyme, basil and chives.

Cooking Methods

Steaming and blanching infuses foods with water, offsetting the heat of summer. Cooking can be light and quick so as to protect a food's vitality and freshness. Steam, sauté or simmer foods in liquid briefly to gently cook vegetables. Of course, meat and fish need to be thoroughly cooked. Think of poaching or steaming meats with herbs and spices. Use less oil and more water for cooking. Raw foods are perfectly fine, but be sure not to eat too much cold and raw food, especially if you have digestive issues — summer will end and you will need to be ready for autumn.

Foods to Avoid

Avoid extremes of hot and cold foods — balance is very important during the summer months. We need to maintain our vitality, be active and stay cool while still protecting internal warmth. Reduce or avoid foods that contribute to heat buildup in the body, including:

- Ice cold foods and drinks, which require increased digestive energy to warm up and can weaken the stomach's digestive process.
- Greasy, fatty and creamy foods that are heavy and counter to the exuberance of the season.
- Processed or baked goods that are overly drying, such as baked goods, chips, crackers.
- Stimulants such as coffee, alcohol and spicy foods, which are also hard on the heart and liver. They create internal heat and can aggravate inflammation as well as exacerbate mental and emotional irritation. Moderate the intake of these foods.

Late Summer and Seasonal Transition: The Pivot

Although late summer is not a true season, it is a distinct period as we continue to experience the heat of summer, ripened fruits and vegetables and other harvested foods. It is a time of transition, which is most noticeable as the Earth pivots and the sun's influence starts to wane. We feel autumn in the air, even though the leaves are still firmly planted on branches. We feel this transition as we do others at the end of each season: as we move from the coolness of autumn to the cold of winter, as we feel the days lengthening in winter and sense the beginnings of new life emerging in spring, and as we leave spring to enter the full heat and sunshine of summer.

These transitional periods at the end of each season are related to the influence of the Earth element (see the Five Phase Theory in Chapter 2, page 33). These are important times to promote harmony and equilibrium through rebalancing activities and foods. In the classical texts of Chinese medicine, the Earth element, which the Five Phase Theory attributes to late summer, is embedded in the later period of *each* of the four seasons. In the *Neijing Suwen*, it states that "the influence of earth's energy is present in all the seasons." The notion of the earth season being "late summer" is a later interpretation based on the central location of China's August rain season in the lunar calendar. The Earth element represents the transformative energy inherent at these later stages as we move from one season to the next.

Organ Systems

The earth time of the season and year is when the energy of the stomach and spleen predominates. In Chinese medicine, the stomach and spleen network is responsible for the breakdown, transformation and absorption of our food. A healthy stomach–spleen network is the foundation for nourishment and vital *qi* — the center and pivot for all activity in the body. Its healthy functioning governs absorption, transformation of food into nourishment and the capacity to transform nourishment effectively. The stomach breaks down the food we eat and the spleen is the center of transforming what we eat into fundamental energy for the body (for more information, see Chapter 7, page 114).

The stomach–spleen network benefits from moderation, balance and adherence to the natural cycle of life's rhythms, which are inherent in regular eating, sleeping and physical activity. Eating consistent meals, at regular times, brings tremendous benefit by

"Earth permits sowing and reaping. Earth is sweet."

— *Practical Chinese Medicine*

Did You Know?

According to the *Neijing Suwen*, the continual interchange of seasons occurs 18 days prior to the change of each season. Attuning to the subtle changes that occur within and around us as the season starts to shift is a perfect time to rebalance. Simplify eating to reinforce and support your digestive network, shore up internal resources and transition and ready yourself for the next season's imperatives.

fostering your internal rhythm. Erratic and inconsistent eating is a tremendous stress on the system, causing variations in blood sugar levels, as well as dips in energy and focus, and even feelings of anxiety. The stomach–spleen network is the center of nourishment, and needs it regularly. The stomach is adversely affected by excess dryness. The spleen is adversely affected by excess and dampness. Therefore, it becomes more important to find balance in dietary choices to maintain a healthy equilibrium — not too dry, not too damp.

Physical Activities

This is a time to bring more balance into the center of our bodies instead of expending larger amounts of our energy outward. We can engage in this pivotal shift with physical activities that include rhythmic movement and balance, such as bicycling, dancing — in particular, partner and line dancing, which ask us to be in harmony with one another — swimming, walking or doing tai chi, qi gong or yoga.

Flavors and Foods

The *sweet* flavor benefits the center of the body and is found in many whole foods. In Chinese medicine, the sweet flavor found in whole foods such as grains, beans, nuts and seeds, some meats and carbohydrate-rich vegetables is considered to be bland and sweet. The *full* sweet flavor is found in sweeteners and a more cooling and *empty* sweet is found in a wide variety of fruits. The simplicity of a *bland* sweet flavor inherent in whole foods not only nourishes the functions of the stomach and spleen but also promotes the body's capacity to rid the body of excess dampness. The sweet flavor is nourishing, brings balance and harmony and supports our body's capacity to transform and utilize the food we eat without creating stagnation.

Tip

Even though the sweet flavor is the predominant flavor of many whole foods, it must be balanced in our meals and daily eating by a variety of other flavors (sour, salty, bitter, and pungent) to promote healthy digestion, absorption and elimination. An excess consumption of the sweet flavor, even in whole grains, creates an overload on the system that can result in stagnation (dampness). Remember, the spleen does not like dampness. So an excess of dampness inhibits the spleen's capacity to transform, absorb and eliminate. For more information on the types of sweetness, see page 50.

There is a wide assortment of foods that can be included at this time of year to benefit the stomach and spleen, including corn, millet, rice, sweet (or sticky) rice, oats, carrots, cabbage, fennel, winter squash, shiitake mushrooms, soybeans, adzuki beans, almonds, chestnuts, lotus seeds, peas, spinach, poultry, lamb, venison, carp, bass, mackerel, sardines, apples, dates, figs, grapes and licorice root.

Cooking Methods

Simple cooking methods are recommended, including blanching, slow, gentle braising, steaming, boiling and simmering to make the digestion of foods easier.

Foods to Avoid

- Excessive dairy and sugar, which obstructs the spleen's functioning.
- Greasy and creamy foods (think ice cream, milkshakes and rich sauces), which clog up the digestive function and encourage the body to retain what it cannot break down.

Autumn: Drying and Cooling, Moving Inward

Autumn's sky is bright with the fire of leaves just before they dry up and fall. Our vital *qi*, brightened by summer skies, now begins its movement inward as we ready ourselves for winter. Autumn is a time for gathering ourselves for the year ahead. We move indoors. It is a great time to restructure what we do and want to do, creating time and space for reflection and planning. In late summer, we nurtured balance and harmony. Now, as the climate cools we begin to dress more warmly, contract our outward activities a bit more and turn our intention inward so we do not drain our vital energy.

This is an important time of change, just as spring is, requiring our care and attention. As much as spring was the pivot from yin to yang, autumn is the pivotal season from yang to yin. Our energy is retreating from the surface and is more contained within. It is important during this time to begin attend to nourishment and hydration that can protect us from the cooler and dryer air of the autumn, as well as the colds and flu that flourish in this season.

Organ Systems

Autumn is the time of the lungs and large intestine. The lungs directly interact with the environment through the air we breathe.

"The three months of autumn are in charge of withering and of decelerating the momentum of growth."

— *Gao Lian, poet and medical scholar*

After food, breathing is the second way we build our *qi* after we're born (called postnatal *qi*). The lungs are responsible for distributing our *qi* throughout the body. From a Chinese medicine point of view, the lungs coordinate all basic movements of *qi* in the body: ascending, descending, taking in and going out. We rarely take the time to pay attention to our breathing, however, or know how to use its potential to release stress or build vitality.

Take a moment right now to pay attention to the movement that happens in your chest and belly as you breathe in and breathe out. As we breathe in, the air moves down to our lungs, moving the diaphragm downward as the chest and belly expand. The opposite happens as we breathe out — the air moves up and out as the belly and body soften and release. Notice the sensations in your body and know that the oxygenation of cells is also a form of nourishment.

Physical Activities

"Go to bed earlier and get up with the chickens."

— *Huangdi Neijing Suwen, The Yellow Emperor's Classic of Medicine*

Physical activities can be more subtle and nuanced in autumn. Practice breathing exercises, such as mindful breathing or deep breathing, to build awareness of the power of breathing to oxygenate and relax our bodies. Gentle movement or exercise that emphasizes coordinating your breathing and movement — yoga, tai chi, qi gong, pilates or other mind-body techniques — will help you focus on bringing attention inward. Regular meditation, even for short periods, also supports the movement within, giving time and space to be quiet, focus and reflect.

Flavors and Foods

In autumn, we need to protect our internal yin, and we do this by adding in a bit of the **sour** flavor, a yin flavor. The sour flavor stimulates the saliva and production of body fluids to moisten internal tissues and membranes so the nose and lungs are protected from the cooler and drier autumn air. Layering in this flavor also balances external dryness to promote a moist and warmer interior. Sour foods also contain, contract and astringe, promoting the body's capacity to produce and contain body fluids. Choose foods that are lubricating in their action on the body, such as spinach, okra, persimmon, almonds, seeds and soybeans (if you tolerate them), to create a healthy internal balance to the external environment.

Autumnal foods also include grapes, apples, plums, pears, persimmons, pomegranates, lychee, rose hips and various nuts and seeds, such as almonds, peanuts and sesame seeds. We should also add beans, such as adzuki, for their lightly sour and sweet flavor, tofu, sourdough breads, vinegar, olives and a variety of mushrooms, including shiitake, oyster and cremini. Include foods that are more warming, including animal foods (chicken, lamb, beef), whole oats, millet, rice, onions, leeks, Chinese spring onions (scallions), garlic, ginger and cinnamon, as well as sprinkling some black, white or red pepper into dishes, especially if you feel cold inside. The pungent and warming qualities of spices increase circulation of body fluids and help to gently activate digestion.

Cooking Methods

Cook for longer times at lower temperatures. This is a more yang style of cooking and stimulates warmth within the body. We want to add more yang to our food without drying it out. Fermented foods are useful in replenishing beneficial gut bacteria supporting the large intestine and the health of the microbiome. Think of foods like sauerkraut, pickles, yogurt and even fermented grains such as those used in sourdough (see also Sautéed Banana Crêpes on page 322). Baking, blanching, frying, roasting, boiling and simmering are also useful during the autumn season, while adding more seasoning brings warming yang into your cooking to balance the movement into the yin time of year.

Foods to Avoid

To build internal energy and vitality while maintaining inner warmth, avoid foods that are overly dispersing and cooling.

- Foods that are overly fatty, greasy and oily (french fries, deep-fried foods).
- Foods that are excessively cooling and raw or cold dairy foods, which can burden the spleen and inhibit effective digestion.

Did You Know?

The microbiome is defined as the collective genomes of the microbes and more than 100 trillion microorganisms (composed of bacteria, bacteriophage, fungi, protozoa and viruses) that live inside and on the human body. According to the Human Microbiome Project, which is an initiative of the National Institutes of Health that facilitates human microbiome research, we have about 10 times as many microbial cells as human cells.

Did You Know?

When the spleen cannot transform food and absorb nourishment, the following symptoms show up: digestive disturbances, lethargy and stubborn weight that is difficult to lose. In Chinese medicine, this is considered internal dampness, which impedes the yang and *qi* of the spleen.

Winter: Returning to the Roots

"During the three months of winter, heaven and earth shut down and go into a state of storage. Water turns to ice and earth splits open, and the yang *qi* of nature stays unperturbed."

— *Gao Lian, poet and medical scholar*

Even though winter appears to be the most barren time of year, it is one of the most important and active periods for growth and regrowth. Underneath the earth's surface, all life is regenerating itself. Hidden from our view, the roots of trees and plants, bulbs and seeds are resting and regenerating; the yang is resting deep in the yin of the earth. The cold winter freezes all the elements and turns them to ice and slows down all movement.

During winter, the *qi* and yang move from the surface to the innermost foundation of our bodies. It is a time for us to deeply rest, to contemplate, reflect and restore. It is the most yin time of the year and demands that we protect our most precious yin *and* yang. This is when we adjust our bodies to go to bed early and rise a bit later with sunrise (not always doable if you live farther north, where the sun can rise as late as 8 a.m.). It is a time to support our inner descent, protecting ourselves from the outer cold winds by nourishing our inner yang and protecting our yin.

Organ System

This is the time of year for the kidneys, the origin of all yin and yang. The kidney yin is the root of physical yin (blood and essence), kidney yang is the root of all yang, and the kidneys are the root of all *qi*. In Chinese medicine, the kidneys are considered the "palace of all yin and yang in the body." The kidneys house our ancestral *qi* and *jing* (our genetic makeup or constitution) and govern reproduction, birth, development and aging. Any long-term chronic illness demands a tremendous amount of energy from the body and can weaken the kidney *qi*.

Physical Activities

This is the most yin time of the year and a crucial time to nourish our innermost being so that we can emerge upward in spring with plentiful *qi*. The slow and steady movements of tai chi, walking mediation, qi gong or restorative yoga (rather than a more energetic or hot form of yoga) engage the body and mind in movement without overexertion. Because it is also a good time for reflection, activities like journaling and meditation are ideal.

What is Walking Meditation?

In walking meditation, the physical act of walking becomes the focal point, similar to how the breath and the awareness of breathing is the focus in sitting meditation. The simplicity of walking meditation helps develop focus, calm and is grounding. To practice, start by turning your attention toward the physical sensation of walking, one foot in front of the other, for 10 to 30 paces. Then turn and continue, back and forth for 10 to 15 minutes. Walk slowly or change the pace and breathe. Walking meditation opens the senses to allow us to focus on what we see, the sounds we hear and the sensations of the feet coming in contact with the ground as we walk.

Flavors and Foods

The **bitter** and **salty** flavors support the descent of *qi* downward and inward. The salty flavor is cooling and supports kidney function, promoting the elimination of fluids through urination while at the same time supporting the distribution and dissemination of body fluids throughout the body, which serves to keep the tissues hydrated. The bitter flavor, which is cooling, also descends the *qi* and purges excess heat buildup. Much as we like to sit by a fire to warm up, too much heat is dangerous and can dry us out, potentially injuring our yin. Incorporate the cooling bitter flavor to balance out the warming foods during these cold winter months. Limit the addition salt on your food; instead, balance saltier foods with a bit of bitter foods, which helps to prevent a buildup of internal heat. Even though the salty and bitter foods support the descent and consolidation of vitality into the kidneys, these are not flavors we should use in excess. We still need to include all the five flavors and a variety of foods from all the food groups in our diet. We can use salty and bitter frequently as condiment flavors.

During winter, when a plethora of fresh and local foods aren't available, we literally reach into the earth to extract nourishment from the many tubers and roots we eat at this time of year. It is important to strengthen our inner yang, and we can rely on the energy stored in roots and hardy vegetables, grains, beans and legumes and meats, as well as preserved and canned foods, to get us through the winter.

Foods that have a salty flavor and are beneficial during the winter are seaweeds (sea vegetables), seafood, millet, miso, tamari, barley, pork, ham, oyster, duck, salty condiments and the addition of high-quality sea salt (see page 159 for more salt options) in cooking. Bitter foods that support the kidney in the winter season include chicory, endive, escarole, black tea with spices (as in chai or ginger tea), dandelion leaves, chicory root (roasted chicory root and barley are often used as a coffee substitute), roasted dandelion or burdock roots, walnuts and black sesame seeds.

Of course, salty and bitter both have a cooling nature, which can be balanced through cooking methods as well as with herbs and spices that warm the body, such as cinnamon, star anise, chile peppers, curry, cloves and nutmeg. Lamb and venison are warming meats. Small amounts of tonic wines taken in the morning can nurture yang *qi* and warm the whole body.

Cooking Methods

This is the time of year to cook to generate warmth without drying or overheating the body. The longer stovetop or slow cooker methods, as well as roasting, baking, and simmering stews, heartier soups and bone broths, which extract essential nourishment, are most beneficial in promoting internal warmth. Pay special attention to balancing these longer and slower cooking methods with soups, steaming, water sautéing or simmering in water to protect the internal yin and avoid drying out.

Foods to Avoid

As much as we need to nurture yang and inner warmth, maintaining yin balance is key. The seesaw is now tilted toward the cold environment, so it will take more warming and yang to bring us to balance. Avoid or reduce the following:

- Excessive use of spicy foods, which can dry up inner fluids.
- Too many grilled foods, which contribute to inner heating.
- Raw and cold foods, which deplete inner yang.

Reflection: Measure Your Relationship with the Seasons

Each season offers us the opportunity to change. In spring we renew, in summer we rejoice, in seasonal transitions we rebalance, in autumn we regroup and in winter we recharge. These extraordinary shifts provide a natural occasion that we can respond to, by changing our food choices, activities or inclinations. We rarely take the time to reflect upon our experiences in the seasons. Take a few moments now to do just that and note your preferences in temperature, light, activity and food.

- *Which season do you most enjoy?*

- *Do you know why?* Is it the rituals associated with holidays? The beauty of impending spring, when there is a multitude of possibilities? The abundant vitality of summer that drives you outdoors?

- *Do you prefer the cooler temperatures and shorter days of autumn and fall,* when you can be indoors reflecting and being quieter?

- *What season is it right now as you read this book?* Check in with your energy level and your health.

- *Think about the energy of this season* and take a moment to ask yourself if you feel in synch with it.

- *Flip to the description of the season you're currently in* and jot down a few foods that you could reduce or avoid. Add in some of the foods and cooking styles recommended. Also, see the recipes section, starting on page 206, for more inspiration.

Chapter 6

The Kitchen, Your Laboratory

"Cooking — of whatever kind, everyday or extreme — situates us in the world in a very special place, facing the natural world on one side and the social world on the other. The cook stands squarely between nature and culture, conducting a process of translation and negotiation."

— *Michael Pollan, Cooked: A Natural History of Transformation*

What we cook and who we cook for has a tremendous influence on our lives. The act of cooking can strengthen our connection to nature, to ourselves and to others while increasing our vitality and affecting our health. Cooking is creative and transformative. Cooking can be calming and therapeutic. The act of choosing fresh ingredients and the process of chopping and assembling them into a meal can be a source of nourishment for the cook. It is an opportunity to immerse ourselves, to focus all our attention on the task at hand while cutting out the noise of the day.

Cooking may not be that for you yet — it may still feel like a task — and you may not be the cook you want to be. Perhaps you're a little intimidated by it all. But it is certainly possible to change this relationship. It is possible to bring dishes together that are not complicated but still offer all the desired benefits. Think of it this way: the raw ingredients that sit on your counter, in your fridge and in your pantry are simply waiting for water and the flame on your stove to be transformed into delicious dishes — that's it!

If you're receptive to the idea of changing how you eat, along with exploring and expanding your food preferences, keep reading. You'll learn when a dish needs a pinch of salt or a spice or a splash of sour. You'll also learn to trust your sense of smell and sight to determine when a dish is done just right. Be open to the different scents, new flavors and various textures along the way.

Note: You'll have ample opportunities to get started and try out recipes for every season, starting on page 206.

Cooking to Transform Health

I have wonderful childhood memories of being in the kitchen, which was often filled with delightful aromas, the clanking of pots and pans and the scurry of people. My mother cooked, baked and liked trying new recipes. I fondly remember sitting on the counter waiting to lick the cake batter bowl or helping Mom grind the cranberries and oranges for the relish she prepared for Thanksgiving. I often helped my grandmother roll out the strudel pastry, after we'd gone to the Lebanese market to pick up some rose petal jam to add to the apples, nuts, honey and spices for the filling. Passover at my aunt and uncle's was resplendent with formal plate settings and silverware along with the special foods of the holiday. And, most wonderfully, I remember sitting around the large round table during meals, brimming with banter about the world or sharing jokes and stories of the day. We were nourished in that kitchen, not only in body but also in spirit. To this day, I still love spending time cooking with family and my siblings, even on vacation.

Perhaps this hasn't been your experience from an early age. One of my patients, whose upbringing did not promote a healthy association with food, now struggles with eating well. Some members of her family have had problems with their weight or their health: they either struggle with obesity or obsess about fitness and eating "right." Today, as an adult, she finds it difficult to nourish herself. She has never learned to cook and her diet has been filled with foods high in trans fats, sugar and salt. That is what she learned and that is what her body has become accustomed to. Now she is learning how to change her food patterns and find new ways to care for herself, little by little. She is stymied, however, by not knowing what and how to cook and challenged by physiological habits that are hard to break.

Whatever your past experiences with food and eating, whatever your beliefs about your capacity to change habits, you *can* change and you *can* learn to cook in a simple way that stimulates health, one step at a time.

Preparing the Cook

If there is one thing I have learned from cooking is how to be more patient, more present with what I am doing and how to practice and master new skills even though a dish may not work out the way I had hoped. The first step in learning to cook is preparing the kitchen and yourself. Have you ever walked into the kitchen after a long day, only to find the counters crammed with stuff and the sink filled with grimy dishes? This is not a great way to get started.

> **Did You Know?**
>
> Change is incremental. Each day builds a new experience and habit. It takes 21 days to change a habit, so stick with it. And, if you don't succeed, note how you feel.

Making sure that your kitchen is clean and ready to go so you can focus on cooking is key. Believe me, a cluttered kitchen arena does not support an uncluttered mind when it comes to cooking.

The key is to bring presence and patience to the exercise. Being present and focused slows you down as you wash, prep, cut and cook. It focuses your efforts toward the end goal of creating a pleasurable eating experience.

After a long day of work, I love to cook. It frees my mind and affords me the opportunity to focus on one thing alone — bringing out the flavor and texture of foods to create a bookend to a full and active day. After a busy day filled with many different chores, cooking demands that I be present with what I'm doing and focus on the tasks at hand, to be patient as I wash, chop and put foods together in their own time. Cooking affords me the chance to practice all of the above each and every day.

So take a deep breath and check in with yourself before you get to work. You might need some time to yourself before feeding others. Nourish the chef first, either with a cup of calming tea or a 15-minute walk to clear your head.

Getting Started

Focus on some preliminary steps that can help you improve your initial cooking experience.

- Start by making sure your cooking space is clean and free of unnecessary clutter. It's difficult to prepare food that imparts clear *qi* when the *qi* of your own kitchen is encumbered and obscured by dirty dishes and counters. Take a few moments to organize, clean up and wipe down your space.

- Pull your hair back and wash your hands.

- Take stock of your ingredients at hand as well as the necessary equipment you will need to make the meal. Get your favorite knives out and make sure they're sharpened. A sharper knife, used properly, means easier preparation and less risk of cutting yourself.

- Clean as you go. This keeps your cooking area clear and minimizes your work after cooking.

- Wash your vegetables. For leafy greens, fill a large bowl or sink with water to thoroughly rinse and clean greens. A salad spinner is an excellent way to dry leafy greens before you either cook with them or prep them for a salad. Root vegetables and tubers can be scrubbed with a sturdy vegetable brush.

- If you'd rather have some partners in the kitchen, engage your child, partner or a friend, to be your sous chef and assist with washing vegetables, cutting, assembling or cleaning up.

Enhancing Your Cooking Experience

Now that you've organized the kitchen, cleared the counters and stocked the shelves, it's time to approach the kitchen and get cooking.

Take inventory of what you have to work with. You'll want to make sure you have the necessary ingredients on hand to prepare meals before you start cooking. Be sure to stock your pantry, refrigerator and freezer with foundational foods you can draw upon when they're needed so you feel less stressed in the kitchen. You might choose to make it a weekly chore. For example, I have a friend who sits down and plans the week's menus for her family and then shops for ingredients on Sunday to ensure that her kitchen is ready for the week ahead. (See Chapter 9 for inspiration on what to add to your grocery list.) Or if you're more like me and prefer some improvisation in the kitchen, you might choose to have a broad variety of fresh ingredients on hand so you can work with what you have in your fridge and pantry.

Time is a big consideration because cooking takes time. Set aside some time to make your week flow more smoothly by preparing for the next meal a day ahead. Here are some ideas: while you're preparing for the night's dinner, cut and chop extra vegetables for the next day's meal. Or choose a day on the weekend that affords you more time to prep for a few days ahead or to cook a soup or a dish you can reheat during the week. On the days when you're rushed and hungry but just don't feel like spending time cooking, don't make it complicated — create a simple meal that requires little effort. Oh, and after you finish meal prep or dinner, enlist some assistance to do the dishes! Every cook needs a little help.

Reflect for a few moments before cooking on the people you're cooking for: children, teens, a partner, elderly parents or just yourself. What we eat today replenishes the energy we have expended and also prepares us for the days to come. Here are a few other things to consider:

- **Energy:** Is everyone tired? Do they need a meal that enhances and protects vital energy?
- **Stress:** Has everyone been running around, and do they need to have something that calms and centers them?
- **Physical activity:** Was the day filled with intense physical activity, which requires a certain type of nourishment, or was it restful and relaxing?

> **Tip**
> Set yourself up for success when you're cooking for optimal health. Learn how to discern food labels, fill your fridge with whole foods and stock a healthy pantry to make meal planning an attainable endeavor. See more in Chapter 9, page 144.

In a single family, it's not unusual for different life stages to be present at the same table, and this scenario means that different people will need different types of nourishment. While it might sound overwhelming for the novice cook, it takes only a bit of time and effort to cook one meal with many options, either by using a variety of cooking methods for the same meal (more on this later in this chapter) or by adding a choice of condiments (see recipes on page 422).

What Kind of Cook Are You?

- Do you enjoy cooking? How often do you cook? Do you consider it a chore?
- Do you need a recipe to cook so you know where you're going? Or are you an improviser working with what you have at hand?
- How do you choose your recipe — with what is available? With what you are hungry for?
- Do you know how to create what you want?

Taking a few moments to think about what and how you will cook will make a big difference in the result. Here are a few additional thoughts to enhance your cooking skills:

- Consider the season, whether it is warm or cold outside, and adjust to eating fresh, seasonal foods.
- Use your senses to cultivate your cooking. Does the meal you're making smell ready? Does it look ready? Aromas, colors, texture and sounds (yes, sounds, such as the sizzle and bounce of oil when it converges with the moisture of foods in sautéing or stir-frying vegetables or the whizzing from a pot with ingredients that might be drying up or close to burning) will guide you as you cook.
- Timing is *almost* everything. Make sure you time the meal so it is ready within minutes of serving. Make sure you know when to add ingredients and how long to cook them so the meal has the right consistency and flavor.
- Experiment — your kitchen is a type of laboratory and place of discovery. Recipes can be thought of as guides, so feel free to substitute a vegetable, add nuts or seeds and adjust amounts and types of spices and herbs. You will learn more about what works and what pleases you over time.

Supporting Health with Different Cooking Methods

How you cook a meal not only changes how the food tastes, but it can also influence how it makes us feel: invigorated, calm, balanced, satisfied, among other emotions.

All cooking methods share one common fact — they are the conduits for the transformation of food. Cooking raw ingredients also renders them more digestible. When the element of fire is applied, whether on a grill, on the stovetop or in the oven, it enhances dryness, warmth and succulence while bringing delightful flavors to the eater. Water-based cooking, by steaming, boiling or blanching in soups and long-simmered stews, melds many flavors together while putting moisture back into your system when you're feeling hot and dried out; it will infuse your cells with nourishment that can be easier to break down and digest. Fermented foods activate digestion. Drying, curing and smoking condense and intensify flavor and nutrition.

In Chinese medicine, it is believed that different cooking methods — a quick sauté, long slow stewing, braising or boiling — can affect the potency of food and create a balance of yin (moistening and cooling) and yang (drying and warming) to support health. To achieve this, we are asked to pay attention to our energy levels, the season, our internal state of health and our body's internal temperature when choosing the cooking method that best serves us and our family.

Let's take a look at the different cooking methods and their therapeutic impact.

Boiling and Simmering

Actions: Boiling and simmering moisten, add water and remove minerals in food. These methods infuse food with yang *qi* and warmth. They also quickly transmit and infuse heat into food.

Beneficial seasons: All seasons. Can be useful in spring, summer and during any of the seasonal transitions to add hydration back into the system.

Benefits those who feel dry, warm or hot. Also those seeking to simplify their eating for a period of time.

Technique: Bring water to a rolling boil, which is 212°F (100°C) at sea level. If you live at a high elevation, boiling point will occur at a lower temperature. You can be sure that water is boiling when bubbles begin to vigorously break the surface. After the boiling begins, immerse the food you want to cook and turn

Did You Know?

Short-term boiling, for 5 to 10 minutes, does not cause much change to thermal nature. Long-term boiling or simmering infuses food with more yang *qi*.

the heat down to a simmer. Pasta needs to be boiled. Asian-style noodles such as rice, udon or soba, need to be simmered in the water after they have come to a boil.

Recipes to choose from:

Tilapia and Arugula Soup, page 251
Borscht, page 253
Vibrant Summer Vegetables with Tofu Dressing, page 266
Spinach and Egg Drop Soup, page 334
All teas, various pages

Steaming

Actions: Steaming is a relatively quick cooking method, depending on the food and the size of the pieces. One can steam vegetables, tofu, fish and even cakes! Steaming is a moistening cooking method that brings out flavor in foods.

Beneficial seasons: Since steaming is a very neutral and balanced cooking method, it is beneficial in all seasons.

Benefits those who prefer raw food but cannot digest it well. Steaming begins the breakdown of foods to make them more digestible. If you need a simple and balanced meal, choose steaming for some of your dishes.

Technique: Place a metal or bamboo steamer atop a saucepot half filled with water. You can also place foods on a dish or plate (not an open basket) and steam the same way. Bring the water to a boil. The force of the steam releases a large amount of energy when it condenses onto a cooler material — the energy of the boiling water is doubled when you employ the steam to cook a food. Steaming can also occur in a closed dish in the oven.

Recipes to choose from:

Quick-Pickled Radish Tops over Steamed Red Radishes and Cauliflower, page 228
Steamed Artichokes with Cashew Sauce, page 232
Trout Steamed with Green Peas and Lemony Herbed Rice, page 379
Savory steamed egg custard, recipes in most seasons, various pages

Blanching

Actions: Blanching heightens the color of vegetables and preserves the integrity of food in a short time. This method is used to initiate the breakdown of a food. The blanched food can then be added to a quick stir-fry or sauté where you want to maintain a crunchy texture.

Beneficial seasons: A balanced cooking method beneficial in warmer seasons.

Benefits those who prefer raw food but are seeking to avoid cold and raw foods. People who run hot might also benefit from this neutral cooking method.

Technique: Place the vegetable in boiling water for only 1 or 2 minutes.

Health Tip
Blanching improves digestibility by breaking down the raw component of vegetables. (Blanching is not generally used for meats.)

Recipes to choose from:

Thai-Style Textured Salad, page 255

Cauliflower with Basil Sauce, page 310

Edamame, Roasted Cherry Tomato and Blanched Escarole Salad, page 353

Curly Endive and Apple Chopped Salad with Candied Walnuts, page 388

Braising

Actions: Braising adds warmth and a rich quality to foods. It combines fire, through browning or frying with oil, with the addition of small amounts of liquid.

Beneficial seasons: Braising is a very balanced way to cook foods and is therefore beneficial in any season.

Benefits those who seek their food to be enriched. If you run hot, choose more vegetable-based braises. For those who tend to experience more cold and yang-deficient conditions, feel free to cook with more warming foods and spices.

Technique: Place a small amount of oil in a hot pan and quickly brown vegetables or meats. Braising occurs once a small amount of water or broth is added in which the foods can slowly cook for a short or longer period.

Health Tip
Braising is typically done with meats, but braising vegetables imparts a rich taste to them. For meats, season first and then brown in oil prior to cooking in a closed pot, either on the stove or in the oven at low temperatures for a long time. For vegetables, add herbs or spices during the browning phase or at the end of cooking.

Recipes to choose from:

Braised Taro and Baby Vegetables with Citrus Oil, page 233

Braised Tomatoes and Sweet Potatoes with Eggs, page 260

Salmon on Ginger-Braised Kale with Toasted Pine Nuts, page 338

Braised Fennel, page 345

Braised Duck with Lotus Seeds, page 380

Bitter Melon with Shrimp, page 385

Sautéing

Actions: Sautéing comes from the French word *sauté*, meaning "to jump." That is indeed what your food will do when it is sautéing — it will jump as you move it around in the pan. As you sauté, the high heat activates, invigorates and seals in the flavor and freshness of food. It is a yang, activating and warming method of cooking.

Beneficial seasons: Spring is the season to cook food quickly, sealing in the freshness, but sautéing works in all seasons.

Benefits those who need to feel more activated and uplifted.

Technique: Heat the pan over medium-high heat for a few minutes. Add a small amount of oil, just enough to cover the bottom of the pan, and heat for about 10 to 30 seconds (be careful not to allow the oil to smoke) before adding ingredients. Sautéing is a dry method, meaning that no water is added, which imparts flavor quickly to foods.

Water Sauté Technique: Heat a pan or skillet on the stove with 3 to 6 tbsp (45 to 90 mL) of water or broth over medium-high heat. When water starts to steam, but just before boiling, add ingredients and stir frequently. Cover or leave uncovered. Add liquid as needed to keep ingredients from sticking or burning. Moderate the amount of crispness you want by adjusting the cooking time.

Recipes to choose from:

Sweet Potato Noodles with Spring Greens and Shredded Lamb, page 225
Sautéed Broccoli with Tangy Ginger Dressing, page 234
Pungent-Herb Breakfast Fried Rice, page 249
Bitter Melon and Ground Pork, page 269
Cauliflower with Basil Sauce, page 310
Sautéed Celery and Cabbage Ribbons, page 311
Sautéed Banana Crêpes, page 322
Hijiki and Carrot Sauté with Ginger, page 392
Sautéed Prawns in Rice Wine, Garlic, Ginger and Leeks, page 420

Pan-Frying

Actions: Pan-frying enriches foods by cooking on high heat with oil.

Beneficial seasons: Since frying is a more yang and warming cooking method, it is best used in autumn and winter.

Benefits those who run cold or have a hard time gaining weight (this is considered yin deficient). It is not recommended as a regular cooking method for anyone with fevers, common coughs or circulatory or cardiac issues, which are considered hot and excessive conditions.

Technique: Turn heat to medium-high and thoroughly heat the pan. Add oil and food(s) into the pan. Do not disturb until food is browned on one side before flipping.

Recipes to choose from:

Pan-Fried Vegetable Cakes, page 292

Lox Eggs with Winter Vegetable Hash and Pungent Greens, page 293

Chicken and Chestnut Fried Rice, page 339

Mushroom and Adzuki Bean Breakfast Fried Rice, page 372

Broiling and Grilling

Actions: Quick direct heat, or fire, dramatically increases the warming and yang *qi* of foods while reducing the moisture content. These methods enhance the flavor of the foods being cooked, imparting a richness in taste and texture. Studies from the National Cancer Institute in the United States, however, have shown that meats exposed to temperatures over 300°F (150°C) increase the potential for HCA (heterocyclic amines) and PAH (polycyclic aromatic hydrocarbons) to form, increasing the risk for cancer. For this reason, broil or grill meats only on occasion and be careful not to burn them.

Beneficial seasons: No season is considered more beneficial.

Benefits: No true health benefit. Grilling and broiling are warming and can be quite delicious. They are not recommended for people who already have chronic heat conditions or excess conditions.

Technique: Season the food you will cook with herbs, spices and oil. Cook either directly over (or under) the heat or wrapped in aluminum foil.

Recipes to choose from:

Rosemary Grilled Fish with Lemony Greens and Pilaf, page 258

Herb-Grilled Chicken, page 261

Grilled Squid, page 304

Grilled Romaine Lettuce with Anchovy Sauce, page 352

Tip

Choose high-quality oils and fats that can sustain high heat: avocado, coconut or ghee.

Health Tip

These methods can be beneficial with vegetables. Meats, for the most part, are already warming and add more intense heat. Grilling foods that are already warming in nature is not recommended for people who are prone to heat symptoms. Try vegetables or fruits instead, which are either neutral or cooling in their thermal nature.

Baking

Health Tip
If you have a tendency toward feeling hot or have heat-related symptoms, be sure to moderate your use of the baking method. Of course, a baked dessert can be a nurturing and well-deserved treat from time to time!

Actions: Baking is drying and warming. It enhances the sweet flavor, reduces moisture and fortifies yang. For anyone who suffers from a cold condition, baking can be very useful because it brings more yang *qi* into all foods.

Beneficial seasons: Baking in heat and adding yang *qi* to foods is most beneficial in cold winter months, as well as the colder and wetter months of autumn.

Benefits those who are vegetarians or vegans, who often feel cold and whose diet may not supply them with enough warming and yang *qi*. Baking can moderate the effect of cooling foods, such as tomatoes or fruits. Because baking imparts true heat deep into foods, it is beneficial for people who often feel cold.

Technique: Whole foods, such as vegetables and fruits, can simply be baked with added spices and herbs. Foods can be put together into casseroles and baked in an oven at varying temperatures between 350°F (180°C) to 400°F (200°C). Be sure to let the oven come to full heat before putting in the foods. If baking a cake or cookies, be sure to pay attention to the recommended timing and check for doneness — ovens vary in how they conduct heat.

Recipes to choose from:

Baked Spiced Rhubarb, page 241
Cardamom-Roasted Plums with Pistachios, page 284
Apple Honey Cake, page 319
Crunchy Seed Cookies, page 364
Cranberry and Apricot Crumble, page 365

Roasting

Actions: Roasting — cooking over an open fire or within the confines of a pan in the oven — is considered a dry-heat method of cooking. Suffice it to say, roasting foods have a drying and warming effect on the body, enhancing yang as well as flavor.

Beneficial seasons: Roasting is usually most beneficial in the autumn and winter. However, there are also appropriate times when you may need extra warmth and more fortifying foods to roast in spring, summer and during transitional times of each season.

Benefits those who may generally feel cold or energy (*qi*) deficient.

Technique: Roasting is usually done in an open pan at oven temperatures between 325°F (160°C) and 400°F (200°C). Meats and vegetables are the foods generally roasted, and aromatic herbs and spices can be added to enhance flavor. Vegetables are usually brushed with either oil or animal fat and salted before roasting.

Recipes to choose from:

Simple Roasted Asparagus, page 236
Pan-Roasted Honey Carrots with Aromatic Spices, page 343
Roasted Beet Salad with Pickled Mustard Greens, page 349
Roasted Sweet Potato Salad, page 354
Roasted Peanuts with Tangerine Peel, page 355
Roasted Chunky Root Vegetables with Tangy Tahini Dressing, page 394

Long- and Slow-Cooked Broths and Soups

Actions: Long-cooked soups — those that are cooked for 6 to 36 hours — are considered medicinal soups. Extracting key minerals and nourishment in the liquid of long-cooked or slow-cooked broths, which simmer between 2 hours for congees and 36 hours for bone broths, affords easy digestibility and requires little action by the body to break down and absorb nourishment. Key ingredients can include vegetables, sea vegetables, meat and meat bones, and fish and fish bones, as well as specific herbs (both medicinal and culinary) to add flavor and healing potential. These long-cooked soups will benefit *qi* and blood, yin and yang, depending on the combination of food, herbs and spices. They are a delicious form of medicine.

Beneficial seasons: All.

Benefits those who are tired, cold, have low appetite and poor digestion, or in Chinese medicine terms, those that are *qi*, blood or yang deficient. Such soups and broths are most beneficial for those recovering from a long illness who still feel fatigued, and for women after giving birth. They are also excellent for older people, children and those who have digestive or malabsorption problems.

Technique: Add ingredients into a large pot and cover with plenty of water. Bring to a boil, turn the heat to low and cook for 2 to 36 hours. Or place ingredients and water in a slow cooker and cook on low as the recipe directs. Check the pot every hour to ensure that the ingredients are well covered and add water as needed.

"In the business of harmonious blending, one must make use of the sweet, sour, bitter, pungent and salty… The transformation which occurs in the cauldron is quintessential and wondrous, subtle and delicate."

— I Yin, legendary chef, in Lu Shih Chhun Chhiu (Master Lu's Spring and Autumn Annals)

Did You Know?

Soups and broths are the precursor of medicinal teas and porridge, most notably congee (rice soup), which was first mentioned in the Chinese medical classic *Shang Han Lun (Treatise on Cold Damage)*, circa 220 CE. Congee can also be made with other grains, usually millet or barley.

Recipes to choose from:

Pickling and Fermenting

Pickling and fermenting are among the oldest and easiest methods of food preparation. Throughout the world, there are traditions of brined and fermented pickles, each with its own unique flavor palate, depending on the herbs and spices added to the brine or ferment.

People eat fermented foods all over the world. Fermented foods include some common treats such as chocolate, sourdough bread, yogurt, alcohol, coffee and tea, as well as fermented vegetables, fruits, grains and meats, seafood, eggs and dairy.

Fermentation can occur with the addition of salt or a "starter," such as previously prepared sauerkraut, kimchi or miso, or koji (*Aspergillus oryzae*). A starter is used to make sure that beneficial bacteria and yeasts are most prevalent and the end product is safe.

When preparing fermented foods, cleanliness is very important. Wash the produce, clean the equipment thoroughly and rinse well. Use a starter that smells good (not musty or cheesy) and looks good (not an off-color such as pink and with no apparent mold). Follow the recipe to make sure that the starter, if used, or the salt comes into proper contact with the food to be fermented. In some recipes, the starter or salt will be layered with the food; in others, there will be enough moisture to submerge the food in the starter's liquid or liquid generated by the salt. Don't cut down on the amount of salt — in some recipes, it is necessary for a traditional flavor, and in others it is necessary for controlling the growth of unhealthy bacteria and yeasts. If the recipe directs you to submerge the food under liquid, make sure you follow this instruction to ensure continued fermentation. Keep the food no warmer than room temperature to avoid rot and the growth of unwanted pathogens. The recipes in this book generally have a brief fermentation period so you can eat the food sooner; because the foods include a starter, you will still be consuming live probiotics and benefit from some predigestion. The food will continue to ferment slowly if you store it in the refrigerator. Discard (and avoid tasting!) any fermented food that develops an off-color such as pink or black, any food with mold, and any food that becomes slimy (most food becomes more tender and supple as it ferments, so that's fine). If the fermented food is too salty for your taste, drain thoroughly and try using it as a condiment.

Pickling

Actions: The use of water, salt and vinegar means pickling is generally a more cooling and yin method of food preparation.
Beneficial seasons: Any.
Benefits those who have a compromised digestive or immune system that needs some support.
Technique: There is minimal cooking in only a few cases; in other cases, simply a container, some salt and possibly herbs is all that is needed.

Recipes to choose from:

Tea-Pickled Eggs, page 312
Pickled Mushrooms, page 427
Kombu Vinegar Pickle, page 428
Fragrant Pickled Peaches, page 429
Miso Daikon Pickles, page 439
(See other recipes in Condiment Recipes, page 422)

Tip

Pickles are usually made by brining, but some are fermented. The pickles listed below are brined. The fermented pickles are in the fermenting section.

What's on Your Table

Nora Ephron, the wonderful writer and filmmaker, once said, "The most important thing that I learned from Lee [Bailey] was something I call the Rule of Four. Most people serve three things for dinner — some sort of meat, some sort of starch, and some sort of vegetable — but Lee always served four. And the fourth thing was always unexpected."

In many countries around the world, the table is laden with a variety of dishes for people to choose from. Creating a meal with options means that you can pick and choose what to eat while being sure there's enough to feel satisfied. Whenever you serve a meal, you can bet that no one at the table will eat *exactly* the same thing. Some of you might lean on more vegetables, while others might prefer one dish over another, so it is a good idea that you have enough to choose from. Condiments are a unique and easy way to add flavor, palatability and variety. Spend some time creating an assortment of condiments (see Condiment Recipes, starting on page 422) to have on hand, and you and your family will be able to customize meals.

Fermenting

Did You Know?

Some familiar fermented foods include chocolate, bread, alcohol, coffee and tea.

Actions: As author and educator Sandor Katz says in *The Art of Fermentation*, fermentation is "the digestive action of bacterial and fungal cells and their enzymes. Food may be preserved, but its composition is altered by the organisms involved.... Minerals become more bioavailable and certain difficult-to-digest compounds are broken down." Fermentation renders foods more digestible by the action of microorganisms which "predigest" foods such as soybeans and milk products. In addition, fermentation can generate additional nutrients, such as B vitamins and micronutrients. For example, natto, a fermented soy product, creates natto-kinase, a micronutrient known to help break down fibrin in blood vessels and reduce high cholesterol. Indeed, the most profound benefit of eating fermented foods is the ingestion of beneficial bacteria necessary for a healthy gut and immune system. Fermented foods such as yogurt, sauerkraut and some pickles, which are still "alive," add beneficial bacteria, yeasts and enzymes to the gut, aiding the digestive process and diversifying the gut bacteria necessary for a healthy immune system. Eat fermented food daily in small amounts for the best effect. Your gut will be happy.

Beneficial seasons: Any and all seasons.

Benefits everyone. If you have a serious digestive disturbance, please check with your health-care provider. Some people have trouble with the live yeasts in some fermented foods.

Technique: Fermenting is a relatively easy process for home cooks who preserve seasonal foods while adding tremendous flavor to them. There are many methods of fermenting, but the most common is the simple addition of salt to a food that is then kept submerged under liquid in a covered container in a cool dark place for a period of a few days to a few years. The food ferments due to the natural bacteria and yeasts it picks up from the air during preparation.

Recipes to choose from:

Drying and Smoking

Drying and smoking were methods first adopted by ancient peoples to preserve foods that would sustain them over long, cold winters. Most foods are dried and smoked with the addition of heat, either from the sun, from embers from a fire or from the low heat of a dehydrator.

There are no recipes for drying or smoking in this book.

Actions: Nutrients are concentrated and the thermal nature is warming. Use these foods in moderation and only for special occasions.

Beneficial seasons: Recommended during colder seasons when fresh foods are less available.

Benefits those who need more concentrated nourishment and require supplementation of *qi* and vitality in the winter. Avoid eating these foods in excess due to the concentration of nutrients.

Deep-Frying

Deep-fried foods are not recommended for enhancing health; therefore, we do not include them. If you have any cardiac, circulatory, liver, gallbladder or blood sugar issues or are overweight or obese, you should avoid deep-fried foods altogether. They contribute to stagnation, heat and stubborn fat buildup in the body. If you are generally in good health, it's acceptable to have a special treat of deep-fried foods occasionally (meaning a few times a year) to celebrate or take part in a special holiday. So when you do, make sure you have the best and enjoy every bite!

Health Tip

It is beneficial to include a side of pungent food (radish, horseradish, pungent greens) to aid the digestion of fried foods and fat.

Microwaving

Microwave ovens and microwaving are ubiquitous in the modern world. According to the United States Bureau of Labor Statistics, 90 percent of U.S. households own a microwave.

Microwaves may be quick, but they do nothing for developing a healthy relationship to cooking and food. As the adage goes, "All good things take time." So take time to cook. Just the same, here is some information on microwaving food.

Tips

We do not recommend microwave cooking to advance health.

If you want a hot lunch, resist the urge to bring cold food to work and microwave it. Consider heating your lunch on the stove in the morning and storing it in a good-quality thermos before leaving for the day or eating the food at room temperature if it's safe to do so.

Actions: Microwave ovens emit microwaves produced by an electron tube called a magnetron. The microwaves are reflected off the interior walls of the oven and absorbed by the food, causing water molecules in the foods to vibrate and produce heat that cooks the food. Foods are cooked quickly, which is convenient.

Other Therapeutic Methods of Cooking

Cooking with Alcohol

The alcohol used in cooking is generally rice wine, or red or white grape wine in Western-style cooking. For our purposes, we used mostly rice wine in this book's recipes. To create tonic wines, certain herbs or foods are soaked in rice wine, brandy or vodka, creating a type of tincture that is taken in very small amounts.

Actions: As alcohol is warming, pungent and sweet, it scatters cold while warming the body, moves *qi* and blood circulation and can dissolve stagnant energy in the body. It moves the energy upward in the body and out to the limbs. It adds warmth to dishes as well as deepening flavor. Because of its *qi*-moving capacity, it can also serve to lift the spirit and ease tension.

Beneficial seasons: For medicinal use, this method is best in the colder seasons to add warmth. However, it is useful in any season when used prudently.

Benefits those who have cold conditions or poor circulation. It's excellent for older people as well. Do not use alcohol if you have cardiac problems or alcohol dependence.

Technique: Rice wine is added in the cooking process (see below for how and when).

Some traditional ways it is used in Chinese medicine:
- Soak foods in 1 cup (250 mL) of wine a few hours before cooking.
- When boiling foods, add some wine before removing from heat.
- Crush $3\frac{1}{2}$ ounces (5 tbsp/75 mL) of gingerroot and squeeze out the juice. Mix the juice with rice wine and heat in a small pan until warm. Drink to induce perspiration.

Cooking with Cooling Foods

All meals need a balance of yin (cooling or neutral) and yang (warming) dishes. This renders a feeling of satisfaction after eating.

Actions: Using cooling foods in cooking can balance the warming aspects of a meal.

Beneficial seasons: All seasons.

Benefits those who have a hot nature, are easily irritated or easy to anger, suffer from hypertension or general liver *qi* stagnation with heat. Cooking with cooling foods can ease and calm the liver.

Technique: Look at the nature of the foods and herbs you are using and adjust or add accordingly — most methods are suitable including braising, steaming, sautéing, grilling.

Cooking with Warming Foods, Herbs and Spices

Everyday warming herbs and cooking spices you already have in your pantry have a powerful energetic effect on the foods you cook with them. Do not underestimate their potency both in flavor and effect.

Actions: Besides the delightful flavors they add, these ingredients also promote digestion and warm your digestive center.

Beneficial seasons: All seasons

Benefits those who have a sluggish digestion or often feel cold. Also recommended for vegans or vegetarians to boost internal warmth and yang.

Technique: Varies with recipes.

Health Tip

Warming foods and spices can aggravate hot symptoms and conditions, including irritability, pent-up tension and frustration, spring allergies, and red and itchy skin eruptions. If you experience any of the above, moderate the intake.

Recipes to choose from:

Hato Mugi and Cinnamon Twig Congee, page 244

Creamed Cauliflower Soup with Aromatic Chive Condiment, page 330

Chicken and Chestnut Fried Rice, page 339

Fall Herbs and Cinnamon Tea, page 356

Nourishing Lamb Stew with Butternut Squash and Dang Gui, page 382

Keep it Simple

As one of my favorite Chinese medicine teachers once said to me, "The simpler the formula, the more potent." Be intentional and judicious with herbs and spices in your cooking. Try only one or two to start with so you can connect to the flavor and effect of the spice. One way to get to know them is through infused teas, a staple in many countries to help digestion, ward off colds and ease tension and stress.

Chinese Medicinal Food Cures

In Chinese herbal medicine, vinegar, salt, alcohol, honey and fresh ginger juice are added to foods and herbs to alter and direct the therapeutic and healing action of those ingredients. These methods of preparing and cooking herbs and foods are known as the ancient practice of *pao zhi* (processing medicinals) and have been used for centuries. Below are some ways to use these therapeutic foods in everyday situations.

Rice Vinegar

We know that rice vinegar can be used as a seasoning, but it also has health benefits. Vinegar promotes digestion, moves stagnation and eases discomfort caused by eating fish or greasy foods. In Chinese medicine, it is also known to help increase blood circulation and is used to treat nosebleeds.

Suggested use: Slice 8 ounces (250 g) fresh radish, either red radish or daikon radish. Cover with rice vinegar and soak for a few hours. Eat as a salad that aids digestion.

See Pickled Umeboshi Radishes recipe, page 434.

Fresh Ginger Juice

Health Tip
If you often feel hot or sweat easily, avoid excessive use of ginger.

Ginger is known for its positive effect on nausea, indigestion and the common cold. Added to food, ginger juice increases the warming and yang nature of those foods. Ginger juice directs movement outward to the surface of the body, helping to expel cold.

Suggested use: Add to soup before it is removed from the heat.

See Scatter-the-Cold Congee recipe, page 324. You can use the scallion and gingerroot topping on this congee in 1 cup (250 mL) of hot water for the first sign of a cold.

Salt

Health Tip
If you suffer from water retention, avoid excessive use of salt.

Salt moistens and softens. Using salt in dishes helps food move downward. It is beneficial in relieving abdominal pain and constipation.

Suggested use: Place $1/2$ teaspoon (2 mL) of salt in a glass of warm water and stir until completely dissolved. Drink before eating, to relieve constipation due to heat.

Honey

Honey's sweetness is often used in the preparation of foods and herbs. Preparing food with honey increases the warming and nourishing aspect. It moistens and lubricates the lungs and large intestine and can ease the symptoms of a cough or soothe a sore throat.

Suggested uses:

- Place 3 tablespoons (45 mL) of honey in a pan and heat over low heat until runny. Add water to cover and stir. Add warmed honey to food and cook together until the liquid starts to become dry and sticky. *See Kumquat Electuary Tea recipe, page 399.*
- Make a hole on the side of a pear or an apple. Pour in some honey and steam until tender. Crush and eat the fruit. (Great for a dry sore throat.)

Health Tip

Avoid honey if you tend to experience loose stools, phlegm or food stagnation.

Experiment and Practice

Experiment with different cooking methods in your kitchen. Remember: patience, presence and practice. You will get the hang of it — and enjoy the variety and satisfaction these cooking methods will bring to your table. As you may have noted, balance is key to eating in a healthful way. By creating a meal that incorporates different cooking methods, you bring choice and balance to your table.

Reflection: Which Cooking Method is Right for Your Meal Today?

- *Are you cold?*
  Try baking, roasting, slow-cooked soups or adding alcohol or warming herbs and spices to your cooking.

- *Are you too hot?*
  Try steamed or lightly boiled foods, salads, cooking with cooling foods, cooling soups and beverages.

- *Are you agitated and moving too fast?*
  Try a slow-cooked stew, long-cooked soup or simple vegetable dish.

- *Are you lethargic?*
  Try a sautéed dish.

- *Are you tired?*
  Try slow- and long-cooked soups or stews and add qi-building herbs.

- *Are you feeling down?*
  Try sautéing and adding pungent and fragrant herbs and spices to your cooking.

Chapter 7

The Digestive System: The Key to Health

"A man does not live on what he eats, but on what he digests."

— *Proverb*

"You are what you eat." You've heard the saying many times. While it has some truth, it is more accurate to say that you are *what you digest and absorb*.

One of the first questions I ask patients when they first come to see me is, "How's your digestion?" The answers I typically get focus only on the very end of the digestion process — what was eliminated — and disregard the early phases of an intricate and complex process that begins even before we take our first bite and continues long after we've eaten. In Chinese medicine, the digestive system is the cornerstone to whole-body-mind health. We have always regarded the health of the gut as vital in the regulation and operation of all systems. While we identify digestive dysfunction or disharmony with obvious symptoms such as bloating, gas, heartburn, mild nausea, diarrhea or constipation, we may not correlate digestion with seemingly unrelated symptoms, including headaches, foggy thinking, poor energy or appetite, anxiety, lethargy, joint pain or inability to lose or gain weight.

The Role of Digestion

Increasingly, Western medicine is recognizing the importance of "gut health" and its relationship to whole-body-mind health. However, the conventional methods for diagnosing and treating illness generally fail to use gut health as a means to diagnose ailments that may seem unconnected to digestion and absorption. Nor does it routinely address adjusting diet and eating habits as a way to improve and regulate digestion and all it affects.

In conventional Western medicine, doctors routinely look at the role and functioning of specific organs — such as the pancreas, liver, gallbladder, small intestine, large intestine and stomach — when examining digestive functioning. Furthermore, the practice of medicine is compartmentalized into specialties, and specialists focus on a particular area of the body to diagnose illness. A gastroenterologist will examine digestion, for example, while an endocrinologist will look at hormonal function. However, the endocrinologist examining a patient's hormonal problem does not typically correlate digestive functioning with the problem at hand.

From its origins, Chinese medicine has put digestion at the center of health, with specific understanding about its relationship to other body systems. The system of diagnosis in Chinese medicine utilizes the perspective of yin and yang, *qi* and blood to examine a digestive disorder in relation to other symptoms and imbalances. Symptoms such as hormonal issues, fluctuating energy levels and frequent headaches, for example, are considered in relation to concurrent digestive symptoms and addressed with food, herbs and acupuncture. In other words, the practitioner regards various physical, mental and emotional symptoms as manifestations of possible digestive distress or imbalances.

The Digestive Process

Digestion is initiated when we start thinking about eating. At the first thought of food, the brain sends a signal to the mouth where it begins to produce enzymes in the saliva, preparing the body for food. Chewing further stimulates the process when we take that first bite. From mouth to anus, as food travels along the alimentary canal, aka the digestive tract, it will go through a number of processes to mechanically break it down and nourish the body. Once food has been chewed and liquids swallowed, it lands in the stomach — the most acidic part of the body — where gastric glands in the stomach secrete acids and enzymes to transform the food into chyme, a pulpy, digestive fluid. The chyme then slithers through the sphincter into the small intestine and nutrients begin to be absorbed. Here, enzymes from the pancreas, and bile created by the liver and stored in the gallbladder, join in to further digest foods, with each organ contributing to the separation and absorption of the resulting chyme and transporting its nourishment through the intestinal wall into the blood vessels. Finally, the residue of undigested fiber and other waste moves down to the large intestine, where beneficial bacteria tackle the undigested material and condense the residue into fecal matter that is excreted through the anus.

> **What's the difference?**
>
> DIGESTION = breakdown of food
>
> ABSORPTION = assimilation into the blood and cells of the body

Digestion, from the Western perspective, is indeed the process by which whole foods, made up of proteins, carbohydrate, fats, vitamins, minerals and fiber, are gradually broken down (digested) to their simple forms. The protein is digested to become amino acids, the carbohydrates to glucose, and fat to fatty acids. In healthy digestion, these breakdown processes move into the blood (absorption), where they travel to nourish all the cells of the body. In Chinese medicine, the production of amino acids and glucose is closely associated with the production of blood, and the circulation of fatty acids is associated with the nourishment and movement of *qi*.

Another View: The Stomach and Spleen = Earth

This diagram (below) represents the Five Phases: red-fire at the top (summer: heart/small intestine), white-metal at the right (autumn: lung/large intestine), black-water at the bottom (winter: kidney/bladder), green-wood at the left (spring: liver/gallbladder), yellow-earth in the center (earth: stomach/spleen/pancreas).

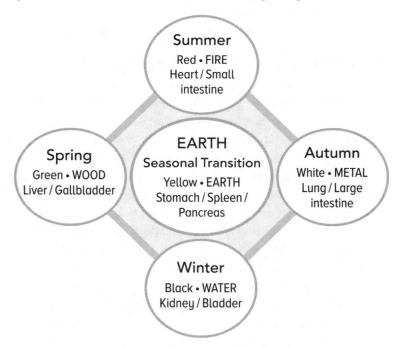

Summer
Red • FIRE
Heart / Small intestine

Spring
Green • WOOD
Liver / Gallbladder

EARTH
Seasonal Transition
Yellow • EARTH
Stomach / Spleen / Pancreas

Autumn
White • METAL
Lung / Large intestine

Winter
Black • WATER
Kidney / Bladder

Without going into the details in full, the diagram above shows the specific role of the stomach and spleen. Located at the center, they represent the Earth element, which can be further understood to be the realm of each individual's physiology and nourishment. In Chinese medicine, the stomach and spleen are seen as a unit of digestive functioning that embodies both yin and yang. Suffice it to say, the balance and health of digestion is built upon the health of the stomach–spleen network, which is considered the cornerstone of nourishment. The stomach, which is the main vessel for the breakdown of foods, needs the spleen to transform food into nourishment and distribute it through the body. Together, they are seen as central to the production of *qi* and blood — energy and substance. If the breakdown of food is suboptimal (stomach), so will be the body's capacity to distribute and absorb nourishment (spleen).

The Stomach

The stomach is considered the most important of all yang organs. Working with the spleen, its yin organ pair, the stomach is considered the root and origin of postnatal *qi*, which fuels our energy on a daily basis. The stomach's role of breaking down food through a type of "fermentation," known as rotting and ripening, is key to the spleen's role of transforming and transporting nourishment throughout the body.

To further the breakdown of foods, the stomach needs a moist and damp environment to ferment and digest food so it can send the slurry mixture to the small intestine. The yang stomach relies on the balance of yin (fluids and cooling) for its optimal functioning: it is what science has identified as stomach acid (hydrochloric acid), pancreatic enzymes and certain components of pancreatic juices, liver bile and other gastrointestinal fluids. The vitality of digestion is often expressed in Chinese medicine as the strength of one's *digestive fire*, equated with the production of these gastrointestinal fluids. The "cooking pot" of our digestion, the stomach, requires a balanced internal climate that is neither too hot nor too cold and with ample amount of digestive fire (stomach acid) to promote this process.

Stomach Environment

Certain foods provide and nourish the necessary fluids for this process. Promoting a moist (yin) internal stomach environment is therefore beneficial. Foods that are overly heating and drying can cause stomach yin deficiency. Inversely, cold and icy foods inhibit and slow down the stomach's digestive function. Deficient stomach *qi* (digestive fire) can lead to low appetite, stomach discomfort, a feeling of whole-body weakness, loose stools or indigestion. Excess stomach heat, due to an overconsumption of hot, spicy and drying foods, can lead to stomach pain, constipation, desire to drink cold liquids, dry mouth and lips, and extreme thirst.

Did You Know?

In Chinese medicine, all organs are paired with another and they act together in what is called an organ network or pair. The digestion pair includes a yang organ (stomach) and yin organ (spleen).

"The stomach tends to favor tranquility and cheerfulness, while the spleen favors music."

— *Ancient Chinese saying*

Did You Know?

Cold foods straight from the refrigerator and foods that are cold in thermal nature — such as juices, fruits, yogurt, ice cream and raw foods — weaken digestive fire and injure the spleen's capacity to transform and transport nourishment.

The Spleen

As we have seen, the spleen's main role is to assist the stomach in the process of digestion, as well as to help distribute nutrients throughout the body. Western medical science acknowledges that digestion requires an extraordinary amount of metabolic energy. Similarly, Chinese medicine looks to *qi* to help the spleen function well. Healthy spleen *qi* can effectively extract nourishment from foods into what Chinese medicine refers to as "food *qi*," which is central to the formation of blood and *qi*.

Spleen Environment

Did You Know?

The spleen, an organ tucked between the stomach, pancreas and left kidney, is considered a storage container and filter for blood, as well as the largest lymph node in the body. Even though it is not a physical part of the digestive system, it is connected to the blood vessels of the stomach and pancreas.

In contrast to the stomach, which needs a moist environment to function optimally, the spleen needs warmth and dryness to effectively transform and refine food into nourishment. The yin spleen organ therefore needs a dry, warm and yang environment to function well. That is, the stomach, a yang organ, needs yin to support its balance and function; inversely, the spleen, a yin organ, needs yang for its optimal functioning. An excessive intake of foods that are cold, iced or creamy, rich and fatty will impede and weaken its function. Symptoms that may indicate a weakened spleen *qi* include fatigue, a feeling of heaviness in the limbs, an inability to focus or concentrate, or conditions of excess phlegm or mucus. In addition, weakened or deficient spleen *qi* means that the spleen cannot effectively transform and transport nourishment, which then ends up being deposited throughout the body in the form of phlegm, fat, plaque or mucus and stagnating.

Finding Balance

The harmonious functioning of the stomach–spleen network is keenly affected by our choices of foods and lifestyle habits. Conversely, this network's disequilibrium is often not straightforward and people may experience conflicting symptoms, such as lethargy and cloudy thinking (dampness) with food stagnation and heartburn (heat). These symptoms are usually a combination of excess (heat, dampness and stagnation) and deficiency (cold and feelings of weakness).

Unfortunately, digestive distress is so common that many have come to accept it, soothed by intermittent abstention from certain foods and medications that fail to solve underlying problems. The foods we eat and the dietary habits and lifestyle activities we practice can benefit a healthy stomach–spleen network to promote regularity and balance and limit stress on the digestive system.

Healing with food can clear out excess and supplement deficiency to help the body find equilibrium.

Beneficial Foods

Foods that strengthen and nourish digestion are characterized by a bland sweet flavor found in many of the whole foods we eat on a daily basis. Most of these beneficial foods will neither heat us up nor cool us down excessively, as digestion is impaired by overabundant intake of either hot and spicy foods or icy and cold foods. The foods below are considered mostly neutral or warming in nature. It does not mean that these are the *only* foods to eat — they do not represent the full scope and balance of what we need to eat every day — but these foods do comprise the center of a healthy diet that benefits the stomach–spleen network. They are also familiar to many cultures worldwide.

Whole grains: short-grain brown rice, sweet (glutinous) brown rice, oats, buckwheat

Beans, pulses and legumes: chickpeas, soybeans, adzuki beans, peas

Vegetables: all winter squashes, carrots, cabbages, peas, fennel, pumpkin, sweet potatoes or yams, shiitake and other mushrooms, green beans, lotus root

Nuts and seeds: peanuts (which are technically considered a legume), chestnuts, almonds

Animal foods: beef, chicken, duck, pork, lamb, all broths of beef and chicken, eggs, trout, salmon, catfish

Fruits: red dates (jujubes), sweet cherries, peaches, red grapes, raisins, apples, figs

Beverages/teas: Many warm beverages, including fennel tea, ginger tea and licorice tea, tonic liquors that include digestive herbs (such as ginger and cardamom wine; see Winter Recipes, page 366) or foods that nourish stomach and spleen, and Mushroom Immune Broth (see page 329).

Sweeteners: raw unpasteurized honey, pure maple syrup, rice syrup, date or coconut sugar

Spices: fennel seeds, cardamom, star anise, gingerroot, nutmeg, coriander, cinnamon, nutmeg, peppercorns

Culinary herbs: rosemary, thyme, chives, vanilla

Medicinal herbs: Chinese yam (dioscorea), lotus seeds, astragalus root, codonopsis

Did You Know?

Stomach *qi* normally moves downward as it breaks down and digests food. When stomach *qi* is rebellious, it flows upwards, causing nausea, belching and possible vomiting.

Detrimental Foods for the Stomach and Spleen

The stomach and spleen depend on a balance of yin and yang. Avoid these foods to achieve a healthy balance:

- Too many raw and cold foods, such as foods straight out of the refrigerator and iced drinks, and the overconsumption of cooling foods, including cucumbers, tropical fruits, watermelon, salads (especially during the winter), sorbet
- Too many creamy and greasy foods, including an excess of dairy products — milk and milk products such as yogurt (especially if it is sweetened), ice cream, cottage cheese, kefir
- Hot and spicy foods
- Too much sugar and too many sweet foods. Too many desserts and candy
- Too much coffee or hard liquor (which is very warming)
- An excess of grilled foods
- Regular consumption of deep-fried foods
- "Damp" foods: If you live in a damp climate, it is important to counter the exterior dampness by minimizing the intake of damp-producing foods, such as dairy products, sugar, refined carbohydrates and cold, greasy and creamy foods.

Eating Rhythms and Habits

Besides the type of foods we eat, our dietary habits exert an influence on the health and functioning of the stomach and spleen. Appetite has its own rhythm, similar to energy levels that wax and wane from morning until night. Listening and responding to hunger is important.

But one of the more important habits we can foster is the consumption of regular meals at regular intervals during the day. In Chinese medicine, we stress the value of eating at regular times to honor natural rhythms and energy flow. This is one of the most common recommendations I make in clinical practice to help with issues of energy and mood. Eating at certain times, pausing to eat, and then not eating for 3 to 4 hours allows our stomach to digest and empty and fosters the spleen's capacity to transform, absorb and distribute nourishment effectively. If we eat constantly, our digestive system is taxed and overworked. If we ignore hunger and don't eat, our digestive system overworks as well by extracting whatever nourishment it can to fuel body and brain. Have you ever noticed that when you don't eat, you can have a hard time focusing or summoning your energy? A lack of regular nourishment impedes our cognition and energy flow.

In addition, eating while working or scrolling through social media feeds, eating while driving, eating while walking, or eating when we are upset or angry interferes with digestion. When eating, simply eat.

Finally, nighttime is when our body needs to rest and that includes digestion; eating late at night is a stress on digestion.

Detrimental Food Habits

- Eating when angry, upset or depressed
- Not chewing food thoroughly. Digestion starts in the mouth.
- Overeating, feeling too full. Stop eating once you feel 80 percent full.
- Not eating enough to satisfy hunger or restricting eating
- Frequent dieting and changing diets continuously, which require the stomach to keep adjusting
- Inappropriate and frequent fasting
- Excessive mental strain without regular exercise
- Skipping breakfast. The optimal functioning of the stomach–spleen network occurs between 7 and 9 a.m.

Did You Know?

It is important to stop eating before you feel full — it takes about 20 minutes for the body to sense fullness.

Did You Know?

Chinese medicine has long recognized how too much mental strain stresses digestion and absorption by diverting nourishment and blood (yin) from the gut to fuel the brain. Modern research and science also associates the effects of mental burden on the gut–brain axis. Both systems of medicine advocate regulating stress and strain to regulate digestion and support absorption. For thousands of years, Chinese medicine has treated this problem with herbal formulas made into teas.

Treating Common Digestive Problems

Many common health problems are rooted in the functions of digestion and absorption. These problems are well addressed by a change in diet using the principles of yin and yang to stimulate production of *qi* (vital energy) and blood (substance and nourishment). The chart below lists some of the most common digestive issues, along with their Chinese medicine diagnosis, possible causes and dietary solutions for stimulating healing and balance.

Symptom(s)	Chinese Medicine Diagnosis	Possible Causes	Solutions
Fatigue or general exhaustion	Spleen and stomach *qi* deficiency	• Poor nourishment, irregular meals, skipping meals, too many cold, raw or cooling foods, excessive amounts of carbohydrates. • Creamy and rich foods. • Drinking cold drinks and drinking liquids with meals.	• Eat breakfast and regular meals. • Eat brothy soups, congees or vegetable-based meals. Include carbohydrate-rich vegetables, pumpkin, sweet potatoes. • Eat cooked foods. • Include pungent and aromatic cooking herbs and spices such as nutmeg, fennel seed, ginger, cinnamon. Include sweet and bland and the pungent (but not spicy) flavors, including fennel, leeks, brown rice (short- and long-grain), pumpkin, squash, onions. • Include lean meat and fish. • Include warming fruits such as raspberries, peaches and cherries.
Fatigue after eating	Spleen *qi* deficiency and spleen dampness	• Eating while rushed or without chewing completely. • Consuming too many refined carbohydrates. • Overeating, eating late at night. • Irregular eating, poor nourishment, too much sugar, too many cold, raw or cooling foods, too much dairy, all of which contribute to and weaken the spleen function and digestion. • Stress and emotional upset.	• Eat warming foods with the pungent flavor, such as alliums, mustard greens; herbs such as basil, cilantro, thyme, parsley; spices such as cardamom, nutmeg, anise seeds, cumin, coriander. Include adzuki beans, celery, Chinese spring onions (green onions).

Symptom(s)	Chinese Medicine Diagnosis	Possible Causes	Solutions
Poor appetite	Spleen *qi* deficiency	• Irregular eating, poor nourishment, too much sugar, too many cold, raw or cooling foods, too much dairy, all of which contribute to and weaken the spleen function and digestion. • Stress, emotional upset and worry, chronic illness.	• Eat regular meals. • Include foods that are more warming in thermal nature, pungent and sweet in flavor. Include long-cooked broths that are easy to digest with meat or fish (trout, salmon or tuna, beef, chicken or lamb). • Include congee or soft-cooked whole grains. Include hato mugi in rice dishes. • Include fruits that are more warming such as cherries, plums, peaches, red dates, red grapes. Include sweet carbohydrate vegetables such as pumpkin, sweet potato, carrot or cabbage. Include pungent spices such as cinnamon, ginger, fennel, cardamom, nutmeg, small amounts of black pepper or Sichuan peppercorns, rosemary, thyme or oregano. • Nuts and seeds including pine nuts, pistachio, brown sesame seeds. • Small amounts of honey can be used as a sweetener.
Excessive appetite Bad breath	Stomach heat	• Too many hot and spicy, fried and grilled foods. • Excessive coffee and alcohol consumption. • Consuming poor-quality fats. • Over- or undereating. • Excess long-term stress.	• Eliminate hot and spicy foods. • Include vegetables with a cooling nature such as spinach, eggplant, okra, greens in the chicory family: endive, escarole, frisée, radicchio.
Food cravings	Disharmony of stomach and spleen	• Fatigue, overwork or overexertion. • Eating late at night, snacking and eating too often. • Unbalanced eating, with too many salty, fatty or sweet foods.	• Eat regular meals. Include a balance of the five flavors, as well as good-quality oils, small amounts of meat and fish, with more dark leafy vegetables. Include pungent and bitter flavors, as well as sweet vegetables such as pumpkin, squash, sweet potatoes, whole grains, to satisfy cravings for sweet.

Symptom(s)	Chinese Medicine Diagnosis	Possible Causes	Solutions
Heartburn	Stomach heat and stomach yin deficiency	• Irregular eating habits, eating late at night, eating too fast without adequate chewing. • Eating too many spicy hot, greasy, fatty or deep-fried foods. • Excessive coffee or alcohol consumption.	• Eat soothing and cooling foods such as soups and congees. Include cabbage, napa cabbage, spinach, okra, mushrooms, avocados, tofu (if soy is tolerated). • Incorporate cooking methods such as steaming, blanching, water sautéing or fermenting to boost gut flora.
Bloating and poor digestion	Spleen yang deficiency and spleen dampness	• Overeating, eating too quickly. • Eating foods you are sensitive to and cannot tolerate or digest (for example, gluten, sugar or dairy). • Eating while emotionally upset.	• Include fennel seeds or fennel seed tea, ginger tea, crataegus (Chinese hawthorn) fruit (*shan zha*) tea, anise seed tea, carrots, coriander, steamed cabbage, ginger-infused vinegar, or plain rice vinegar or apple cider vinegar. • Most importantly, slow down your eating and be sure to chew well.
Diarrhea	Possible mild food poisoning or spleen *qi* deficiency or spleen dampness	• Eating foods that are rancid, poisonous or spoiled. • Poor-quality nourishment, skipping meals. Too many refined carbohydrates and sugary foods. • Too many greasy or fatty foods. Too many cold, icy and/or raw foods.	• For acute issues, drink warm or temperate fluids as in soups, congee, broths or teas. Include cooked carrots, sweet potatoes or yams.
Constipation	Stomach heat and yin deficiency or spleen *qi* deficiency	• Too many hot and spicy foods or cold foods, including hot chile peppers and garlic.	• Include soft and cooked vegetables, spinach, carrots, mushrooms. Include peaches, persimmons, bananas. • Eat seeds such as flax, hemp, sesame, and pine nuts. • Chew well.
Nausea, belching	Rebellious stomach *qi*	• Foods the body cannot digest well, causing fermentation and rotting in the stomach. • Eating too quickly. • Eating while upset, anxious or worried. • Food poisoning leading to vomiting.	• Drink Ginger and Tangerine Peel Tea (see recipe, p. 238). • Include pineapple or pineapple juice (if you suffer from feeling cold, add a small amount of grated gingerroot to the juice). • Add spices such as cloves, nutmeg, marjoram.

Center of Health

As we said at the start of this chapter, you are what you eat, digest, transform and absorb. When the digestive system is functioning well, we hardly notice it and we feel robust and resourceful. We might take guidance from Chinese medicine in the way it considers the stomach and spleen as Earth, the center of health and functioning. If we care for our Earth element, we will be nourished well. Small signs and symptoms of distress are signals that it may be time to adjust what and how you are eating. So take time to tune in to what your stomach–spleen network — your rhythm machine — is telling you on a continual basis, whether it is to remind you when to eat or that you need more or different fuel for everyday activities.

What can you do today to make a difference in how and what you eat? Start with one or two things you can do successfully. Each step toward the health of your stomach–spleen network builds your *qi* and blood — a process that is cumulative and central to overall functioning.

Reflection: How Are Your Eating Habits?

Before you sit down to eat your next meal, take a moment to think about the following:

- *How did I start my day of eating?* Did I sit down to a warming breakfast?

- *Am I simply focused on eating?* Or did the TV, computer or phone distract me?

- *Am I chewing enough?* (Chewing food more thoroughly will make digestion easier.)

- *Is my plate balanced with the five flavors* (sweet, sour, salty, pungent and bitter) and the five colors (green, red, yellow or orange, white or beige, black or blue)?

- *Did I eat regular meals today?* If not, do I need to learn how to manage mealtimes? (See Chapter 6, page 94.)

- *How do I feel after eating?* Do I feel comfortable? Satisfied? Do I have an adequate amount of energy? (To start, remove food obstacles and clear out your pantry, see Chapter 9, page 144.)

- *Do I have any minor digestive disturbances?* What are they? (Take stock and get some help. Those first signs of distress can be remedied with help from a trained health-care provider or dietitian/nutritionist and a shift in what and how you eat.)

- *Am I eating mindlessly because I'm anxious, upset or depressed?* Recognize that you may need some other type of nourishment that may not be extracted from food.

Chapter 8

Food Recommendations for Common Health Problems

"The five types of foods have specific effects and properties. When combined with the principles of the seasons, the five elements … one can utilize the methods of dietetics as an adjunct tool to nourish, convalesce and treat."

— *Huangdi Neijing Suwen, The Yellow Emperor's Classic of Medicine*

Note

If you are dealing with a serious health problem, such as ulcerative colitis, diabetes, chronic pain or high blood pressure, always consult your physician or a trained and licensed health-care provider, who can work with you over time to create a dietary plan to address your symptoms as well as conditions that can become more severe if left untreated.

By now we know that in the tradition of Chinese medicine, treating illnesses includes dietary recommendations to assist healing. The same applies to common health problems, from seasonal allergies to coughs and colds to high blood pressure to insomnia, for which Chinese nutritional therapy has been shown to be an effective antidote.

While the practice of Chinese medicine is individualized based on a person's unique makeup and symptoms, incorporating or eliminating certain foods in the diet can influence and support healing. But whether you are seeking to strengthen your immune system, reduce allergies or lower blood pressure, making dietary changes for only a few days or a week is not enough time to experience long-lasting results. Transforming body chemistry isn't a quick fix — it takes at least 8 to 12 weeks, and making changes to eating behaviors and adjusting food preferences is a process of experimenting, practicing and learning to integrate these changes into your daily life.

Common Health Conditions

Seasonal Allergies

Seasonal allergy symptoms most often plague sufferers in the spring, summer or fall. From a Chinese medicine perspective, seasonal allergies result from the body's susceptibility to invasions of wind heat or cold or possible spleen *qi* deficiency. Symptoms can include regular sneezing, itchy eyes, headaches, foggy thinking, a stuffy nose or sinus congestion, hives, acute asthma attacks, achy joints or digestive distress (bloating, heartburn, diarrhea or gas) and can range from mild and bothersome to severe reactions that hinder everyday functioning. To treat seasonal allergies with diet, Chinese medicine considers eliminating foods that are too warming, hot or cold (depending on a person's condition) and those that diminish spleen *qi*.

See Chapter 9, page 144, for a complete breakdown of common foods to avoid and/or eliminate for optimal health.

The Chinese and Western perspectives on inflammation and allergies are quite similar, though they use different language. Western medicine views foods that are inflammatory in nature as activating the histamine response and potentially causing "allergic" symptoms. Thus, by reducing inflammatory foods, the symptoms can be reduced. In Chinese medicine, these same inflammatory foods are seen as aggravating health conditions from the perspective of increasing heat, cold, dryness or dampness and contributing to stagnation, excess and deficiency.

I have witnessed hundreds of patients change their diets and reduce or clear up seasonal or perennial allergy symptoms by eliminating aggravating and inflammatory foods. In general, with most seasonal allergies, it is recommended to reduce and avoid these common inflammatory foods: wheat and wheat products,

Did You Know?

Histamines are chemicals, made by the body, that cause inflammation in various cells, from the mucous membranes of the nose and lungs to the lining of your gut, as a way to force out an "invading" substance.

soy, refined sugar, dairy, corn, peanuts, eggs, chocolate, caffeine and alcohol, as well as artificial preservatives like monosodium glutamate (MSG) and artificial sweeteners, such as aspartame, for a period of 8 to 12 weeks.

For allergy symptoms that include itchy eyes, sore throat or red skin rashes that feel hot, the warmer weather can worsen them.

Avoid: Heating spices, such as any kind of pepper, chile, garlic or cinnamon. Frying or grilling foods. Too much fruit and fruit juices, yogurt, cold and raw foods or sour and fermented foods.

Foods and herbs to include: Cooling foods, including chrysanthemum, nettles, mint, lavender, dandelion, hato mugi (Job's tears) or green tea. Include pungent vegetables such as radish, turnip, leafy green vegetables with a pungent flavor such as nettles, chives, arugula and vegetables with a sweet flavor such as spinach, peas, asparagus (sweet and bitter, baby carrots and beets, as well as seaweeds, which are cooling and detoxifying. Include foods to stimulate and activate digestion, such as ginger. Include astragalus root, Chinese yam and brown rice to strengthen stomach–spleen *qi*.

Suggested recipes for allergies

Essential Seed and Nut Porridge (all seasons, various pages)

Spring Tonic Congee, page 212

Tofu and Snow Pea Breakfast Fried Rice, page 214

Quick-Pickled Radish Tops over Steamed Red Radishes and Cauliflower, page 228

Spring Greens and Lotus Root Sauté, page 235

Spring Nettle and Fragrant Flowers Tea, page 237

Ginger and Tangerine Peel Tea, page 238

Mushroom Immune Broth, page 329

Arame Sauté with Carrots and Broccoli, page 342

Common Colds

In Chinese medicine, "catching" a cold is the result of changing climate and exposure to wind (*feng*). Since a cold initially affects the surface of the body with feelings of heat (fever) or cold (chills), along with body aches and stiffness, sneezing, sore throat or mild cough, the treatment seeks to push the "pernicious" influence of wind and cold out with pungent herbs and foods. Chinese medicine has treated the common cold and flu-like symptoms this way for thousands of years.

Whether it is viral or bacterial, how a cold is treated will vary, depending on symptoms. For example, an acute sore throat accompanied by symptoms that can include one or more of the following; a feeling of burning in the throat, fever or heat symptoms with the beginnings of a cough and profuse mucous will be treated with foods — such as radish, turnip, napa cabbage and figs — and herbs that help clear heat, toxins and phlegm, as well as those that will help soothe the throat, such as peppermint, honeysuckle buds and lily bulb. On the other hand, treatment for a common cold with chills, no fever, stuffy nose, stiff neck and muscle aches would include pungent and warming foods and herbs that dispel the cold, clear toxins and release the pathogens from the body.

Common colds with symptoms of heat, known as wind heat invasion, can include a burning sore throat, fever, dryness and thirst, sweating, runny nose and nasal congestion, thirst and a slight cough with yellow phlegm.

Avoid: Overeating. Spicy, greasy, fatty or creamy foods, cheese, red meat, chicken and shrimp. Grilling, frying or the heavy use of oil and fat in cooking.

Foods and herbs to include: Lightly cooked vegetable broths or soups and congee. Cooling pungent foods and herbs such as radish, turnip, peppermint, honeysuckle buds and chrysanthemum. Eat animal foods in broths or soups that include a plethora of vegetables.

Suggested recipes for common colds with heat symptoms:

Spring Greens Tonic Soup (without the herbs if you have mucus and phlegm), page 220
Herbed Nettle and Asparagus Risotto, page 222
Spring Nettle and Fragrant Flowers Tea, page 237
Strawberry-Rose Fruit Salad, page 240
Clear-the-Heat Mung Bean Congee, page 244
Arame Salad with Lemon and Chives, page 265
Vibrant Summer Vegetables with Tofu Dressing, page 266
Pineapple Chrysanthemum Kanten, page 279

Common colds with symptoms of cold, known as wind cold invasion, can include nasal congestion, chills, sneezing and runny nose, headache or body aches and coughing with clear phlegm.

Avoid: Raw and cold foods, iced or cold drinks, dairy, refined carbohydrates and sweets.

Foods and herbs to include: Gingerroot, cinnamon, Chinese spring onions (scallions or green onions), parsley, carrots, parsnips, small amounts of chives or garlic.

Suggested recipes for common colds with cold symptoms:

Scatter-the-Cold Congee, page 324. (You can also put the topping for the congee in hot water to help disperse cold symptoms.)
Hato Mugi and Cinnamon Twig Congee, page 326
Clear-the-Lungs Tea, page 356
Fall Herbs and Cinnamon Tea, page 356

If you find yourself **susceptible to common colds** or are around others who often catch colds, such as small children, including tonic foods in your diet weekly (when healthy) can help boost immunity.

Suggested recipes to boost immunity before you get a cold:

(Eat one or two of these recipes every week during cold and flu season.)

Chinese Yam Congee with Lotus Seeds and Hato Mugi, page 288

Miso Soup, page 296

Nourish the Qi and Blood Tea, page 313

Red Date, Almond and Cinnamon Liquor, page 315

Mushroom Immune Broth, page 329

Duck Broth with Tatsoi, page 375

Trout Steamed with Green Peas and Lemony Herbed Rice, page 379

Dang Gui and Astragalus Tea with Ginger, page 421

Constipation

Did You Know?

Digestion starts in the mouth with chewing. More chewing means your food is broken down further and is easier to digest. Be sure to chew food well, up to 35 times per bite.

Generally speaking, Chinese medicine identifies three primary types of constipation. Liver *qi* stagnation, sometimes caused by stress or travel, can turn to heat and cause difficult evacuation and dry stools. Deficiency of *qi* and yang diminishes the peristalsis action of the large intestine and most commonly affects older people, people recovering from long-term illness or surgery and postpartum women. Finally, constipation can be a result of yin deficiency, usually in older people, with symptoms of dry stool, dryness in the mouth and throat, and dry skin.

To treat excess constipation caused by liver *qi* stagnation and heat:

Avoid: Baked goods, crackers, hard cheeses and excess meat and fatty foods, which are more difficult to break down and eliminate. Beans, which are drying (except for soybeans and soy-based products like tofu, which are more lubricating). Caffeine, such as in coffee or caffeinated teas, which can be too drying.

Foods and herbs to include: More vegetables and fruits with fiber, such as celery, spinach, cucumbers, napa cabbage, mung beans, tomatoes, bananas, rhubarb, apples, pears, plums. Seeds and nuts, such as black sesame seeds, coconut, hemp seeds, flax seeds, pine nuts, pistachios. Tofu, apple cider vinegar and fermented foods such as sauerkraut, miso, natto and yogurt, to increase healthy gut flora.

To treat *qi* or yang deficiency–type constipation:

Avoid: Baked goods, crackers, hot and spicy foods. Reduce roasted bitter foods such as coffee, tea and chocolate.

Foods and herbs to include: Steamed vegetables (which add more moisture back into foods), congee, soups and fermented foods (to increase beneficial gut flora). Spinach, okra, sweet potatoes, fennel, carrots, seaweed. Nuts and seeds, including black sesame seeds, flax seeds, hemp seeds, almonds and peanuts. Tofu, oats, rice, bananas, plums and pears.

To treat yin deficiency–type constipation:

Avoid: Baked goods, crackers, hot and spicy foods. Reduce roasted bitter foods, such as coffee, tea and chocolate, which are warming and drying.

Foods and herbs to include: Steamed vegetables (which add more moisture back into foods), congee, soups and fermented foods (to increase beneficial gut flora). Seaweed, eggplant, cucumbers, black sesame seeds, peanuts, bananas, pears, apples, apricots, plums and prunes.

Suggested recipes for constipation:

Essential Nut and Seed Porridge (all seasons, various pages)
Simple Roasted Asparagus, page 236
Sesame Seed–Crusted Eggplant, page 270
Nourishing Vegetable Treasures, page 300
Sautéed Banana Crêpes, page 322
Roasted Sweet Potato Salad, page 354
Autumn Fruit Salad with Rose Syrup, page 360
Walnut Chai, page 401

Coughs

Coughs can vary in their intensity (weak or strong), quality (dry and unproductive or phlegm-filled) and duration (acute for days or a few weeks, or chronic, lasting more than 1 month). Coughs can arise from exposure to wind, cold, dryness, dampness and heat or due to internal disharmony from a poor diet, smoking or excess intake of spicy foods, fats and alcohol.

Avoid: Fatty, greasy, sugary, spicy or fried foods. Warming foods: shrimp, prawns, meat, peppers, chile peppers, garlic, alcohol and coffee. Avoid smoking.

Foods and herbs to include: Gingerroot, mulberry leaves, lily bulbs, thyme tea with honey, honey and aniseed tea, dried schisandra, pears, dark leafy greens, almonds, pine nuts, sesame seeds, congee with the addition of orange peel and ginger.

Did You Know?

If a cough persists for more than a couple of weeks, with phlegm that is yellow or green accompanied by fatigue, or if you have a dry cough that exceeds 3 weeks, consult your doctor to rule out a more serious complication.

Cough with Hot Phlegm

If phlegm is either yellow or greenish, the Chinese medicine diagnosis would be hot phlegm, which can indicate infection.

Avoid: Warming and spicy foods, such as garlic, all hot peppers and hot pepper sauces, dried ginger, lamb, shrimp, chocolate, coffee and alcohol.

Foods and herbs to include: Neutral or cooling foods, including pears, anise seeds, radishes, turnips, mustard greens, napa cabbage, sprouts, persimmons, green tea, seaweeds.

Suggested recipes for cough with hot phlegm:

Quick-Pickled Radish Tops over Steamed Red Radishes and Cauliflower, page 228
Borscht, page 253

Cough with Phlegm, without Heat Symptoms

If a cough is accompanied by clear and thin mucus, the Chinese medicine diagnosis is cough with phlegm, which is aggravated by a damp climate or weak spleen *qi*.

Avoid: All cooling, cold, raw foods, dairy products, sugar and refined foods.

Foods and herbs to include: Pears, apricots, kumquats, dried orange peel, fresh or dried ginger, mushrooms, radishes, carrots, millet, rice, oats, pine nuts, almonds, mustard greens and onion.

Suggested recipes for cough with phlegm:

Plain congee with 1 to 2 tsp (5 to 10 mL) of grated orange peel
Ginger and Tangerine Peel Tea, page 238
Steamed or sautéed mustard greens
Vegetarian Dashi, page 297
Mushroom Immune Broth, page 329
Carrot Burdock Kinpira, page 344
Velvety Pears with Anise Seeds, Lemon and Honey, page 361
Kumquat Electuary Tea, page 399

Dry Cough

A dry cough is typically categorized as a stubborn and weak cough with little or slightly sticky phlegm.

Avoid: Foods that are drying, including spicy and heating foods, baked goods, crackers and chips.

Foods and herbs to include: Moistening foods that are neutral and cooling. Cooking methods that are moistening, such as boiling, steaming and braising. Watercress, mushrooms, radishes, carrots, pears, bananas, oranges, peaches, figs, honey. Anise seeds, walnuts, black sesame seeds, almonds, pine nuts. Tofu, soy milk, poached eggs, seaweed, lotus root, chrysanthemum flower tea and lily bulbs.

Suggested recipes for dry cough:

Spring Greens and Lotus Root Sauté, page 235

Simple Roasted Asparagus, page 236

Essential Seed and Nut Porridge with Feta (leave out the feta) and Fresh Fruit, page 247

Goji and Lily Bulb Beneficial Congee, page 325

Mushroom Immune Broth, page 329

Spinach and Egg Drop Soup, page 334

Velvety Pears with Anise Seeds, Lemon and Honey, page 361

Cocoa Crumble on Sliced Oranges (leave out the cocoa crumble, which is too warming), page 406

Type 2 Diabetes

Type 2 diabetes is a serious chronic disease in which either the pancreas can no longer produce insulin (the hormone necessary for regulating blood sugar) or the body cannot effectively use the insulin produced by the pancreas. In Chinese medicine, a diagnosis of diabetes or high blood sugar (known as prediabetes) can begin as a yin-deficiency pattern that can later manifest as a heat syndrome that further damages *qi*, yin and yang. Changing the diet is tantamount to minimizing symptoms and progression of type 2 diabetes.

Avoid: Overeating. Poor-quality fats, fatty, greasy and creamy foods, processed meats and refined carbohydrates, sugars, alcohol (high sugar content) and all artificial flavorings and sweeteners. Avoid highly spiced, sweet and excessively salty foods. Reduce portion sizes and skip second portions. Reduce intake of raw foods, which puts stress on the stomach's digestive capacity. Eat meals at regular intervals; avoid eating after 7 p.m. and heavy meals at night.

Did You Know?

Bitter melon has been shown to be effective in helping regulate blood sugar. It contains bioactive compounds that help regulate blood sugar. Bitter melon's cold nature and bitter flavor help to clear heat caused by underlying yin deficiency. If you are trying to get pregnant, are pregnant or nursing avoid eating bitter melon.

Foods and herbs to include: Cooling or slightly warming foods, including spinach, turnips, millet, fresh corn, tofu, mung beans, Chinese yam, black-boned (Silkie) chicken, duck, small amounts of fermented soy and dairy (if tolerated). Eat the five flavors in a healthy variety of vegetables, nuts and seeds, beans, animal food, fruits and condiments. Include pumpkin, mushrooms, broths, soups and congee, as well as a variety of condiments to increase palatability (see Condiment Recipes, page 422). Lightly cook your vegetables and fruits.

Fatigue

Fatigue, or low energy, is a common complaint often caused by a lack of sleep or poor sleep hygiene (including staying up too late), overwork, overexertion, irregular eating, poor food absorption, trauma, physical and emotional stress, ongoing chronic illness or pain. If you suffer from unremitting fatigue, seek help from a health-care provider to understand possible causes — an underlying medical condition such as endocrine imbalances, poor digestion and absorption, thyroid dysfunction, depression or a virus could be a contributing factor. If you suffer from chronic fatigue that makes it difficult to get out of bed in the morning or if you become severely exhausted after exertion, it is vital to get help from a health-care provider.

From a Chinese medicine perspective, liver *qi* stagnation, which occurs commonly with stress and overwork, can inhibit energy (*qi*) circulation, causing fatigue and possible depression. Liver *qi* stagnation can lead to spleen *qi* deficiency and result in internal damp conditions that further impede spleen function, evidenced in feelings of lethargy, poor appetite and foggy thinking. Dampness can lead to heat conditions or yang deficiency, with symptoms that include feeling cold, particularly in the extremities.

Avoid: Eating late at night. If you feel cold, avoid raw and cold foods, which can be difficult to break down and inhibit digestive function. If you are suffering from fatigue and burnout and are easy to irritate or anger, avoid foods that are spicy and heating.

If you are suffering from fatigue with a feeling of lethargy and heaviness, avoid rich and heavy foods, dairy products, sugar and refined carbohydrates.

Foods and herbs to include: Neutral or warming foods, such as brown rice, sweet (glutinous) brown rice, millet, oats, buckwheat and amaranth. Animal foods include beef, lamb and chicken, as well as trout or salmon, mussels or shrimp. Vegetables include winter squash, pumpkin, fennel and onions. Warming fruits include cherries, raspberries, peaches and red grapes. Depending on underlying causes, and if there is no chronic virus, astragalus root, cordyceps, red dates and goji berries can be beneficial. Include pungent and aromatic herbs and spices such as rosemary, thyme, nutmeg, cardamom, star anise, fresh or dried ginger, cinnamon and black pepper. Include sesame seeds, pine nuts, peanuts and pistachios. Honey can be fortifying. Eat meals at regular intervals during the day to fuel the body and regulate blood sugar. The recipes at right are tonic in nature and can be beneficial in boosting vitality.

Suggested recipes for fatigue:

Spring Tonic Congee, page 212

Nourish the Qi and Blood Tea, page 313

Red Date, Almond and Cinnamon Liquor, page 315

Boost-the-Qi Chicken Soup, page 332

Warming Winter Squash Soup, page 376

Braised Duck with Lotus Seeds, page 380

Nourishing Lamb Stew with Butternut Squash and Dang Gui (especially beneficial for those who feel cold), page 382

Qi Tonic Vegetable Broth, page 417

High Blood Pressure

Chinese medicine has used food, herbal therapy, acupuncture, qi gong and bodywork to treat high blood pressure for thousands of years. Treatment and recommendations are based on whether the diagnosis is due to ascending liver yang — sometimes accompanied by dampness and phlegm — or deficient liver or kidney yin. Symptoms that accompany ascending liver yang include headaches, dizziness, red eyes and face and dry mouth. A liver yin deficiency could bring on dizziness, feeling light-headed, insomnia, dry eyes and hot flashes. Symptoms associated with kidney yin deficiency can include difficulty sleeping, poor memory, dizziness and tinnitus. Finally, a feeling of pressure in the chest, fatigue, dizziness, difficulty losing weight and a feeling of heaviness may signal issues with dampness and phlegm. Diet therapy can be applied to clear out excess (dampness, phlegm and heat) or to nourish yin.

Avoid: Spicy and very warming foods such as garlic and hot peppers. Alcohol, caffeinated tea and coffee are too stimulating and can aggravate heat and damp conditions as well as diminish yin. If symptoms include phlegm and dampness, avoid icy and cold foods, sweets, fatty meats, dairy products, fruit juice and tropical fruits.

Foods and herbs to include: Cooling and heat-clearing vegetables and fruits, such as celery, dandelion greens, mung beans, spinach, tomatoes, radishes, seaweeds, soybeans, black sesame seeds, mulberries, plums, lemons, red grapes and apples. Include calming herbal teas made with chrysanthemum, lavender, rose buds and petals, mint, chamomile or dried schisandra. Deep-sea fish.

High Cholesterol

We need healthy cholesterol for hormonal, nervous system and brain functions. Cholesterol is key in the production of sex hormones, bile and vitamin D. However, the accumulation of cholesterol can obstruct arteries and be a precursor of atherosclerosis and cardiac disease. The condition can be due to a variety of reasons, including genetic predisposition, long-term stress (which obstructs the smooth flow of *qi* and blood), lack of physical exercise, smoking, excess consumption of alcohol, a diet (which includes an excess of saturated and poor-quality fats, refined foods and sugar). Chinese medicine considers high cholesterol a damp condition and a yin pathogen that congests the arteries and vessels with plaque deposits.

Avoid: Poor-quality fats, refined carbohydrates and sugars.

Foods and herbs to include: To stimulate digestion and clear excess stagnation and damp accumulation, include bitter foods and herbs such as chicory, escarole, bitter melon, dandelion greens, artichokes and green tea. Include mushrooms, legumes and beans (mung beans, soybeans), which are nourishing and clear out excess damp. Include fish, nuts and seeds, and olive oil. Seaweeds have been found to have a positive impact on reducing cholesterol, are filled with beneficial and soluble fiber, and are detoxifying.

Suggested recipes for high cholesterol:

Sweet Potato Noodles with Spring Greens and Shredded Lamb, page 225
Steamed Artichokes with Cashew Sauce, page 232
Ginger and Tangerine Peel Tea, page 238
Mung Beans Cooked in Green Tea, page 245
Arame Salad with Lemon and Chives, page 265
Wakame Salad, page 307
Tame-the-Tension Tea, page 314
Grilled Romaine Lettuce with Anchovy Sauce, page 352

Insomnia

Insomnia is medically defined as difficulty in falling or staying asleep and can be acute or chronic. If you have trouble sleeping at least three times a week, you may be suffering from chronic insomnia. In addition to producing an enormous amount of physical and emotional stress, lack of sleep can cause symptoms of fatigue, low energy, trouble with concentrating, mood swings and decreased mental and physical performance. Losing just 1 hour of sleep a night adds up to losing 1 full night of sleep a week!

In Chinese medicine, insomnia is considered an imbalance of yin and yang due to overexertion, overwork, anxiety, depression, hormonal imbalances and yin deficiency — a common condition in peri- and menopausal women. Insomnia is also linked to eating late at night, which can aggravate poor digestion and cause food stagnation.

Avoid: All spicy and heat-aggravating foods, including fatty, greasy or very pungent foods, especially in the evening. Avoid alcohol, caffeine, overeating or eating late at night.

Foods and herbs to include: Red grapes, red dates, longan, lotus seeds, Chinese hawthorn (crataegus) fruit, tea with orange or tangerine peel and ginger, radishes and turnips. Calming herbal teas such as chrysanthemum, lavender, rose buds and petals, mint, chamomile and dried schisandra.

Suggested recipes for insomnia:

Simple Roasted Asparagus, page 236
Borscht, page 253
Nourish the Qi and Blood Tea, page 313
Tame-the-Tension Tea, page 314
Quinces in Schisandra Syrup, page 362
Mushroom and Adzuki Bean Breakfast Fried Rice, page 372
Mulberry and Goji Berry Chutney, page 459
Walnut and Black Sesame Sprinkle, page 451

Mood Swings

Mental and physical health are inextricably intertwined when we consider overall well-being. Chinese medicine views minor mood swings, which are not of a psychiatric nature, as dependent upon the smooth flow of liver *qi*, a sound and stable heart (home to the *shen*, or spirit) and a strong foundation of spleen and kidney *qi*. Food recommendations, along with treatments such as acupuncture, herbs, qi gong and bodywork, are intended to calm the spirit, nourish blood and move *qi*.

Suggested recipes for mood swings:

Steamed Artichokes with Cashew Sauce, page 232

Spring Nettle and Fragrant Flowers Tea, page 237

Tilapia and Arugula Soup, page 251

Nourishing Vegetable Treasures, page 300

Maple Tapioca Pudding with Toasted Nuts, page 318

Boost-the-Qi Chicken, page 332

Spinach and Egg Drop Soup, page 334

Roasted Winter Squash, page 347

Avoid: Foods that cause spikes in blood sugar, such as sugary foods, refined flours and carbohydrates. Sugar substitutes and food additives. Foods that congest liver *qi* flow, such as cheese, red meats, alcohol, stimulants, too much caffeine or foods that are fatty, greasy and fried. Avoid skipping meals.

Foods and herbs to include: Foods and herbs that are neutral to warming or slightly cooling in nature, such as lotus root, romaine lettuce, asparagus, artichokes, radishes, celery, plums, seaweeds, lotus seeds and dried longan. Include foods with omega-3 fats such as those found in fish, nuts and sesame seeds. Whole grains such as amaranth and quinoa. Herbs that move liver *qi*, such as chrysanthemum, rose buds and petals, mint, fennel seeds, dang gui, white peony, goji berries and tangerine peel.

Obesity and Difficulty Losing Weight

The causes of obesity and an inability to lose weight are complex and depend on many factors. From a Chinese medicine perspective, the cause is a breakdown in the functioning of the "Earth element," that is, the stomach–spleen network, which can be categorized as a spleen *qi* or spleen yang deficiency. Being overweight and obese is a damp condition that causes the body to retain substance, in this case weight.

Avoid: Constant snacking, eating late at night, skipping meals and frequent dieting. To avoid overeating, reduce portion sizes, skip second portions and stop eating before full. Sugar and sweet foods, processed and salty, fatty, greasy, creamy or fried foods. Too many cold and raw foods, which impair the stomach–spleen function.

Did You Know?

Your family doctor can offer lab testing to analyze your blood sugar levels to determine whether you are prediabetic or if your thyroid is functioning properly. An underactive thyroid can cause unexplained weight gain.

Foods and herbs to include: Salmon or trout. Include bitter greens such as dandelion, escarole, chicory and romaine lettuce to stimulate digestion and clear dampness. Include pungent foods and spices such as radishes and turnips, gingerroot, citrus peel, cardamom, nutmeg, vanilla, anise, fennel seed, rosemary and thyme. Include other vegetables such as seaweeds, burdock root, carrots, cabbage, fennel, sweet potatoes, winter squash and pumpkin. Include vinegar to stimulate digestion.

Suggested tea recipes for obesity and to stimulate digestion:

Ginger and Tangerine Peel Tea, page 238
Corn Silk Tea, page 272
Basil Tea, page 273
Ginger and Mint Tea, page 397

Suggested aperitif recipes to support and stimulate digestion:

Plum Drinking Vinegar, page 276
Cardamom and Ginger Digestive Liquor, page 359
Fragrant Pickled Peaches, page 429

Suggested recipes for supporting weight loss:

White Fish and Celery Congee, page 246
Arame Salad with Lemon and Chives, page 265
Five-Flavor Sautéed Cucumbers, page 268
Hibiscus-Poached Peaches, page 282
Salmon on Ginger-Braised Kale with Toasted Pine Nuts, page 338
Carrot Burdock Kinpira, page 344
Braised Fennel, page 345
Roasted Beet Salad with Pickled Mustard Greens, page 349

NOTE: See Spring Recipes (page 210) for more recipes that stimulate renewal and cleansing. Once you have made changes and are losing some weight, you can look at Seasonal Transition Recipes (page 286) for meals to nourish stomach and spleen function.

Perimenopausal and Menopausal Symptoms

Perimenopause is a normal and important transitional phase of a woman's life that can begin in her 40s and last for up to 10 years. Chinese medicine recognizes this period as a time when a woman's blood and "dew" yin, or moistening and body fluids begin to wane, contributing to symptoms of vaginal dryness, lower libido, drier skin and hair, and joint problems. The transition can be smooth or include mood swings as well as increased irritability, anxiety, depression, sleep issues, hot flashes, night sweats, headaches and aggravated PMS symptoms.

In Chinese medicine, perimenopause and the transition into menopause is ruled by the kidney channel. Symptoms can be due to kidney yin or yang deficiency complicated by liver *qi* stagnation, dampness and phlegm.

Suggested recipes for perimenopausal and menopausal symptoms:

Essential Nut and Seed Porridges
(all seasons, various pages)
Spring Greens Tonic Soup, page 220
Qi-Moving Rose Liquor, page 239
Strawberry-Rose Fruit Salad, page 240
Tame-the-Tension Tea, page 314
Creamy Cabbage Salad, page 387
Walnut and Black Sesame Sprinkle, page 451
Mulberry and Goji Berry Chutney, page 459

Avoid: Too much caffeine or alcohol. Foods that are drying, spicy, hot and pungent (especially if you suffer from hot flashes or sweats) and damage the moistening and cooling yin of the body. Minimize cheeses, baked goods and crackers and fried, fatty or greasy foods. Avoid eating late at night or skipping meals. Be sure to stay hydrated during the day.

Foods and herbs to include: Nuts and seeds, which nourish the yin and are lubricating: almonds, walnuts, sesame seeds, chia seeds, hemp seeds and cashews. Chinese medicinal herbs such as red dates, goji berries, lotus seeds, Chinese yam, astragalus, dang gui, white peony, longan, corn silk, chrysanthemum flowers, peppermint and rose buds or petals. Shiitake, oyster and maitake mushrooms and seaweeds.

Suggested recipes for PMS and painful menses:

Essential Seed and Nut Porridge
(all seasons, various pages)
Spring Nettle and Fragrant Flowers
Tea, page 237
Qi-Moving Rose Liquor, page 239
Roasted Eggplant and Tomato with
Peanut Sauce, page 256
Arame Salad with Lemon and Chives,
page 265
Grilled Squid, page 304
Nourish the Qi and Blood Tea,
page 313
Maple Tapioca Pudding with Toasted
Nuts, page 318
Silkie Chicken Soup with Lotus Seeds
and Red Dates, page 416

Premenstrual Syndrome (PMS) and Painful Menses

In Chinese medicine, a woman's essence is blood (in men it is the semen). The menstrual cycle and accompanying symptoms depend on the smooth circulation and balance of blood (essence and moistening yin) and *qi* (warming and drying yang). Symptoms of *qi* and blood imbalance with PMS indicate possible stagnation of *qi*, stasis of blood and can include minor to severe mood swings, breast tenderness, headaches, fatigue, increased physical stress and tension, crying spells, increased irritability, water retention, food cravings, changes in bowel function (either constipation or loose stools) and low back pain. Painful menses (cramps) are also rooted in the issues that contribute to PMS.

Avoid: All cold, greasy, fatty, creamy (ice cream) or deep-fried foods. Foods with a cold nature or foods directly out of the refrigerator, including ice cold drinks. Refined sugars and high-sodium or spicy foods. Alcohol and caffeine.

Foods and herbs to include: Dark leafy greens and wild greens, which are high in minerals, to clear the heat and benefit the liver meridian. Seaweeds, in small amounts, for their minerals and detoxifying actions. Include herbs that relieve tension, such as mint, chrysanthemum, rose buds and petals and lavender. Culinary herbs and spices that are aromatic, warming and support digestion, such as Chinese chives, cumin, fennel seeds, cardamom, nutmeg, basil and cinnamon. Include animal foods such as salmon, trout or halibut, chicken and lamb. Include soybeans, tofu, nuts and seeds in moderation.

Stress and Tension

According to Chinese medicine, the liver regulates the smooth and harmonious flow of *qi* in the body, thus affecting the smooth movement of muscles and joints. The liver is very sensitive to emotional and physical stress. Stress and tension activate the sympathetic nervous system, sending adrenaline coursing through the body, constricting blood vessels and muscles, increasing heart rate and preparing the body for survival. With ongoing stress, the liver *qi* and blood flow is also constrained and can cause muscle tension in the upper body. Muscle tension can bring on headaches, while stress can incite feelings of frustration, impatience and irritability. There can also be symptoms of chest tightness, difficulty sleeping or restless sleep, frequent nightmares, anxiety and the physical need to release tension through frequent sighing, as well as digestive distress such as poor appetite, indigestion, bloating and irritable bowel symptoms.

Avoid: Overeating, eating late at night and eating when upset or angry. Foods that congest the liver, such as fiery and spicy foods, as well as excess alcohol and coffee.

Foods and herbs to include: Dark leafy greens, nuts and seeds, seaweeds (in small amounts daily), lightly fermented foods and salads. Sweet vegetables and herbs that calm and regulate liver function, such as mint, rose buds and petals, lavender, basil, turmeric, cardamom, rosemary, gingerroot and dill. To drain and purge any heat buildup, include bitter foods such as dandelion or other bitter wild greens, artichokes, asparagus, romaine lettuce, chicory and escarole.

Suggested recipes for stress and tension:

Essential Seed and Nut Porridge with Strawberries and Honey, page 213

Herbed Nettle and Asparagus Risotto, page 222

Qi-Moving Rose Game Hens, page 226

Quick-Pickled Radish Tops over Steamed Red Radishes and Cauliflower, page 228

Spring Greens and Lotus Root Sauté, page 235

Spring Nettle and Fragrant Flowers Tea, page 237

Qi-Moving Rose Liquor, page 239

Raspberry Coulis and Peaches with Maple-Spiced Pecans, page 280

Part 3

East Meets West in the Kitchen

Chapter 9

Transforming Your Health: Restocking Your Pantry

"Our bodies are our gardens, to the which our wills are gardeners."

— *William Shakespeare*

Clearing and changing the terrain of a kitchen serves to create an optimal environment to nourish your life. It can be compared to transforming a yard to generate a bountiful garden. After choosing an area with enough light and circulation, it is time to weed, clear out the debris and pick out the stones. Then the soil is amended, usually with compost and other sources of nutrients. Only when this is complete do you seed and plant. Finally, to see the garden flourish, you provide it with water and tend to its fledgling growth every day. Every garden needs a good foundation, and so does a healthy kitchen.

Clearing Out the Kitchen

If you're ready to improve your own and your family's health, start by clearing out the pantry and setting yourself up for success. It is time to get rid of foods that are simply "weeds" in your pantry, those foods that take up space but that have no appreciable value. There is no more surefire way to sabotage your efforts to improve your diet than to have junk food readily available for those times when fatigue, stress or upset makes you lack or lose the will to refrain from grabbing the first munchies you see.

Let's be clear. There is very little possibility that your health will change or improve if your kitchen is filled with processed junk food that has little vitality and nutritional value. So let's carve out a path to good health and start by discarding all those addictive foods you just can't stop eating (you know what they are!) and all those packaged products that are highly refined, high in sugar, made with ingredients you can't pronounce and include trans-fatty acids (trans fats), chemical additives and flavorings, as well as those foods that have been sitting on your shelf for more than a year.

Where Do I Begin?

First things first: remember what you want to accomplish. If you're seeking more vitality and better health, it is very important to eat whole foods and the best-quality foods you can find. Equally important is to avoid or limit exposure to additives, preservatives and high levels of pesticides, sugar, salt and fat. Of course, most of us will have a hard time avoiding harmful elements *all* the time. That's because some processed foods, whether these are canned tomatoes, pasta, noodles, dried fruits or nuts, are stocked in our pantry. Sometimes, however, even the simplest processed foods, the ones that don't seem harmful, can be laced with added substances, some benign and others more corrosive, that are used to enhance foods and lure us into purchasing them.

So what exactly are you eating? And is it real food? The labels on packages of processed foods can tell us a lot about what's inside, but they can be also misleading, so it's buyer beware. For example, labels on the front of packages might tout 100% natural, 100% whole grains, gluten-free, low-fat or "healthy," among other claims designed to "sell" the so-called health benefits of a food. Low-fat may mean high in sugar to make up for the lost flavor while gluten-free may simply mean nothing more than the product itself is naturally gluten-free. Look further to the list of ingredients and nutrition facts table (also known as the nutrition information panel) on the back or the side of a package that can tell an entirely different story. Here's where added flavors and ingredients used to enhance a food's color, texture, flavor and shelf life are revealed — a possible sign that the food is not fresh. These additions may make packaged foods more "tasty," but they do nothing to change the terrain of your health and infuse your body with *qi* (vitality) and nourishment.

The ingredients list, which is separate from the nutrition facts table, lists the exact ingredients used to make the food product, in descending order by weight. If the list contains ingredients you do not recognize or would not use in your own cooking, such as textured vegetable protein, high-fructose corn syrup, monosodium glutamate (MSG) or trans fat, you most likely

> ### Did You Know?
>
> Look for foods colored from whole ingredients such as beets, annatto, paprika, turmeric, spinach, blueberries, matcha powder or carrot. Real flavor comes from real food, herbs or spices.

do not need that food on your shelf. Of course, not all additives are created equal. Some are more problematic than others, so do your best to reduce your exposure to them. If you know what you're looking for, you can make better food choices.

What's In a Label?

Here are some guidelines when comparing labels to better assess a food's health benefit:

- **Stick to a short list:** Look at the length of the package's list of ingredients. If the list is longer than five or six ingredients, examine it more closely for added sugars, trans fats, sodium levels, preservatives, food coloring or "natural" flavorings. American author and food activist Michael Pollan has some very simple and useful rules when it comes to making choices about what you eat: "Avoid food products containing ingredients that a third-grader cannot pronounce," and "Don't eat anything your grandmother wouldn't recognize as food."

- **Pay attention to added ingredients and where they sit on the ingredients list:** Ingredients are listed from most to least, so whatever is at the top indicates a great amount of that ingredient. Sugar and sweeteners are tricky to assess — some sugars are found naturally in a food, such as yogurt and dried fruit. Then there are the 56 different names for the sweeteners found in 74 percent of the packaged food supply, according to SugarScience at the University of California San Francisco. You might be surprised to see sweeteners in the most unusual places, too. The next time you pick up a small packet of salt at a take-out window or restaurant, turn the package over and you could see dextrose, a sugar extracted from corn, listed in the ingredients list! So pay attention to all labels. If you want sweets in your life, it's best to get them in whole foods themselves, such as fruits and vegetables, and a simple dessert made with one natural sweetener (such as maple syrup, honey, organic unrefined sugar or coconut sugar, which is also low-glycemic).

- **Know how much salt you're consuming:** You need salt to maintain a balance of body fluids and for daily bodily functions, but not in the quantities found in many processed foods, where it is typically added to make such foods tastier. Sodium content on a label can be misleading. Even if the listed sodium count may seem low (for example, 140 mg per 1-cup/250 mL serving

Did You Know?

Avoid added or artificial sweeteners, including the following, often seen on labels: corn syrup, dextrose, sucrose, invert (or inverted) sugar, fructose, crystalline fructose, sucrose, maltose, white granulated sugar, high-fructose corn syrup, maltodextrin, trehalose, saccharine, aspartame, alitame, sucralose or cyclamates.

for broth), you can easily consume three times as much when you consider the serving size, which is generally quite small. The U.S. Department of Agriculture (USDA) recommends no more than 2300 milligrams of salt per person a day, yet according to the U.S. Food and Drug Administration (FDA), Americans consume an average of 3400 milligrams a day. If a lot of your food comes out of packages, it is quite easy to go over the recommended limit — without even knowing it. To help reduce your sodium consumption, reduce your packaged and processed foods, prepare and cook your own food with a moderate amount of salt, and do not add salt to food at the table.

- **Avoid hydrogenated and trans fats:** Fats are important and necessary to our health, but hydrogenated and partially hydrogenated fats (trans fats) are not. Some saturated fats occur naturally, such as those in avocado and coconut. Unlike good fats such as polyunsaturated and monounsaturated fats, trans fats are synthesized, partially hydrogenated and added to foods to influence texture, prolong shelf life and heighten the flavor. That's why it can be hard to resist those french fries or fried onion rings. Added animal shortening is an indicator that the food you are about to put in your mouth contains trans fats. Here is a list of processed foods where trans fats can hide, according to The Cleveland Clinic:

  - Commercial cakes and pies (especially with frosting)
  - Frozen biscuits
  - Microwaveable foods, including breakfast sandwiches
  - Popcorn
  - Margarine or shortening (butter is better!)
  - Frozen dinners
  - Commercial crackers
  - Cream-filled candies
  - Doughnuts
  - Fried fast foods, including french fries and onion rings
  - Some ice creams
  - Non-dairy creamers
  - Frozen or creamy beverages
  - Commercial frozen pizza

Did You Know?
Studies have shown that trans fat consumption increases the risk for stroke and diet-related chronic diseases, such as heart disease and type 2 diabetes.

So ditch foods with trans fats — it's time for an oil change. Find out how to get healthy fats in your daily meals by eating nuts and seeds, avocados, organic free-range eggs, more fish and unrefined organic extra virgin olive oil, coconut oil or ghee.

- **Whole grains are nourishing, important and beneficial, but make sure that's what you're getting:** Not all labels are clear on what "100% whole grains" really means. Here's where to start: if the grain is whole, it will be listed in the ingredients list as either whole-grain wheat flour, brown rice, whole oats, whole barley, buckwheat, bulgur or organic whole-grain corn. If the label includes words such as "wheat flour" or "bromated wheat flour," it is refined and devoid of whole grain. Beware of the terms "fiber-rich" or "added fiber." Some foods being sold as whole grain have been known to include added cellulose — essentially sawdust — which has been found in bagels, conventional corn and flour tortillas, breakfast cereals, packaged cookies, whole wheat bread, packaged cupcakes and frozen crusts, including those on pot pies. If you want whole grains in breads, look for the specific whole grain listed, such as whole wheat, whole spelt, whole rye, millet or corn.

- **Know your additives:** Natural food additives you might use in the kitchen when canning or preserving foods include vinegar, salt and herbs or spices to enhance flavor and texture and aid in food preservation. These are truly natural additives. Artificial chemical additives are added to processed foods for much the same reasons. The FDA has not definitively ruled on the health risks of many common additives found in processed foods, such as artificial food coloring, natural flavoring and other chemical additives, but some studies indicate that food additives can play a role in the health and symptoms of individuals, especially children, with increased incidence of allergic reactions, respiratory issues, headaches, joint pain, foggy thinking, digestive disturbances, mood swings and fatigue. Get to know your food additives — what they are and why they are used.

The Path to Healthy Eating

Now use the above guidelines to go through your kitchen cupboards, refrigerator and freezer, assess what's in them and toss anything that isn't 100% whole food! Then you're on your way to a healthier life. Once you've cleared out the old, you can begin to restock your pantry with nourishing, healthy whole foods that are rich in all of the five flavors (sweet, salty, sour, pungent and bitter) as well as the five colors (green, white, red, yellow and black) we discussed earlier (see Chapter 3). You can derive much flavor directly from foods — use the recipes at the back of the book to learn how to cook with herbs and spices to enhance the flavor and energy of your food.

Food Additives

Below is a list of some of manufactured food additives that you may find on the labels of food products, many of which include:

- **BHT (butylated hydroxyanisole)** and **BHA (butylated hydroxytoluene)** are added to foods and cosmetics to preserve the fats and oils. Often found in potato chips, preserved meats, chewing gum, cereals and beer.

- **EDTA (ethylenediaminetetraacetic acid)** is added to canned foods, cereals and vegetable oils to preserve color and the food itself.

- **MSG (monosodium glutamate)** is a chemically derived flavor enhancer often added to Chinese foods, canned vegetables, soups and processed foods. Glutamate is the naturally occurring flavor in kombu (a seaweed) and is more commonly referred to as the umami (savory and earthy) flavor. MSG has been used as a flavor enhancer for decades and is "generally recognized" as safe but its use remains controversial. Some people can have adverse reactions to it, however, with headaches, flushing, sweating and facial pressure or tingling.

- **Sodium nitrites** and **nitrates** are added to processed lunch meats, bacon, sausages and hot dogs to help retain a brighter color and prolong shelf life. In 2010, scientists at the World Health Organization's International Agency for Research on Cancer specified that nitrates and nitrites are possible carcinogens.

- **Olestra**, a manufactured fat substitute created during the low-fat craze in North America, is found in potato chips.

- **Hydrolyzed vegetable protein (HVP)** is used to add flavor to packaged soups, snacks, meat products, sauces, ready-to-make bouillon and snack foods.

- **Artificial sweeteners** and sugar substitutes, such as aspartame (Equal) or sucralose (Splenda), are used in a variety of foods and drinks often marked "sugar-free" or "diet."

- **High-fructose corn syrup (HFCS)** is a highly refined and concentrated sweetener and a major source of added calories in America. It entered the food supply in the 1980s and is a significant contributor to the rise in obesity. It hides in many foods, including bread, flavored yogurts, soft drinks, salad dressings and cereals.

- **Trans-fatty acids** or **trans fat** (see page 147).

- **Food dyes** Blue #1 and #2, Red #3 and #40 and Yellow #6 and #5 (tartrazine) are commonly found in soft drinks, fruit juices, macaroni and cheese, carbonated beverages, salad dressings and even pet foods. Many of these artificial food dyes are linked to behavioral problems in children and, according to the Center for Science in the Public Interest (CSPI), have been known to have carcinogenic effects.

- **Sodium sulphite** is a preservative used in wines and other foods. According to the FDA, approximately 1 in 100 people are sensitive to sulphites in foods. Symptoms can include headaches, rashes and breathing problems.

- **Sulphur dioxide** is found in beer, soft drinks, juices, wine, vinegar, dried fruits and vegetables, and potato products.

- **Potassium bromate** is an oxidizing agent used to increase the volume and add an appealing white color in some bread and rolls.

Shop Right

Here are a few strategies for picking healthy essentials the next time you visit your grocery store:

- Shop the perimeters of your supermarket, where the fruits, vegetables, meats, fish and dairy products are stocked.
- Explore the organic and bulk foods section for grains, nuts, legumes and spices.
- Talk to your grocer about the foods they carry — ask if meats are grass-fed, when meat and fish are delivered (to get the freshest product), and which produce is grown either sustainably (little pesticide or herbicide use) or organically. Sometimes you can even ask to taste certain produce.
- Read the labels carefully before making any purchases.

The Dirty Dozen

Buy the following organic if possible:

1. strawberries
2. spinach
3. nectarines
4. apples
5. peaches
6. pears
7. cherries
8. grapes
9. celery
10. tomatoes
11. sweet bell peppers
12. potatoes

Organic Foods: Are They Important?

The vitality, or *qi*, you cultivate starts with how food is grown and raised. It's next to impossible to nourish a body healthfully when the foods you eat are loaded with chemicals, pesticides, herbicides, antibiotics and toxins. The best-quality food might come from our own kitchen garden, a local farmstand or farmers' market, a food co-op or a local grocery or produce market. You want to find and choose food that is fresh, vibrant and grown organically or sustainably to ensure you are not exposing yourself or your family to pesticides, fungicides and herbicides. At times, organic foods will cost more, so you may have to make choices about which organic foods you choose to eat (see sidebar, left). Think of your food purchases as health insurance — the better the quality of the foods you eat, the healthier you will be. It may take some time and effort in the beginning, but do your best. Choose organic vegetables, fruits, grains, nuts, seeds and meats when possible. Try sourcing quality foods at local grocery stores and through local farmers, buying clubs and food co-ops; if these are not readily available, consider starting your own buying club or food co-op. Taking a greater interest in sourcing food gives you an opportunity to build relationships with the merchants and farmers who sell their foods. When you get to know your market, your farmer and the source of your food, it can be invigorating and enjoyable and provide a sense of pride that you're bringing home the most vibrant foods.

Dirty Dozen and Clean 15

The Environmental Working Group (EWG) Shopper's Guide to Pesticides in Produce, updated every year since 2004, ranks pesticide contamination in 48 popular fruits and vegetables. The guide is based on the results of more than 35,200 samples tested by the U.S. Department of Agriculture (USDA) and the Food and Drug Administration (FDA). The latest list of the top 12 fruits and vegetables with high levels of pesticides, known as the Dirty Dozen, includes strawberries, spinach, nectarines, apples, peaches, pears, cherries, grapes, celery, tomatoes, sweet bell peppers and potatoes. Conversely, the Clean 15, the foods least likely to be laden with heavy pesticides, are sweet corn*, avocados, pineapple, cabbage, onions, fresh or frozen sweet peas, papaya*, asparagus, mangos, eggplant, honeydew melon, kiwifruit, cantaloupe, cauliflower and grapefruit. For more information, visit www.ewg.org.

*Note: Corn and papaya that are not organic are probably genetically modified organisms, or GMOs. There is a great deal of controversy regarding GMO foods, so it is important to learn as much as possible about their possible effects on health. Get to know the foods that are generally GMO so you can make a choice in your purchasing decisions.

But I Feel Deprived!

Change is a process that changes as you change. In the beginning, your body may go through a bit of withdrawal. When people give up coffee, they can sometimes experience headaches and fatigue. Stopping sugar or refined carbohydrates may also have its own symptoms, which may start with cravings or more hunger, since sugar can mask hunger. These reactions are real because your physiology is changing and adjusting. You might experience a period of withdrawal from some of your go-to junk food snacks or get some pushback when your family's favorite snack food is no longer in the pantry. Hang in there. After a few days you will feel better and the cravings for those substances can diminish. Think of it as a great opportunity to engage your family in the process of making changes and discovering new foods. But take heart — everyone will get used to it as food preferences start to shift over time. If you learn how to replace those "flavored" foods with *flavorful* foods, your taste buds and preferences *will* change. As Leslie McEachern, my good friend and owner of the groundbreaking, organic and vegan restaurant (now defunct) Angelica Kitchen in New York City, often reminds me, "Discipline is remembering what you want."

The Clean 15

1. sweet corn
2. avocados
3. pineapple
4. cabbage
5. onions
6. sweet peas
7. papaya
8. asparagus
9. mangos
10. eggplant
11. honeydew melon
12. kiwifruit
13. cantaloupe
14. cauliflower
15. grapefruit

Taking Small Steps

If you want to feel better, keep your eyes on that prize. It's well worth it. Making lifestyle changes, especially when it comes to eating, can be a challenging and meandering journey. You may move forward and backward; you may feel better and worse. That's OK. With every step forward, pay attention to how you feel. Are your energy, mood, pain levels or physical discomforts different? And if you slip back into old, unhealthy habits, note the difference in energy, mood and discomforts. Think of it as an educational experience — you are learning about yourself, getting in touch with how food affects you. There's no need to despair or be ashamed. You are changing your relationship with food, or maybe you are simply tweaking or expanding it. It's an adventure, and any adventure is a little bit exciting, and perhaps a bit overwhelming or downright scary. So know that change happens one step at a time. The next step for you may be simply learning how to shop for the best ingredients.

Stock Your Kitchen for Optimal Health

> **Tip**
>
> It's always a good idea to smell bulk items such as nuts and seeds or grains to ensure freshness. The nose knows. Any stale, musty or rancid smell indicates that the food is no longer fresh.

Shopping and eating shouldn't be so complicated. However, a few simple guidelines can be helpful.

Start with paying attention to what foods are in season. In the Pacific Northwest, there are cycles and seasons for strawberries, Copper River salmon, Dungeness crab, asparagus and cherries, to name a few. Talk to your local produce manager and fish and meat purveyor and ask them which foods are the freshest and most flavorful (they might even have a simple recipe suggestion). Foods that are in season are fresh, packed with nutrients and have traveled a shorter distance to get to you.

It also helps to have a shopping list for the week, depending on what meals you plan to prepare. In our home, we have a checklist of staples we use to keep track of what needs to be replenished for when we go to the store (it also helps to contain spending).

As any new habit takes shape, it gets better with practice. Start simple and work your way on to becoming a food shopping pro. Of course, from time to time you might bring home a rotten apple or something that you realize is not as fresh as it seemed in the store, but that is all part of the learning. In the following section, you'll find a basic shopping list to ensure your home is stocked with the basics you'll need to start preparing and eating nutritious, flavorful meals. (See Resources on page 466 for more on where to purchase herbs, grains, fresh produce and meats, as well as useful cooking utensils.)

Now it's time to shop and stock. Let's get started!

Must-Have Ingredients

In the kitchen, we like creating and making meals that family and friends will enjoy eating, so it's important to have foods that can be put together easily. Having a variety of foods and core ingredients on hand may ignite an inspired meal when you least expect it. Stocking your pantry with certain grains, beans, nuts, seeds, condiments and spices ensures that even on those nights when you're tired, whipping up a simple meal will take little effort. Try to cover all the five flavors (sweet, sour, salty, bitter and pungent) as well as foods that are warming or cooling in nature to ensure that you can adapt your cooking to balance your food preferences and health needs.

Did You Know?

According to Chinese medicine, foods and herbs have qualities that either warm or cool the body. For more information, see Chapter 3.

Sample Pantry

Here is a sampling of some key ingredients in a well-stocked pantry and fridge:

- *Organic whole grains:* brown rice (long- and short-grain), sweet (glutinous) brown rice, brown Arborio rice, brown basmati and jasmine rice, stone ground corn grits or polenta cornmeal, large flake or steel cut oats, buckwheat groats, millet and quinoa
- *Organic beans, pulses and other legumes:* lentils (red, brown and French [Puy]), chickpeas, black beans, black soybeans, adzuki beans, white beans (or navy or cannellini beans)
- *Organic nuts and seeds:* almonds, walnuts, cashews, peanuts, pumpkin seeds, sunflower seeds, sesame seeds (black and white), chia seeds, flax seeds and hemp seeds
- *Flours:* almond and brown rice flour
- *Oils and fats:* organic extra virgin olive oil, avocado oil, toasted sesame oil and ghee
- *Salt:* high-quality sea salt (not iodized), kosher salt (for pickling) and tamari or coconut aminos (as a substitute for soy sauce, if you are sensitive to soy)
- *Vinegars:* raw unpasteurized organic apple cider vinegar, plain (unseasoned) rice vinegar and dry rice wine like sake

- *Herbs and spices:* cinnamon, nutmeg, star anise, pure vanilla extract, cumin, turmeric, Sichuan peppercorns, coriander seeds, dried basil and dill. You could grow some tender perennials in your garden or windowsill, such as thyme, rosemary, sage and chives, or garlic, providing you with fresh or dried herbs and seasonings all year round.
- *Medicinal herbs and foods:* goji berries, gingerroot, astragalus root, dried shiitake mushrooms, hato mugi (Job's tears), miso, green onions, dried roses petals and hips, dried nettles leaves, dried peppermint or spearmint
- *Seaweed:* kombu, nori, dulse, wakame, arame and hijiki
- *Refrigerated fresh foods:* Fresh produce — including leafy greens, green onions, onions, sweet potatoes, gingerroot, carrots, avocados, lemons and a variety of fresh fruits and root vegetables — will last for a week or more in the refrigerator. Also keep on hand organic eggs, miso paste, fresh tofu, fish sauce, prepared mustard, tomato paste, anchovies, pickles and sauerkraut.

Whole Grains

- Brown Arborio rice (excellent alternative for congee)
- Brown basmati rice
- Brown jasmine rice
- Brown rice, long- and short-grain
- Buckwheat groats
- Hato mugi (Job's tears) (you will most likely need to purchase this at an Asian grocer or online)
- Millet
- Quinoa
- Red rice
- Rolled oats: large flakes
- Sweet (glutinous) brown rice
- Whole-grain stone ground corn grits or polenta

Your Pantry Shopping List

Most people get into a "shopping rut" and reach for the same foods over and over again while failing to include some foundational foods in the pantry. The following list is a comprehensive guide on what to buy when you visit the grocery store to ensure that you have an inventory of healthful ingredients on hand. Of course, you won't need to buy everything on this list. Make a few choices from each category and challenge yourself to try something new every time you visit — maybe one new grain or spice a week, with lots of inspirations from the recipes in this book. (For more information about some of the lesser-known ingredients here, see Chapter 10.)

Whole Grains

Buy your whole grains in the bulk section of your grocery or health food store or food co-op. Selecting grains, legumes, nuts and seeds from bulk gives you the flexibility to only buy what you need and save money. Store them in tightly closed glass jars in a cool dry place. Always rinse your grains well before using by swirling them around with cool, filtered water and straining a couple of times until the water runs clear.

Beans, Pulses and Legumes

Dried beans, pulses and other legumes can be found in the bulk section of the grocery or health food store or food co-op. You can also find good-quality packaged dried beans. Look for organic or sustainably raised beans. Beans should have a slight shine on them to indicate freshness. Store them in tightly closed glass containers in a cool, dark, dry place. Many legumes need to be soaked for at least 8 hours, except for any type of lentils or dried split peas. After soaking, drain out the soaking water and rinse your beans well before using by swirling them around with cool, clean water and draining thoroughly.

Beans, Pulses and Legumes

- Adzuki beans
- Black soybeans
- Cannellini or white beans
- Chickpeas
- Lentils: brown, green, red and French (Puy)
- Mung beans
- Split peas — green and yellow

Nuts and Seeds

Raw nuts and seeds can be found in the bulk section of the grocery or health food store or food co-op. It's optimal to store nuts and seeds in a glass jar (plastic leaches the oils out of the nuts) in your refrigerator (you can even freeze them!) or in a cool, dark, dry place to protect the volatile oils inherent in nuts and seeds. The freshest nuts will be those in their shells — when hulled, nuts and seeds begin to lose their nutrients and can easily become rancid (not good!). If you can, taste or smell the nuts before buying. If they taste stale, sour or bitter, don't buy them. If the nuts have a fishy or unpleasant odor, chances are they are rancid. Look for organic or sustainably grown nuts and seeds, since the fats tend to store pesticides and toxins. Fresh nuts and seeds are extraordinarily nourishing and beneficial for the immune system, digestion and elimination and the nervous system.

Nuts and Seeds

- Almonds
- Cashews
- Chestnuts
- Chia seeds
- Flax seeds
- Hazelnuts
- Hemp seeds
- Peanuts
- Pecans
- Pine nuts
- Pistachios
- Pumpkin seeds
- Sesame Seeds: unhulled brown and black
- Walnuts

Grab Some Nuts

Nuts rich in essential fatty acids, fats that can't be made by the body and must come from the diet, and fat-soluble vitamin E are valued as a restorative and nourishing food in the tradition of Chinese medicine. Nuts enhance the immune system, protect and nourish the nervous system and are one of the best ways to include beneficial fats and oils in your diet. Seeds, in Chinese medicine, are considered fundamental nourishment for the kidney *qi* and yin. Include some nuts and seeds in your daily diet to receive the benefits of high-quality oil and fats for your health. Eaten in large amounts, however, their benefits can be reversed and they can cause digestive problems.

Oils and Vinegars

Oils

- Avocado oil
- Coconut oil
- Ghee
- Organic extra virgin olive oil
- Toasted sesame oil

Always purchase unrefined cold-pressed oils in a dark glass bottle or metal can in small quantities (never buy oil sold in plastic bottles). Unrefined oils are pressed at a temperature lower than 160°F (75°C). These oils will retain their original taste, color and aroma. Refined oils are processed with high heat, altering their color, clarity and flavor. Oils can also break down when exposed to heat or light, changing their color, odor and taste. Look for oils that are organic or sustainably grown and processed. Olive oils are generally used for dressings and cooking with lower heat. Avocado and coconut oil, as well as ghee (clarified butter), are more stable and thus suitable for cooking on higher heat. Toasted sesame oil is best used for sauces, dressings or as a finishing flavor, as it does not have a high smoke point.

Vinegar was referred to in the classic Chinese herbal text, the *Shang Han Lun*, as *ku jiu*, or "bitter liquor," and it is thought to have some medicinal properties beyond its culinary contribution. Vinegar is warming, sour and slightly bitter, which can move and break up congestion and improve circulation.

Vinegars

- Apple cider vinegar
- Rice vinegar (unseasoned)

Traditionally made vinegar is brewed over a period of months to a year. Look for vinegars that are organic and naturally brewed without the addition of chemicals. In some cases, as in raw unfiltered apple cider vinegar, the cider will not be clear and particles will have settled to the bottom of the bottle. The list at left contains some of the common vinegars used in this book. Adding herbs or spices to impart varied flavors and actions can also modify the effect vinegars have on the body (see the Condiment Recipes, page 422, for some vinegar recipes).

Flours

Flours

- Almond*
- Brown rice
- Oat

*Almond flour or finely ground meal, from blanched or unblanched almonds, are often interchangeable. The almond meal is typically more coarsely ground, adding more texture to a baked good.

Only gluten-free flours are used in the recipes in this book, so they are suitable even for people who are sensitive or intolerant to gluten. (Besides, everyone should be able to enjoy a dessert!) Both almond and rice flours impart a unique texture and flavor. Look for almond or brown rice flours in plastic bags in the baking or natural foods section of your grocery store. If you want to buy them in bulk, do so only if you know there is a good turnover for bulk items. Flours can easily go rancid or become mildewed if exposed to moisture. At home, store them in a sealed glass jar in a cool dark location or in the refrigerator. Well sealed, almond, rice and oat flour will keep for up to 6 months in the pantry and 1 year in the refrigerator.

Teas

When buying loose leaf tea, look at and smell it before you buy. The aroma should be refreshing. Green tea should be a vibrant shade of green, rooibos a dark red and oolong or black tea dark and uniform in color and shape. Brewed green tea has a light green-yellow clarity to it. Rooibos is a deep brownish red and oolong, a lightly fermented tea, is lighter in color than a typical black tea when brewed. Of course, there are many options for hot teas that are free from caffeine. In Europe, these are referred to as infusions or tisanes, indicating that the "tea" is made with herbs, flowers or roots instead of tea leaves. In the list at right, you will see some of the common herb and flower infusions used in this book.

Teas

- Green tea
- Hibiscus tea
- Jasmine tea
- Lavender tea
- Nettles tea
- Oolong tea
- Peppermint tea
- Rooibos tea
- Rose hips tea

Dried Fruit

Dried fruits are a concentrated sweet snack, delicious to eat as they are, in desserts or mixed with nuts. When hydrated, they can be added to fruit salads or teas. Because they are such concentrated forms of sugar, be prudent in the amount you eat. It can take pounds of fresh fruit to make 1 pound (500 g) of dried fruit. They are generally found in the bulk section of a grocery store or sold in packages. Look for unsulphured and sorbate-free dried fruits with no added sugar or oils.

Dried Fruit

- Dates: medjool, deglet, red or jujubes (See Chapter 10 to learn more about red dates.)
- Dried apricots
- Dried barberries
- Dried cherries
- Dried goji berries
- Dried hawthorn fruit (aka Chinese hawthorn or *Crataegus pinnatifida*), not be to confused with hawthorne berries
- Dried mangos
- Dried plums
- Raisins
- Unsweetened dried cranberries

Sulphites

Sulfites (sulphur dioxide) and sorbate are additives used in dried fruit to enhance their color, vibrancy and pliancy. Avoid them if possible — some people react negatively to these additives. (See "Food Additives" on page 149 for more information).

Culinary Herbs and Spices

Culinary Herbs and Spices

- Anise seeds
- Basil, fresh or dried
- Caraway seeds
- Cardamom, pods or ground
- Cinnamon, ground or sticks
- Cloves, whole or ground
- Coriander, fresh, seeds or ground
- Cumin, seeds or ground
- Dill, fresh, dried or seeds
- Fennel seeds
- Gingerroot or dried ginger
- Nutmeg, whole or ground
- Oregano, fresh or dried
- Peppercorns, black, white or red
- Rose buds or petals, dried
- Rose hips, dried
- Sichuan peppercorns
- Star anise
- Thyme, fresh or dried
- Turmeric, fresh or dried ground

Herbs and spices have played a major role in worldwide food cultures since ancient times. Their prized flavors and medicinal actions have been revered, sought after and documented as the engine of exploration and conquest; even functioning as currency and markers of wealth. These herbs and spices have been used to cure everything from the simplest ailment to the most complex disease. Beyond their potent medicinal benefits, spices and herbs elevate cooking — and the best way to get to know the power of their fragrance and flavor is simply to experiment with them. If you can grow some of the more common kitchen herbs in your garden or on your porch, windowsill or fire escape, do it! You will glean great pleasure and delight from their fresh, bright flavors and aromas as well as bringing healthful medicinal value to your table.

When buying fresh or dried herbs and spices from the grocery store, try to buy them in bulk or buy dried herbs and spices from a reputable herb and spice company. (See Resources, page 466, for more information.) For vibrant flavor, use fresh herbs when possible. When purchasing dried spices, purchase from a store where there is high turnover to ensure fresher quality, buy the whole form and grind them at home. The substances in dried herbs and spices are volatile and most potent if you buy whole seeds (such as cumin, pepper, coriander, anise, etc.) and grind them when needed in a small coffee grinder dedicated to herb and spice grinding or with a suribachi or mortar and pestle. Be sure to go through your dried herbs and spices yearly. Herbs and spices that have been on your shelf for more than a year just might need to be composted — they lose their flavor and potency over time.

Fresh herbs and spices can usually be found in the produce section of a grocery store. Dried herbs and spices are found either in the bulk or spice aisle.

Medicinal Herbs

The medicinal herbs and foods listed below are often found at Chinese herbal suppliers or in the dried herb section of Asian grocery stores. If you're buying them at an Asian grocery store, be sure to check the label for sulfites. Many Chinese herb suppliers test their herbs to ensure they are free of sulfites and pesticides, which affect their quality and taste.

Medicinal Herbs

- Astragalus root (*huang qi*)
- Chinese yam (*Dioscorea* or *shan yao*)
- Chrysanthemum flowers (*ju hua*)
- Codonopsis (*dang shen*)
- Dang gui (*dong quai* or Chinese angelica root)
- Hato mugi (also known as Job's tears, coix seed or *yi yi ren*)
- Honeysuckle flower buds (*lonicera* or *jin yin hua*)
- Lily bulb (*bai he*) and dried daylily flowers
- Longan fruit (*long yan rou* or longan)
- Lotus seeds (also considered as a nut) (*lian zi*)
- Red dates (jujubes or *da zao* or *hong zao*)
- Schisandra berries (dried) (*wu wei zi*)
- Tangerine peel, dried (*chen pi*)

Sweeteners

If you are going to sweeten your food (we are talking about desserts), it's best to use natural sweeteners, as opposed to refined sugars that are chemically processed and devoid of nourishment. Sweeteners such as coconut and date sugar, honey and maple syrup lend a deeper and richer flavor to your desserts. Unsweetened apple and grape juice are higher in fructose and should be used less frequently. Just the same, even natural sweeteners should be used judiciously. A little bit goes a long way in bringing a sweet satisfaction to desserts. Sweeteners such as some of these specialty sugars are usually found in the baking, bulk or natural foods section of a grocery store.

Sweeteners

- Coconut sugar
- Date sugar
- Honey
- Palm sugar
- Pure maple syrup
- Unsweetened apple juice
- Unsweetened grape juice

Salt

There is almost no place on Earth without salt, including our bodies. Salt has been a prized commodity throughout the ages and is a valuable ingredient in cooking. Our bodies lose minerals daily and their daily replacement is necessary for health. Using high-quality sea salt contributes to some mineral replacement while imparting a savory and deeper flavor to many foods. Other types of salting with foods, such as tamari, miso, umeboshi plums and sea vegetables, which impart a mildly salty flavor, are also valuable in bringing deeper and richer flavor to your cooking and can be added to the "salt" section of your pantry. Look for organic tamari in the international or health food section of your grocery store.

Salt

- High-quality sea salt
- Tamari (organic, gluten-free)
- Miso (there are many varieties: red, white, rice, barley, chickpea or even dandelion and leek miso)
- Umeboshi plums or umeboshi plum paste

Miso, a salty and fermented bean (soybean, adzuki or chickpea are some common beans used to make miso) and grain (rice or barley) paste, is usually found in the refrigerated section. Umeboshi plums, made by pickling the ume fruit, are found in the international food section or online. Be sure that you're buying pure umeboshi, free of any added food coloring or preservatives.

Dried Vegetables

Seaweeds and dried mushrooms bring "umami" to your cooking. Seaweeds are nutrient-dense and rich in minerals and glutamic acid, the foundation of umami. Their detoxification properties have been used throughout the world and are common to many coastal communities. Seaweeds are usually found in the international or natural food section of a grocery store. In Asian grocery stores, sea vegetables usually have their own section. Dried mushrooms are a specialty item that can sometimes be found at farmers' markets, grocery stores or more cheaply in Asian grocery stores. See Resources, page 466, for more high-quality options.

Now That Your Kitchen Is Ready: Get Equipped

We recommend these kitchen utensils for the recipes in this book and to make meal planning and cooking easy and stress-free:

- **Blender:** Thanks to their powerful motors, food blenders are indispensable when it comes to puréeing soups, dips and sauces. Find a reputable, good-quality, heavy-duty blender that can withstand some tough grinding jobs — it will last for many years and be up to the task of blending and puréeing cooked vegetables, nuts and seeds.

- **Suribachi or mortar and pestle:** Nothing beats a suribachi (Japanese mortar and pestle) for grinding whole seeds and spices. The grooves in the ceramic bowl add friction to the ingredients you are working with and make the vitality you put in through the circular grinding process uniquely satisfying. The Western mortar and pestle can suffice for grinding whole seeds and spices; it is durable and gets the job done but is more laborious because it lacks grooves in its bowl. If you buy a typical mortar and pestle, be sure to get one made

---

Seaweeds*

- Kombu
- Wakame
- Arame
- Hijiki
- Nori
- Dulse
- Agar-agar

*All of these are used throughout the recipes section of this book

- Dried shiitake mushrooms (or use dried porcini, dried morel or dried common mushrooms)

of marble, for its durability and longevity, with a bowl at least 4 to 6 inches (10 to 15 cm) in diameter.

- **Steamer:** Steamers are wonderful for quickly steaming up vegetables, fish or tofu. Many pots have steamer inserts that make steaming easy. The alternative is collapsible metal steamers that can be inserted into pots of varying sizes or bamboo steamers that can be placed atop a cooking pot.

- **Wok:** While a wok is one of the key traditional cooking utensils found in every Chinese kitchen, it isn't essential for this book. Woks are used for quickly cooking foods at very high heat, either with or without oil. In the traditional Chinese kitchen, woks are also used for steaming foods with a wooden steamer. Look for a carbon steel wok with a cover and wok ring, which stabilizes your utensil on the stove. (They do not work well on an electric stovetop.) Your new wok will have a thin coating on it that needs to be washed off. Wash the wok thoroughly and use dish soap and a stainless steel scrubber to clean it. Then rinse and dry over low heat. You will then have to cure it by adding 1 tablespoon (15 mL) of avocado or coconut oil, using a paper towel or spatula to spread it over the entire surface. If cared for properly, woks can last a lifetime. When you have finished cooking in the wok, immediately put it in hot water (no soap) and soak for 5 minutes. Then rinse it and use a scrubber sponge to clear out any food and residue. Return it to the flame to dry it off and your wok is ready for the next meal.

- **Food strainer:** These are different from colanders, which are used to drain noodles or pasta. Fine-meshed strainers are very handy when you want to rinse rice, wash small quantities of greens or herbs, or strain out ingredients from a soup or tea. Some people even use strainers to sift certain flours. Having a variety of strainer sizes give you some flexibility in the kitchen, whether for rinsing the smallest amount of an ingredient like a herb sprig or straining bones from a larger soup or stew. If you were to only purchase one size, a 5-cup (1.25 L) strainer is the most versatile. Look for strainers that have a sturdy handle and are made of stainless steel. A teapot, mug or teacup with a built-in strainer is invaluable for making loose-leaf brewed teas or mixed herbal teas

Now that you've cleared out the pantry and stocked a kitchen with all necessary ingredients, let's get cooking.

Chapter 10

Culinary and Herbal Ingredients

Note

Certain ingredients in this chapter are referred to as "herbs" when they may, in fact, include a plant's roots, rhizomes, stems, bark, leaves, flowers, berries, or fruits. In Chinese medicine, these medicinal plants, as well as their parts, are referred to simply as "herbs" to indicate their health and therapeutic value.

Some of the key ingredients in Chinese medicinal cooking — from legumes and seeds to vegetables and fruits to medicinal plants and roots — may be unfamiliar to you but are considered vital to your diet because of their therapeutic value and, ultimately, their benefit to your overall health. Here, we'll explore these foods further. In the first part, you'll find a list of the more uncommon ingredients used in the recipes starting on the next page, each with a description of its essential flavor, therapeutic properties, use in cooking, storage tips and places to purchase them. The second part of this chapter (starting on page 184) includes a table of common foods and Chinese herbal ingredients categorized according to certain Chinese medicine classifications: their *thermal nature* (the action of a food to warm or cool), *flavor* (sweet, salty, sour, pungent and bitter) and *energetic action* on different organ systems, as well as the food's *therapeutic value* and *use in meals* to treat certain conditions; for example, to calm the mind, soothe a cough or clear excess heat in the body. For more information on Chinese medicine, thermal nature, flavor and therapeutic actions, see Chapters 2 and 3.

You may feel a bit like an explorer in a new land when you're experimenting with some of these foods. Wonderful! By trying out new foods, you'll be venturing into a new world of flavor and texture while stimulating your senses. Try something new and pay attention to how it makes you feel; your body changes, adapts and sends you signals with every new experience. Now let's discover a new world of foods.

Adzuki beans (*Vigna angularis*) are small, dark red dried beans. They have a mild and slightly sweet-and-sour bean flavor, and are most often used in congee on their own and sweetened to make Asian desserts. Beans should look clean, not dusty, and their interior should be light-colored (a dark color may indicate old beans that will not soften when cooked). Store dried beans in an airtight glass container or bag in a dark place: up to 3 months at cool room temperature, 6 months refrigerated or up to 1 year frozen. Beans can be purchased at Asian grocery stores, at health food stores or online.

Apple cider vinegar is apple cider or juice (must) that has gone through two stages of fermentation to become vinegar. It has a fruity, tangy and slightly sweet taste and is most commonly used in salad dressings and marinades, but also to bring out the nutrients in bone broth and add acidity to beans while cooking. The vinegar may be clear or cloudy, depending on whether it has been filtered and pasteurized, and should not smell musty. Store unpasteurized vinegar in a sealed glass container and pasteurized vinegar in an airtight glass container: up to 3 months at cool room temperature or 6 months refrigerated. It can be purchased at most grocery stores.

Arame: see Seaweed.

Asian greens include many members of the *Brassica* genus, including bok choy (also known as mustard cabbage), baby bok choi, Asian mustard greens and napa cabbage. These greens are widely used throughout Asia. They generally have tender leaves and fleshy stalks and vary in size, color and taste, from mild and slightly sweet to aromatic and grassy to slightly bitter and tangy or peppery. A variety of these greens are available throughout different seasons; similar greens can be substituted in most dishes. Asian greens are edible raw but are more nutritious and easily digested when fermented or cooked. Greens should be dry on the surface with no soft or wet spots; if they have lost some internal moisture, they may be slightly wilted, but this is fine. Store loosely wrapped in paper towels or a paper bag: up to 2 days at cool room temperature or 1 week refrigerated. Avoid storing in plastic, as this can cause the leaves to rot. They can be purchased at Asian grocery stores and large supermarkets and may be grown in most regions of North America.

Astragalus root (*Radix astragali*), or *huang qi* ("yellow leader") in Mandarin, is considered a superior Chinese medicinal and is widely used in teas, soups and dishes to boost *qi* and vitality. After harvesting, the root is sliced in shapes resembling tongue depressors or cut into small rounds and then dried. The root should be slightly moist, with a light brown bark on the exterior and a pale yellow hue on the inside. It has a distinct sweet flavor and is warming in nature. In Chinese herbalism, it is known as a consummate *qi* tonic and is most often used to boost vitality. It should be avoided if you have a respiratory infection, as its tonic effects can impede resolution of congestion and "lock the thief in the house." Use it when you feel generally healthy but a bit run-down or to boost the immune system when you're feeling tired after a cold but have no further symptoms. Dried astragalus root can be purchased in the herb section of Asian grocery stores and natural food stores or through a reputable supplier of Chinese herbs. It is best to purchase astragalus root from a reliable supplier of herbs to ensure that it has been tested for pesticides and is sulfite-free.

Avocado oil is pressed from avocados. Avocado oil has a neutral flavor and is used extensively in the recipes that call for high heat, making it suitable for frying. Store in an airtight glass container: up to 3 months at cool room temperature or 6 months refrigerated. Avocado oil can be purchased at health food stores, many large supermarkets and online.

Barberries, or zereshk, are the small, oblong dried red fruit of the thorny bush *Berberis vulgaris*. Many types of barberry are grown as ornamental bushes, but only this variety is edible; the fruit is used extensively in Persian (Iranian) cooking. The plant is native to southern Europe, northwest Africa and western Asia. It is important to note that the fruit is distinctly different in therapeutic value from the root and bark, which is used in Western herbalism. The bark and root have high levels of berberine and are used therapeutically to combat colds and treat inflammatory bowel conditions. Therapeutically, the dried fruits have been used to calm stomach upset, fever and diarrhea as well as to ease inflammation and urinary infection. Barberries have a strong sour flavor and have been used in cooking for thousands of years, for example as the distinguishing ingredient in the Persian rice dish known as zereshk polo (rice pilaf with barberries). In India, barberries are pickled and served as a condiment with curries or in desserts. Barberries can be purchased in Middle Eastern markets or online.

Bitter greens include several members of the *Cichorium* (chicory) genus, including frisée, escarole, endive, chicory. Others include dandelions, broccoli rabe (or rapini) and arugula. They generally have tender leaves and are mild to very bitter. These greens are widely used in salads; in this book, they are generally cooked. When fresh, greens should be dry on the surface with no soft or wet spots and should not be unevenly dark or slimy. Store loosely wrapped in paper towels or a paper bag: up to 2 days at cool room temperature or 1 week refrigerated. Avoid storing in plastic, as this can cause the leaves to rot. They can be purchased at farmers' markets, specialty grocers or large supermarkets and may be grown or gathered wild in most areas of North America.

Bitter melon (*Momordica charantia*), aka bitter gourd, karela or balsam pear, is a green, warty, spindle-shaped gourd, about 8 inches (20 cm) long and 2 inches (5 cm) in diameter. There are two common varieties: one is a darker green with pointier warts and the other has shinier skin and warts in ridges. The first is preferred for its firmer flesh, but either may be used. As its name suggests, bitter melon is powerfully bitter. Most recipes include methods for tempering the bitterness, but it may be a flavor that takes time to get used to. The melon brings out the savory flavor of other ingredients in recipes, however, and you may find yourself an enthusiast! Bitter melon has a long history of use in Asia as a purgative, digestive aid and appetite stimulant and has been used to treat malaria and stabilize blood sugars in people with diabetes. Melons should be dry on the surface with no soft or wet spots and very green in color, not orange or yellow. Store up to 2 days at cool room temperature or a week refrigerated. It can be purchased at Asian grocery stores and may be grown in areas of North America with long, hot summers.

Button mushroom: see Mushrooms.

Cardamom (*Elettaria cardamomum*) comes from a plant in the ginger family. Its dried green pods are small and ridged and filled with fragrant, tarry black seeds. The pods are sometimes steeped or simmered in liquid to flavor a recipe, or the seeds are extracted and added directly to food. The seeds have a warm, gingery, citrusy aroma and flavor. Green cardamom is fragrant and is used as a digestive stimulant. Pods should be medium green, not white (bleached), and sometimes do not have much fragrance until crushed to release the essential oils in the seeds. Store whole pods in an airtight container at cool room temperature in a dark place for up to 2 years; seeds may be stored for up to 3 months. Cardamom is commonly sold in the baking spices section of the grocery store.

Chia seeds are the tiny gray or black seeds of a subtropical sage (*Salvia hispanica*). The seeds are bland but nutritionally dense and have an interesting mucilaginous texture when moistened. Unlike flax seeds, which need to be ground to release their beneficial oils, you can eat chia seeds whole. The seeds should be shiny, with no odor, not dusty- or musty-smelling. Store in an airtight container or bag: up to 3 months at cool room temperature or up to 2 years refrigerated. Chia seeds can be purchased at health food stores, large supermarkets or online.

Chinese chives (*Allium tuberosum*), aka garlic chives, Chinese leeks, yellow chives or *jiu cai* in Mandarin, are a pungent and warming herb known for its versatility in the kitchen. Chinese chives grow upright in spreading clumps in the garden. They have slender flat leaves (whereas Western chives are cylindrical) and may sometimes have green buds or petite clusters of white flowers at their peak, when blooming anywhere from mid to later summer. The flowers are edible and work well as a pungent garnish for a vegetable dish or salad, just be sure to wash them and check for insects. The leaves have a mildly sweet garlic fragrance that adds warmth to many cooling vegetable dishes. In Chinese herbalism, Chinese chives are known for their capacity to impart warmth and disperse stagnation. Look for a slightly shiny green leaf with a crisp stem you could snap off (implying freshness). Store as you would any green leafy vegetable, wrapped in paper towel and stored in a plastic bag in the fridge. It will stay fresh for a few days. You can find them in Asian grocery stores. They are also very easy to grow in the garden or a container.

Shopping Tip

In Asian grocery stores, many packages of Chinese yam will have added sulfites. You want to avoid this preservative, as many people are sensitive or allergic to it. Online and herb suppliers will have more sulfite-free options.

Chinese yam (*Dioscorea opposita*), aka *shan yao* (which translates to "mountain medicine") or *huai shan* in Mandarin, is the starchy rhizome of a vigorous flowering vine that is native to China and easily grown in temperate climates in North America. Chinese yam is sold dried as white, chalky slices. It is sweet in flavor, neutral in nature and considered an essential tonic food in Chinese medicine. It stimulates and invigorates *qi* and is often used in China to help digestion, stem fatigue, soothe a dry cough or curb diarrhea. As a mild food, it can be used regularly in cooking. It is beneficial for all ages and can be used in soups, congee and other grain dishes, and is particularly therapeutic if you're recovering from a long illness and feel run-down. You may find it in Asian grocery stores or through reliable suppliers of Chinese herbs.

Chrysanthemum flower (*Chrysanthemum morifolium*), or *ju hua* in Mandarin, is a fragrant, pale yellow flower that is dried and steeped to make a popular tea that has been used throughout Asia for thousands of years. Chrysanthemum's cool nature and sweet, pungent and slightly bitter flavor disperses heat and calms the body. It is commonly used in Chinese herbalism to "brighten" the eyes and can be part of herbal formulas to soothe burning and itchy eyes in allergy season. In combination with honeysuckle flowers and goji berries (see Tame-the-Tension Tea, page 314), chrysanthemum flowers can is used in Chinese herbal formulas or teas in combination with other herbs to reduce tension and lower stress-related high blood pressure. Its cooling nature also helps in reducing excess yang in the liver, which can give rise to headaches and bloodshot eyes. Include these mild-tasting dried flowers in your assortment of teas for spring and summer. Dried chrysanthemum flowers can be purchased in Asian grocery stores or from reliable suppliers of Chinese herbs.

Cinnamon sticks come from three sources:
1. *Cinnamomum cassia*, aka Chinese cinnamon, Cortex Cinnamomi or *rou gui* in Mandarin, is the outer bark of an evergreen member of the laurel family that is native to China. This is the medicinal cinnamon used in Chinese herbalism and traditional Chinese cooking. As a stick, its appearance is grayish, as it is the outer bark of the plant. It can also be found in grocery stores as a powder marked Chinese cinnamon.

2. Common cinnamon (cassia) — the one with a golden brown color that we commonly use in North American cooking and baking and is easy to find in the grocery store — comes from the same plant but is the inner bark of *Cinnamomum cassia*.

3. True cinnamon, or Ceylon cinnamon, is the inner bark of the *Cinnamomum zeylanicum* (or *C. verum*) tree and has many brittle, thin layers that flake easily. It is sold mostly in Mexican, Southeast Asian and Latin grocery stores. This cinnamon is used in many dishes from Central and South America, North Africa, the Middle East, India, Southeast Asia and Europe to impart a less acrid and more mellow and sweet taste while remaining pungent, sweet and warming in its action on the body.

Cinnamon in General

All cinnamon sticks are about 6 inches (15 cm) long and may be available in the herb and spice section of your grocery store. To decide which variety to use in cooking, consider these factors: If you're creating a truly therapeutic and medicinal dish or seeking a more pungent taste, use the Chinese variety. If you want to add a more mellow flavor to food, choose the true (Ceylon) cinnamon or common cinnamon.

Cinnamon twigs, or *gui zhi* in Mandarin, are the twigs of the plant (*Cinnamomum cassia*) that gives us the common cinnamon bark used in Western cooking. The cinnamon twig is used more often for its therapeutic value, however, not for its culinary contribution. The sweet, warming, pungent twigs are added to Chinese herbal formulas to counter the onset of a cold caused by exposure to wind and cold elements, with symptoms of chills and slight fever. Cinnamon twigs are also used in herbal formulas to treat joint problems. They can be purchased through reliable suppliers of Chinese herbs or online.

Coconut sugar is the dehydrated sap of the flowers of several types of coconut palm trees. It is similar to but different from palm sugar, which is made from the sap of the palm tree. Coconut sugar has an earthy flavor similar to that of refined brown cane sugar. It should smell like caramel or dates, not like coconut, and should have only a few clumps. Store in an airtight container or bag: in a dark place at cool room temperature for up to 2 years. Coconut sugar can be purchased at health food stores, large supermarkets or online.

Codonopsis (*Codonopsis pilosula*), aka bonnet bellflower, poor man's ginseng or *dang shen* in Mandarin, is a common adaptogenic (a natural substance thought to help the body adapt to stress and normalize bodily processes). The crinkly, narrow and apparently shriveled dried root, about 2 to 3 inches (5 to 8 cm) in length, is used widely as a tonic in everyday cooking and medicinal teas to boost *qi* and immunity. It is sweet in flavor and neutral in nature. Where ginseng, one of the most highly valued and expensive of Chinese tonic herbs, is a tonic for the lungs and heart, codonopsis is a tonic for the digestive network that includes the stomach and spleen, what is known in Chinese medicine as the *middle jiao* (essentially, the middle region of the body, which includes the digestive network). It is best used to treat low energy and appetite, weakness, loose stools and shortness of breath. It is used in teas, soups, congees and medicinal tonic wines. Codonopsis root is available through a reliable supplier of Chinese herbs and sometimes in the herb section of Asian grocery stores.

Cordyceps (*Cordyceps sinensis*), aka caterpillar fungus or *dong chong xia cao* in Mandarin, meaning "summer plant, winter worm," is a species of mushroom that has been prized medicinally for its overall tonic effect for more than 1,500 years. Essentially, it is a parasitic fungus that invades the body of a caterpillar (the larvae of a species of moth) to transform it into a type of mushroom. Once you get over this fact, it is a rare, fascinating and powerful fungus. It is warming and has a mild flavor that is sweet, slightly pungent and mildly bitter. It has a mushroom-like, fragrant aroma and looks like either a thin gray finger with a small cap on its tail or long thin vermillion shreds. Cordyceps is traditionally cooked with duck and readily absorbs the sweet flavor of the broth. You may also find it cooked in pork broth along with dioscorea (*shan yao*, or Chinese yam) to boost vitality. It has been called the longevity herb and has a powerful effect on inherent vitality while enhancing libido and endurance and clearing phlegm in the lungs. It can be purchased in the herb section of Asian grocery stores or through reliable suppliers of Chinese herbs.

Crataegus (*Crataegus pinnatifida*, of the *Rosaceae* family) is commonly known as Chinese haw or hawthorn, mountain hawthorn, red-fruited hawthorn or *shan zha* in Mandarin. This variety of *Crataegus* produces a medium-sized, round red fruit with white meat and is not the same as the crataegus berries (hawthorne berries, or haws) that are commonly used in the West. In China, the crataegus fruit can be found everywhere, in Beijing as a sweetened street food, dipped in sugar and served on a skewer, much like a smaller candied apple, or dried and served as a type of very thin fruit leather in Chinese candy stores. As a medicinal herb, it is known for its potency in stimulating and improving digestion, reducing cholesterol and improving heart function. It is commonly used to alleviate indigestion, or as stated in Chinese herbalism, to treat food retention, as it helps to resolve food stagnation after eating a heavy meat meal. It is considered neutral to slightly warming and is sweet-and-sour in flavor, similar to many types of small apples. It can stimulate and improve *qi* and blood flow. It is commonly used as a tea, dried as fruit leather, and used to make wines, syrups and pastes. It is available from reliable suppliers of Chinese herbs, sometimes found in Asian grocery stores or online.

Crimini mushroom: See Mushrooms.

Daikon (*Raphanus sativus longipinnatus*) is a very large white radish that typically grows to 16 inches (40 cm) in length and 2 inches (5 cm) in diameter. It is widely used throughout Asia; with a crisp texture when raw and meaty when cooked, it is appealing in a variety of dishes. The flavor of daikon, as with all radishes, can be fairly sweet and mild or fiercely peppery. Cooking tames any pungency and reveals a gentle sweetness, and daikon also readily absorbs flavor from other ingredients. Daikon should be firm and dry on the surface with no soft or wet spots. If the radish has lost some internal moisture, it may be slightly bendable, which is fine and actually preferable for pickles. Store loosely wrapped in paper towels or a paper bag: up to 2 weeks at cool room temperature, 3 weeks refrigerated or several months in a dry cellar. Do not store in plastic, as this will cause the root to rot or grow mold. It can be purchased at Asian grocery stores and large supermarkets and may be grown in most regions of North America.

Dang gui (*Radix angelicae sinensis*), aka Chinese angelica, *dong quai* and *tang kuei*, is a perennial herb that grows in cold and rainy mountain areas of China. Known as the "female ginseng" or the "gynecological panacea," the strongly fragrant, dried, multi-toned brownish root is usually sold in slices by reliable suppliers of Chinese herbs. It is one of most well-known Chinese herbs for "harmonizing the blood," which in essence translates to nourishing the blood while activating its circulation. It is prescribed routinely for women suffering menstrual irregularities, premenstrual syndrome or endometriosis, as well as perimenopausal and menopausal symptoms. It is warm in nature and pungent in flavor, with a strong aroma. Dang gui is useful in the kitchen, adding flavor and depth to soups, stews, teas, congee and wines to nourish and move the blood. If you suffer from chronic diarrhea or are pregnant, it is best to consult an acupuncturist or a Chinese medicine doctor before using this herb. You will most likely find dang gui through an acupuncturist, a reliable supplier of Chinese herbs or online.

Dulse: See Seaweed.

Fermented foods exist in every culture. People on every continent except for Antarctica from ancient time to the present have used fermented foods. Each culture has unique flavor palates and uses fermentation processes brimming with beneficial microbes and bacteria that benefit health. Some of the more familiar fermented foods people love include pickles, kimchi, olives, cider, coffee, teas, chocolate, cheeses and yogurt, sourdough breads, cured meats, alcohol and vinegar. The unique story of sauerkraut is said to have started in China and traveled along with migrating tribes into Europe, finding its way into Russian, German and Eastern European cultures. Note that some "pickled" foods are preserved in an acid brine such as vinegar and salt with no live microorganisms, while others, including fermented pickles, are fermented in a salty brine. Detailed directions for recipes that are lightly fermented are given in this book and often a little of the liquid from a previous batch is used to help start the fermentation process. Make and seek out live fermented foods that you either make in your own home or find in refrigerated sections of grocery

stores. Fermentation may help to break down dense nutrients, making them more digestible and accessible, in some cases, while generating additional nutrients and micronutrients. The most profound benefit of eating fermented foods is the beneficial bacteria themselves, which are required for healthy digestion, immune function and mental health. Add them to your meals as a condiment, cook with them and drink fermented beverages or their brine. Fermented foods may help with digestion. When purchasing fermented foods, avoid off colors and smells, as well as unintended mold. Different types of fermented foods can be purchased at Asian and Middle Eastern groceries, local farmers' markets, health food stores and large supermarkets.

A World of Flavors

In addition to the health benefits inherent in these foods, fermentation enhances and brings new flavors to common foods. The flavor palate of Eastern Europe, steeped in dill, garlic and salt, renders an entirely different experience from the flavor palate of China, where you find fermented pickles steeped in star anise, cinnamon or Sichuan peppercorns, or the pickles of Latin America, where chile peppers take center stage.

Flax seeds (*Linum usitatissimum*) are glossy yellow or brown seeds similar in size to sesame seeds. Flax seeds are slightly nutty in flavor, very nutritionally dense and have a mucilaginous texture when ground and moistened. To make them more nutritionally available to the body, they need to be ground; otherwise, the vast majority of seeds will end up undigested. The seeds should be shiny, with no odor, not dusty- or musty-smelling. Store whole seeds in an airtight container: up to 3 months at cool room temperature in a dark place or up to 1 year refrigerated. Ground flax seeds (flaxseed meal) can be stored in an airtight container for up to 2 months in the refrigerator or up to 6 months in the freezer. Whole flax seeds and flaxseed meal can be purchased at health food stores, large supermarkets or online.

Ghee is clarified butter, generally made from cow's milk. The butter has been cooked to evaporate the moisture in the milk and separate the milk solids, which are removed and discarded. Purification of the ghee removes all lactose and proteins and yields a delicious nutty browned-butter flavor. It also means that ghee does not require refrigeration. It should not have off-flavors or odors, such as fish or cheese. It can be stored in an airtight container: up to 6 months at cool room temperature in a dark place or up to 1 year refrigerated. Ghee can easily be made from unsalted butter at home or purchased from an Indian grocery store, health food store or online.

Ginger, dried, or *gan jiang* in Mandarin, is made from the same tuber as fresh gingerroot (the rhizome of *Zingiber officinale*), which is dried and usually ground to a powder. This is the ginger you will find in the spice section of your grocery store. As with foods, the processing of herbs changes their nature (the warming or cooling aspect). In this case, dried ginger is much more pungent and spicy than the fresh root. Its nature is purely hot and potent in its power to expel cold and warm the body, so dried ginger is warming and used to dispel an inner feeling of cold and to clear phlegm from the lungs. Like raw ginger, the dried form has a soothing effect on the stomach and digestion, but it is much warmer. Note: Since dried ginger is much more concentrated and warming, it is not recommended if it causes you to feel too hot. Instead, use fresh ginger in small amounts.

Gingerroot (fresh ginger) (*Zingiber officinale*) is known as *sheng jiang* in Mandarin, where *jiang* means "to defend," suggesting its ability to ward off climactic elements of cold that can affect your health. Ginger is one of the oldest, most versatile and valued herbs worldwide, an herbal emissary crossing cultures, countries and time to hold an esteemed place in the kitchen and medicine chest. Ginger grows in tropical or subtropical climates, yet found its way through trade to England, where it was prized for its flavor and medicinal use. The fresh knobby, light brown rhizome can be found in the produce section of most grocery stores. Select ginger that is firm and heavy with shiny, taut skin; skip the ginger that is shrivelled. It has a hot and warming nature and is pungent, spicy and almost sweet in flavor. It has been used for millennia to induce sweating and dispel pathogens (such as viruses), as well as calm nausea and warm the stomach. It is used in Chinese herbal medicine to moderate any mild toxicity of other herbs and increase digestibility. In the Chinese kitchen, ginger forms a large part of the culinary palette. It has been said to reduce the fishy flavor in fish and moderate other strong flavors. If you're hesitant to include ginger in your cooking, try a small amount at first. Many people enjoy ginger and lemon tea (particularly when a cold is looming). It has a unique and zesty flavor that is wonderful when added to teas, soups, stews, vegetables, fruits and desserts and decocted in liquors.

Goji berries (*Lycium barbarium*), aka Chinese wolfberries or *gou qi zi*, are small red berries when dried, similar to but smaller than the Western dried raisin. Their concentrated sweet flavor and neutral nature make them a delicious snack. Goji berries are delicious in snacks mixed with nuts, steeped in herbal infusions and teas and added to wines, and will enhance the flavor of any soup, stew or meat dish. It can be easy to overdo it because they taste so good, but goji berries are a strong therapeutic food, so monitor your intake — a little goes a long way! They are readily found dried in many natural foods, grocery and Asian food stores. They can also be purchased through reliable suppliers of Chinese herbs and online. Be sure to purchase organic goji berries to avoid exposure to pesticides.

A Multitude of Benefits

Legends abound from ancient China on the miraculous anti-aging effects of eating Goji berries. Li Shizhen, the ancient Chinese scholar and herbalist who compiled the *Compendium of Materia Medica (Bencao Gangmu)*, pointed out the effects of eating goji berries on longevity. Chinese herbalists use them to nourish your essence (*jing*) and as a foundation of various fertility formulas. Goji berries are also known to benefit the eyes, counter dizziness and nourish the liver and kidneys.

Hato mugi (*Coix lacryma-jobi*), aka Job's tears, coix seed, aka Chinese pearl barley or *yi yi ren*, has been cultivated for centuries in Asia and Africa as an heirloom grain. It is quite different than the common Western barley — Western barley is considered a glutinous grain while hato mugi is gluten-free. In appearance, it is a smallish, spherical, pearly white seed with a dark brown groove down the center. This small grain is light and delicious, with a firm and almost crunchy texture. It is cooling in

nature and bland and sweet in flavor. It is most often used as a grain dish on its own (but be sure to soak it for at least 1 hour before cooking in a grain dish) or mixed into congee, soups and teas. It has a long history as a Chinese medicinal herb used to disperse internal heat, as a diuretic relieving edema and as a spleen tonic. It is also used to counter joint stiffness when it worsens with damp weather. It also has a beneficial effect on the skin and complexion. You will not find hato mugi in your local grocery store; look for it in an Asian grocery store or Chinese herb shop, or shop for it online.

Honeysuckle flower buds (*Flos Lonicerae japonica*), or *jin yin hua*, "golden silver flowers," in Mandarin, is a fast-growing and abundant vine with fragrant and sweet-tasting blossoms you may already grow in your garden. If you are growing it, try picking the blossoms and suck on their sweet nectar for a summer treat. The dried honeysuckle flower buds are used in Chinese medicine to treat a sore throat that is burning and scratchy. These flower buds have a pungent and sweet flavor that is delightful in a tea. With their cooling nature, honeysuckle buds are especially effective as a summer tea, served either hot, warm or at room temperature, to help with extreme summer heat. You can purchase these dried flower buds in any Asian grocery store or reliable supplier of Chinese herbs.

Hijiki: See Seaweed.

Katsuobushi (*bonito flakes*) is paper-thin shavings of smoked, dried, fermented skipjack tuna or young bonito, which is a cheaper substitute. This Japanese product, used both as a condiment and a flavoring in soup stock, adds umami and a light fish and smoke taste to dishes. The shavings, which look like slightly pink wood shavings, are packaged in plastic packets. Higher-quality flakes are larger and thicker and have a more delicate flavor. They're also sold in smaller packets, since they lose their flavor and texture within a few days once opened. Unopened packets may be stored in a dark place at cool room temperature for up to a year. Katsuobushi can be found in the international food section at some large grocery stores, at Asian grocers and online.

Kombu: See Seaweed.

Lian qiao is the bud of the weeping forsythia bush (*Forsythia suspensa*), which provides one of the telltale signs of emerging spring in temperate climates. This bud, once dried, is tight, a light yellow-green color and one of the key ingredients in Chinese medicine's *yin qiao san* (honeysuckle and forsythia powder), a well-known herbal formula typically taken with the first signs of a scratchy or burning sore throat along with a slight fever. Forsythia buds' bitter, pungent flavor and cooling nature is enhanced when paired with honeysuckle (*Lonicera*) buds. *Lian qiao* is used mostly in herbal teas, which can be decocted and used as a liquid base for congee. It can often be found in the tea or herb section of an Asian grocery store or through a reliable supplier of Chinese herbs.

Lily bulb (*Lilliim brownii*) is known as *bai he* in Mandarin. The bulb's starchy white petals overlapping each other resemble the actual flower that makes up this species of lily. In thermal nature, it is slightly cold with a sweet and slightly bitter flavor. It has been used for thousands of years in China, both in the kitchen and in herbal formulas. Like water chestnuts, the bulb adds a sweet flavor and delicate crisp texture to dishes.

It is often added to stir-fries or soups for its therapeutic value and delightful crunch. In addition to its culinary contribution, it has been used medicinally to calm and tranquilize the mind and soothe a dry cough — a common dish in Chinese medicine to help soothe a cough is steamed lily bulb and pears. Chinese herbalists will often add this herb to herbal formulas when a person has trouble sleeping, is distressed or is suffering from grief. Lily bulb can be purchased in Asian grocery stores and through reliable suppliers of Chinese herbs (look for lily bulb that has not been treated with sulfites).

Longan (*Euphoria longan* (Lour.) steud.) or *Dimocarpus longan*, aka dragon eye fruit or *long yan rou* in Mandarin, is a refreshing and sweet fruit that appeals to both young and old. It is sold fresh and dried in the West. Small and round with a thin dark skin, fresh longan reveals a milky white, shiny, juicy fruit when peeled and is often confused with fresh lychee. In Chinese medicine, the longan is typically used dried, added to herbal teas and soups and steeped in alcohol to render a liquor therapeutic and medicinal. It is warming in nature and sweet in flavor, and it is often used to sweeten dishes. If you have diabetes, however, you should avoid the dried condensed form of this sweet fruit due to its concentration of fruit sugar. In ancient times, the Chinese believed the longan fruit had strong anti-aging properties. Therapeutically, it nourishes the blood, helps calm an anxious mind and acts as an aid for insomnia. Fresh longan is often found in Asian grocery stores or small street produce vendors in Chinatowns. Dried longan can be purchased in Asian grocery stores, reliable suppliers of Chinese herbs or online.

Lotus root, or *lian ou* in Mandarin, is actually the rhizome of the miraculous lotus plant *(Nelumbo nucifera)*, an aquatic perennial that emerges from just below the surface of ponds or shallow lakes and is common throughout Asia. Its edible rhizome and seeds are mild in flavor and distinctive in their therapeutic effect on the body. Its beautiful flower is the subject of legends of purity and transformation. Lotus root is a favorite vegetable throughout Asia and Southeast Asia, with a crunchy, refreshing flavor akin to jicama, another root vegetable. The root resembles smooth, streaked, ivory sweet potatoes that have become attached. When sliced open, the vegetable reveals a circular, lace-like design. Its appealing appearance, texture and versatility make it a wonderful addition to stir-fries, soups and any mixed vegetable dish. To prepare on its own or in a dish, it is best parboiled whole before slicing. It can also be cooked, juiced and made into a refreshing summer drink to cool down. Lotus root's nature is cooling with a sweet flavor when used raw. Its thermal nature changes to warming when cooked and can benefit those who have low appetite or suffer from diarrhea. The juice of the raw root is used as a folk remedy to stop a nosebleed. You can find lotus roots in the fresh vegetables section of Asian grocery stores. The optimal buying season is autumn, winter and early spring. Be sure to select firm, pale, bruise-free roots that are connected to at least one other root. You can store roots in the refrigerator, wrapped in a damp cloth or paper towels and a plastic bag, for up to 1 week. If you're using raw lotus root, it is best to choose small ones. The larger lotus roots with more mature rhizomes are ideal for cooking.

Lotus seeds, or *lian zi* in Mandarin, come from the same plant as the root and resemble round, pale yellow pistachio nuts. The lotus seed brings a light nutty and enriching flavor to teas, as well as a crunchy texture to dishes such as soups, stews and congee. In Chinese cuisine, lotus seeds are also crystallized with sugar as a snack or cooked and sweetened into a paste. The neutral, bland and sweet lotus seeds absorb flavor from the dish to which they are added. They are neither warming nor cooling in thermal nature and have a sweet and slightly astringent flavor. Lotus seeds require soaking for at least 1 hour prior to cooking if added to rice or teas but can be directly added into soups. Therapeutically, lotus seeds nourish the heart, calm the mind, address loss of appetite and treat diarrhea by strengthening the stomach and spleen *qi*. Lotus seeds are available in the dried herb section of Asian grocery stores but are best purchased from a reliable supplier of Chinese herbs to assure that they're sulfite-free. Store them in a glass jar in a cool dark place for up to 6 months or 1 year in the refrigerator.

Miso is a fermented paste made from soybeans, or a combination of grains (rice or barley), or beans and salt, that is combined with the *Aspergillus oryzae* mold, aka *koji*, to initiate the fermentation process. It is aged anywhere from 3 weeks to 3 years and is a consummate food, used to add depth of flavor to broths, stir-fries, dressings and soups. It has been a staple of Japanese cuisine for centuries. While all miso has a savory, salty taste, the flavor of a particular miso is influenced by its ingredients and how long it has been aged. White *(shiro)* miso is milder in flavor and more versatile, while red *(aka)* miso is stronger and typically used for marinades for grilled foods and other recipes where its pungency is tamed. To keep the microorganisms in miso alive, avoid warming it above body temperature. When purchasing miso, look for organic miso that is uniform in color and free of preservatives. Store miso in its original package or in a covered glass container in the refrigerator after opening and it will keep almost indefinitely. Miso may be purchased at Asian grocery stores, health food stores, large supermarkets and online.

Beneficial Bacteria

Because of its long fermentation, miso is rich in probiotics, adding beneficial bacteria to the flora of the intestines to strengthen immunity. In a 2003 article in the *Journal of the National Cancer Institute,* it was reported that women who ate three or more bowls of miso soup on a daily basis reduced their risk of breast cancer in some cases by 50 percent.

Morel mushroom: See Mushrooms.

Mulberry fruit, or *sang shen* in Mandarin, is the fruit of the white mulberry tree (*Morus alba*), one of the few plants in Chinese medicine in which all parts are used: the roots, bark, twigs, leaves and fruits. Indeed, for thousands of years, the Chinese have used the mulberry bark, twigs, leaves and fruit to clear the lungs, treat joint pain, clear a cough and enhance blood and yin. The mulberry leaf is also the food of the silkworm. The mulberry fruit is used in Chinese herbal formulas to treat insomnia and constipation when the underlying cause is blood deficiency. Dried mulberries make a delightful snack, but too many can induce loose stools and a high concentration of sugar, which is particularly unhealthy for people with diabetes. The dried mulberry has a sweet flavor and cold thermal nature. Fresh mulberry fruit is delicate and not typically found in grocery stores but can be grown in home gardens. The trees can be very large and quite productive, so be prepared for lots of mulberries! The dried white mulberry fruit is usually found in Asian, Middle Eastern or specialty grocery stores.

Mung beans (*Vigna radiata*), aka moong bean or *lu dou* in Mandarin, are small dried olive green beans. They have a mild taste and are sprouted for bean sprouts or cooked as a bean in soups, rice dishes or stews. In Chinese medicine and Asian therapeutic cooking, mung beans are known for their diuretic effects and strong heat-clearing properties during hot, humid summers. The dried beans should look clean, not dusty, and their interior should be light-colored (a dark color may indicate old beans that will not soften when cooked). Dried mung beans are often available with skins removed and appear yellow, but recipes in this book use the skin-on (green) beans. Store dried mung beans in an airtight container or bag: up to 3 months at cool room temperature in a dark place, 6 months refrigerated or up to 1 year frozen. Beans can be purchased at Asian grocery stores, health food stores, the bulk section of grocery stores or online.

Mushrooms used in this book include white button and cremini (two forms of *Agaricus bisporus*), morel (*Morchella* species), oyster (*Pleurotus ostreatus*) and shiitake (*Lentinula edodes*). Mushrooms have a characteristic earthy aroma and taste and a meaty texture that is enhanced when cooked. When purchased, mushrooms should be firm and dry on the surface with no soft or slimy spots, though mushrooms that have lost some internal moisture are still acceptable. Store loosely wrapped in paper towels or a paper bag up to 1 week in the refrigerator. Do not store in plastic, as this will cause the mushrooms to rot or grow mold. They can be purchased at farmers' markets, Asian grocery stores and large supermarkets.

Nettles (*Urtica dioca L.*), aka stinging nettles, are one of the most prized early spring wild greens found in meadows and forests in the Western hemisphere. Their upright growth and oval, slightly jagged leaves are reminiscent of the mint family, but the similarity ends there. Nettles can be simply prepared — steamed, added to soups or risottos or infused as a tea. The nature of stinging nettles is cool with a sweet slightly astringent flavor. They are well known for their use in treating common seasonal allergies, have a strong blood-nourishing effect and are detoxifying, blood-building and rich in chlorophyll and trace minerals. You can forage for nettles in meadows and forests, grow them in a garden or find them at various farmers' markets in early spring.

Gathering Nettles

You may have experienced Nettles' "stinging" hairs, which emit a sharp burning and numbing substance, when you have crossed their path or lightly brushed up against them in the woods. When foraging for them (best do it in early spring), be sure to wear gloves and look for young shoots. You simply need to nip the upper sections of the leaves and stems and put them into a bag to take home. As soon as you cook or completely dry them, there is no longer any danger of being stung and you will be rewarded with a delightful flavor similar to that of spinach.

Nori: See Seaweed.

Oyster mushroom: See Mushrooms.

Ras el hanout is the name of a North African spice mixture that originated in Morocco. It translates to "top of the shop" for the high quality of the spices used to make up this subtle and flavorful spice blend. Each combination is unique — it may contain as many as 20 different spices, including fenugreek, cinnamon, cumin, coriander, ginger, cloves, nutmeg, peppercorns and the inimitable rose, which lends a nuanced floral aroma and flavor to the mixture. See Qi-Moving Rose Game Hens, page 226, for a recipe for ras el hanout where the rose and ginger take the lead to emphasize a spicy and floral flavor. Ras el hanout is most often used as a spice rub when cooking meats. If purchasing it premade from a spice merchant, be sure to get the best quality you can in order to experience its true taste. Store the spice mixture in a glass jar in a cool dry place for up to 6 months.

Red dates (*Ziziphus jujuba*), aka jujube fruit, red date or *hong (da) zao* in Mandarin, resemble dried dates except these are red. The sweet dried fruit is common in Chinese cuisine, where it is used to sweeten dishes and in soups, stews, congee and teas as a tonic food to nourish and invigorate your energy. Red dates are a key component of the Eight Treasures tea or congee. The date's sweet flavor and neutral nature make it a common ingredient in Chinese herbal formulas designed as a balancing agent to build vitality and nourish blood. They are used therapeutically to build vitality and soothe insomnia when added to specific dishes or herbal formulas. Seasonally, fresh jujubes are available at Asian grocery stores and can be grown in most temperate regions of North America. Dried red dates can be found in the herb section of most Asian grocery stores or through reliable suppliers of Chinese herbs.

Rice (*Oryza sativa*) is at the center of many traditional Asian diets. It was considered one of the seven necessities of life in ancient Chinese culture, and the symbol for *qi* comes from the vapors of a steaming pot of rice. The sweet and bland flavor of whole brown rice is a foundation for nourishment. Indeed, one could say that there is a rice for every season. Each variety of whole-grain brown rice has a mildly different thermal nature or action on the body. Short-grain brown rice is sweet and neutral in nature: it is perfect all year long. Long-grain brown rice is more cooling, lighter in texture and more suitable in summer. The fragrant basmati rice will activate the senses and nourish and move digestive *qi*. The special brown sweet rice, aka glutinous or sticky rice, is warming and offers more substance in colder months. When buying rice, look for grains that are clean, not dusty, and slightly shiny. If you're buying rice from bulk, make sure it's from stores that have a high turnover rate to ensure freshness. It is always best to store grains in a sealed glass container in a cool dark place.

Rice vinegar is milled glutinous rice that has gone through two stages of fermentation. It has a delicately tangy and slightly sweet taste and varies in color from clear to a golden color; darker vinegars will generally have more flavor. Avoid "seasoned" rice vinegar, as it has added sugar and flavoring. Store in an airtight glass container at room temperature or refrigerated. Because of its high acidity, vinegar can keep for a very long time, but if you need an end date, simply look at the "best if used by" date on the bottle. Rice vinegar can be purchased at Asian grocery stores, many large supermarkets and online.

Rice wine (dry), most widely known as sake, is milled glutinous rice that has been fermented to produce alcohol. It has a slight taste of beer and is colorless, but may be clear or cloudy. You get more or less what you pay for — the cheapest wines are acceptable for cooking, but quality wines for drinking will cost two to three times as much. Store wine for cooking in an airtight glass container: up to 3 months at cool room temperature or 6 months refrigerated. It can be purchased in the United States at Asian grocery stores, many large supermarkets, liquor stores and online (check the regulations for the sale of wines and liquor where you live).

Rose buds or petals (*Rosa rugosa*), or *mei gui hua* in Mandarin, can be used in spice combinations (such as ras el hanout), steeped to make teas, infused in wines and added to meat dishes as well as syrups and desserts. The rose used in Chinese herbal medicine differs slightly from rose petals used in Middle Eastern cuisine, as the former seem sweeter and more fragrant and flavorful. The dried rose buds or petals used in Chinese medicine are warming in nature, fragrant, sweet and slightly astringent in flavor. Rose is used to lift the spirit, ease the mind and relax tension. As long as they are free of pesticides, feel free to use roses that grow in your garden for cooking, spice mixtures, teas and wines. Be sure to purchase dried organic red rose buds or petals, which are more warming, fragrant and go straight to the emotional heart. Dried rose petals or buds can be purchased from reputable spice purveyors, reliable suppliers of Chinese herbs or online. If you grow roses in your garden without pesticides or spray, feel free to pick them and dry the petals or buds on a sheet of paper in a cool dark area for at least 1 week, or until completely dried.

The Flower of Love

All flowers are said to open the senses and lift the spirits, but the rose is considered the queen in doing so. The fragrance of rose is associated in many cultures with the opening of the heart to love.

Rose hips, aka rose haws, are the fruit of the common wild dog rose plant (*Rosa canina*), which are especially used for rose hips. As the flowers fade and the petals drop from this plant, the vibrant red color of its fruit lights up many autumnal paths. Take a bite of fresh rose hips picked straight off the bush and you will discover a sweet-tart flavor with a mild astringent action. Rose hips are most often used to make teas, syrups, jams and liqueurs. High in antioxidants and vitamin C, the rose hip is used in Western herbal medicine to treat the common cold. It is also used to treat rheumatoid arthritis and in the treatment of diarrhea, viral infections and urinary and kidney disorders. Rose hip oil is used externally to add lustre to the skin. Note: Western rose hips are a different variety than the Chinese, *Rosa laevigata* (*jin ying zi* or Cherokee rose), which has a similar effect but is more astringent and is used to treat diarrhea and dysentery, incontinence and excessive uterine bleeding. Dried rose hips are more commonly found in herbal and health food stores and in the bulk section of some grocery stores. You may also find rose hip tea bags in grocery and natural foods stores.

Schisandra berries (*Schisandrae chinensis*), or *wu wei zi* in Mandarin, are an important Chinese herb (remember that in Chinese herbalism, certain fruits, bark, twigs, leaves, stems, rhizomes and roots are all considered "herbs" because of their therapeutic and medicinal value).

Schisandra is known as the "five flavored seed" for possessing all the five flavors (sweet, sour, salty, bitter and pungent) and for its capacity to penetrate, nourish and protect the five yin organs (lung, spleen, kidney, liver and heart). It is considered a tonic and astringent herb. When dried, the dark burgundy berries taste sour on the first bite but reveal unusual and surprising flavors as you continue to chew them. The dried berries are used for their healing benefits in treating coughs, protecting the lungs and beautifying the skin, as well as increasing oxygen capacity to the cells and replenishing vital energy. They are typically used in herbal formulas and added to make teas, wines and syrups. Schisandra is also considered an adaptogenic herb (see Codonopsis, page 167, for more information). According to Chinese folklore, schisandra has the potential to "calm the heart and quiet the spirit." Unlike other berries, such as mulberry, goji or barberries, schisandra is not considered a snacking food. Even though its toxicity is low, its potency is pronounced. You can find this dried berry in Asian grocery stores and Chinese or Western herb stores.

Seaweed or sea vegetables are plants harvested from the sea and generally dried before being rehydrated and eaten. They are sometimes eaten fresh, with a salty, slightly fishy taste and gentle to chewy texture. Sea vegetables have been eaten and used therapeutically by peoples throughout the world. They add depth of flavor to dishes, and their high mineral content is especially beneficial to vegetarians or vegans. Versatile enough to be eaten in a variety of preparations, they are most often associated with Japanese sushi rolls and even desserts. Chinese medicine includes them in herbal formulas to nourish and soften internal cysts and benign masses and reduce swelling. If used only occasionally, buy smaller packages of seaweed, since most varieties will lose their color and flavor when exposed to air and light. Unopened packages may be stored at cool room temperature in a dark place for up to 2 years. Seaweeds can be purchased at Asian grocery stores, health food stores and online from reputable distributors or seaweed companies (see Resources, page 466).

(see Resources, page 466).

Seaweed Varieties

The varieties of seaweeds used in this book include agar-agar (a seaweed used to create gelled dishes such as kanten), arame (used in salads and stir-fries), dulse (toasted, soaked and used in salads and soups), hijiki (used in salads and cooked dishes such as stir-fries), kombu (used as a foundation for broths and cooked with beans and with vegetables), nori (used in condiments, on its own or cooked) and wakame (used in soups and salads). See individual recipes, starting on page 206, for instructions on preparation.

Shiso leaf (*Perilla frutescens*), aka perilla leaf, *jiso* in Japanese and *zi su* in Mandarin, is a member of the mint family and has a taste akin to the aromatic basil leaf. The ruffled leaf is either green or red. It is a quintessential Japanese herb, used in making fermented pickled umeboshi plums and often served with sashimi. In Chinese herbal therapy, it is often used to treat the common cold with a stuffy nose, to move vital energy (*qi*) or to remedy abdominal pain due to fish or crab poisoning. The perilla plant is easy to grow as an annual herb in the garden (be aware: it can spread like mint) or in a container. Look for fresh leaves that give off a fragrant aroma. It is most usually sold fresh in Asian grocery stores but can also be purchased online. It can be purchased dry from reliable suppliers of Chinese herbs.

Shiitake mushrooms (dried) (*Lentinula edodes*) are used in dishes both for their earthy, savory taste and therapeutic value. The highest-quality mushrooms have thick, dark caps with a paler network of lines in a rough starburst shape. The mushrooms are generally soaked before using and the stems discarded, as they are tough and do not have much flavor. Store dried shiitake mushrooms in an airtight container: up to 6 months at cool room temperature in a dark place or 1 year refrigerated. They can be purchased at Asian grocery stores, some large supermarkets and online.

Shiitake mushrooms (fresh):
See Mushrooms.

Sichuan peppercorns, or *hua jiao* in Mandarin, come from the Chinese prickly ash plant (from the *Zanthoxylum family, specifically, Zanthoxylum simulans*) in the citrus family; native to the Sichuan province of western China. Considered a type of berry, the distinctively deep burgundy dried Sichuan peppercorn — which is not related to the conventional peppercorn — is a common ingredient in Sichuan Chinese cooking. It is used to impart a warming and spicy flavor to dishes and forms part of the popular five spice powder. If you bite into a peppercorn, you will be struck by its numbing action on the tongue. Its smoky, fragrant aroma and flavor impart a depth to pickled vegetables and stir-fries. It is also a potent Chinese "herb" used to warm the body, increase circulation of *qi* and blood, stimulate the taste buds and protect the digestive network. The peppercorns make a fine addition to your cooking in moderate amounts if you tend to always feel cold or have sluggish digestion. Avoid Sichuan peppercorns if you have a fever or tend to get agitated easily; they will only serve to heat and dry you out. Look for Sichuan peppercorns that are somewhat shiny in appearance and have a fragrant and slightly spicy aroma. Store in a closed glass container for up to 1 year. Sichuan peppercorns can be purchased in Asian grocery stores or from reliable suppliers of Chinese herbs.

Silkie chicken, or *wu gu ji* ("black-boned chicken") in Mandarin, is a breed of chicken named after the color of its skin and flesh. It has been eaten in China for medicinal purposes for more than 1,000 years. Its flavor is sweet with a neutral nature, neither warming nor cooling, unlike typical chicken, which is warming in nature. Silkie chicken is most often cooked in a soup along with goji berries, dioscorea, tangerine peel, red dates and ginger to nourish women's blood before and after giving birth. With increased migration of Chinese to the West, silkie chicken is in greater demand and is now easier to find in many Asian grocery stores (usually frozen). Treat this meat as you would any chicken in storage and handling.

Solomon's seal (*Polygonatum odoratum*), or *yu zhu* in Mandarin, is a close relative and similar in appearance to lily of the valley (which is poisonous) with its delicate white flowers, but it grows much taller at 3 feet (1 m) high. The plant's rhizome is dried and used in herbal formulas, teas, soups, salves and tinctures. Solomon's seal is valued among North American Native tribes as a "culturally significant plant" for its medicinal value. It also appears in various Chinese herbal formulas and is added as a balancing herb in the tonic soup mix Boost-the-Qi Chicken Soup (page 332). Its mild, sweet flavor is cooling, nourishing the stomach and countering dryness that can be experienced as a dry cough or dry throat.

Dried, it appears as thin, slightly transparent yellowish slivers. When purchasing the dried rhizome, look for rhizomes that are long, soft and yellowish in color. Avoid the ones that are bleached white, which usually means they have been preserved with sulfites. Store in a closed glass jar in a cool dark place for up to 6 months. Solomon's seal is typically available through a reliable supplier of Chinese herbs.

Soybeans (*Glycine max*) are medium in size and fairly round beige or black dried beans. They have a definite bean flavor and are widely used by vegetarians and vegans for their high protein content. Soybeans may be processed to make miso, tofu, tempeh or soy milk or used whole. Dried soy beans should look clean, not dusty, and their interior should be light-colored (a dark color may indicate old beans that will not soften when cooked). Store in an airtight container or bag: up to 3 months at cool room temperature in a cool dark place, 6 months refrigerated or up to 1 year frozen. Beans can be purchased at Asian grocery stores, health food stores or online.

Star anise, aka Chinese star anise or aniseed stars, is the fruit of a Chinese evergreen, *Illicium verum*. The dried fruit is a six- to eight-pointed star, with each point (pod) containing a glossy seed. The pod is more aromatic than the seed and gives a distinctive deep and enriching anise-like flavor to many Asian dishes, particularly in the cuisines of China, Vietnam and India. It is most often used in broths, soups, stews and teas. It is a key ingredient in the Chinese spice combination known as five spice powder, which also includes cinnamon, fennel, cloves and Sichuan peppercorns. Therapeutically, star anise is a warming and aromatic spice that can aid digestion, relieve menstrual or stomach pain due to cold and soothe a cough. Store in a sealed glass jar in a cool dark place for up to 1 year (it will eventually lose its aromatic aroma and flavor). Look for pods that are intact and clean in the spice section of a large supermarket. They can also be found in Asian grocery stores and online.

Sweet potato noodles, typically used in Korean cooking, are thin dried noodles made from the starch of Asian sweet potatoes. The noodles are boiled before being added to other ingredients and are clear and have a slippery texture when cooked; mung bean noodles are the closest substitute. Store noodles in an airtight container in a cool dark place for up to 6 months. They can be purchased at some Asian grocery stores and online.

Tahini is a paste made from ground sesame seeds. It may be made from raw or toasted, hulled or unhulled seeds, but tahini made from hulled toasted seeds tastes the best and does not become rancid as quickly as the paste made from raw seeds. Tahini originated in Middle Eastern and North African cooking and adds body and flavor to dressings and sauces. It should smell rich and mellow, not rancid or acidic. Stir before using to mix in the oil that typically sits at the top of the container. Store container at cool room temperature for up to 2 months or up to 6 months refrigerated. Tahini can be purchased at Middle Eastern markets, some Asian grocery stores, large supermarkets and online.

Tamari is produced from soybeans, salt and water that have been fermented with a specific mixture of bacteria, molds and yeasts. Soy sauce is similar in flavor and texture, but it usually contains wheat.

Tamari has a delicious savory, salty taste and dark color and is used to enhance the color and flavor of other foods. Shop for an organic, GMO- and preservative-free brand, and avoid high-sodium formulations, or simply use less tamari in recipes. Store at cool room temperature for up to 6 months or up to 1 year refrigerated. Tamari can be purchased at Asian grocery stores, large supermarkets and online.

Tamarind is the pod-shaped fruit of a tropical tree, *Tamarindus indica*. The dried ripe fruit is covered by a brittle skin and filled with a slightly sweet and mouth-watering, acidic pulp imbedded with hard seeds. The whole beans are sometimes available, but the recipes in this book use tamarind paste. Even though it is often labeled as free of seeds, some seeds always remain, so the paste must be mixed with water and forced through a sieve to remove them; see individual recipes for details. Tamarind is commonly used in Indian chutneys for its earthy, tart flavor. Store it in an airtight container: up to 2 months at cool room temperature or up to 6 months refrigerated. Tamarind paste is available at Latin American markets (where it will be labeled Tamarindo), East Indian specialty food stores, some Asian grocery stores and online.

Tangerine peel (*Pericarpium Citri reticulatae*), or *chen pi* in Mandarin, is a dried peel that can add the perky tartness of citrus to a dish. The peel is typically dried for at least 3 years, and the longer the drying, the more potent its flavor and therapeutic action. It is often used to stimulate digestive actions and clear coughs with copious phlegm. It is also added to herbal formulas, teas and soups. The peel itself is easy to make at home — simply peel a tangerine, cut out the white pith and set the peel out to dry on a piece of paper in a cool dry place for a couple of weeks. When the peel is dry and hard, keep it in a closed glass jar. If purchased, usually from a reliable supplier of Chinese herbs or an Asian grocery store, look for thin, shiny orangey-red peels. Store in a cool dark place for a few months.

A Treasure

In the Guan Dong province of China, tangerine peel is considered one of the "three treasures" and has a long history of usage as a medicinal.

Taro root is the root of a subtropical plant (*Colocasia esculenta var. antiquorum*), aka taro or eddoes. It has large green leaves and is not to be confused with a type of taro (*Colocasia esculenta*) with large roots that is harder to find and not used in this book. Taro root has an irritant in its skin that is neutralized through cooking, so the recipes in this book specify parboiling before peeling. There is also a level of toxicity in the raw tuber, so it is not recommended to be eaten raw. The roots have a pleasant, bland flavor and when cooked have the texture of a boiled potato. Taro roots can be boiled, steamed, roasted or mashed. Taro roots, also referred to as corms, have been used in Chinese medicine to treat loss of appetite and fatigue due to weak digestion. It is also mashed and applied externally as a poultice to treat boils and cysts. When choosing taro at the store, choose small corms (roots) that are firm and dry on the surface with no black, soft or wet spots. Store loosely wrapped in paper towels or a paper bag for up to 2 weeks at room temperature. Do not store in plastic, as this will cause the roots to rot or grow mold. Taro root can be purchased at some Asian or Latin American grocery stores and markets. If the roots start to sprout, they can still be eaten, but you may want to plant them in a large pot in a warm place and enjoy watching your elephant ear plant grow instead.

Toasted sesame oil is pressed from roasted sesame seeds. Unlike cold-pressed sesame oil, the toasted variety a dark brown color and an earthy, nutty flavor that is commonly used as a flavoring, not as a cooking oil. It is used sparingly to flavor a soup, salad dressing, sauce or stir-fry. Unlike toasted sesame oil, unrefined sesame oil is rich in antioxidants. Oil from toasted sesame seeds does not add or enhance any medicinal effect. Toasted sesame oil can go rancid relatively quickly, so purchase smaller bottles or keep them in the refrigerator. Store in an airtight glass container: up to 3 months at cool room temperature or 6 months refrigerated. Toasted sesame oil can be purchased at Asian grocery stores, health food stores and many large supermarkets, usually in the oils or international section, and online.

Turmeric (fresh) is the rhizome of a sub-tropical plant (*Curcuma longa*) in the ginger family. Its exterior resembles the brown, papery skin of gingerroot, but turmeric has smaller rhizomes with a bright yellow-orange interior. Grated fresh turmeric has a slightly spicy and medicinal flavor with an attractive bitterness. Curcumin, the active ingredient in turmeric, is best absorbed when mixed with beneficial fats and balanced with black pepper. Many people include turmeric in soups, stir-fries and even smoothies. Shop for plump roots with no soft or dark spots. Store loosely wrapped in paper towels or a paper bag for up to 2 weeks at room temperature. Do not store in plastic, as this will cause the roots to rot or grow mold. For long-term storage, peel and grate the turmeric and freeze in an airtight container for up to 6 months.

Turmeric can be purchased fresh at some Asian grocery stores and dried in the spice section of many grocery stores.

Umeboshi plum (*Prunus mume*) aka Japanese apricot, ume, mume fruit, ume plum fruit, or *wu mei* in Mandarin, is part of the *Prunus* family and resembles a small, bland apricot on the tree. The umeboshi noted in the recipes section of this book is a fermented food, processed with the unripe green umeboshi plum and perilla leaf (*Perilla frutescens*), a member of the mint family and a powerful herb used to clear heat, move *qi*, clear food toxicity and ease indigestion. The perilla leaf is what lends the fermented umeboshi plum and paste its deep pink color. Umeboshi is often added to dressings, used in making pickles and prepared as a digestive tea with ginger and tamari. Umeboshi is sour and astringent in flavor and can be used to alleviate a sour stomach, ease hangover symptoms, activate appetite and help with constipation. You may also find umeboshi vinegar and paste or concentrate (called *bainiku ekisu*) in Japanese cooking, where it is used as a digestive aid. The plums and paste are usually found in jars or containers in health food stores, large supermarkets and Asian grocery stores. Purchase umeboshi plum or paste that is pure, made only with added salt and red shiso (perilla) leaves, with no additives, preservatives or food coloring.

Wakame: See Seaweed.

Western greens include some members of the *Brassica* genus, including kale, collards and mustard greens, as well as some milder greens like spinach and Swiss chard. See the recipes section, page 206, for details on which greens to use. While denser, chewier greens can typically be substituted for one another, this is not the case for tender greens. When purchasing greens, they should be dry on the surface with no soft or wet spots. If they have lost some internal moisture, they may be slightly wilted, but this is fine. Store loosely wrapped in paper towels or a paper bag: up to 2 days at cool room temperature or 1 week refrigerated. Avoid storing in plastic, as this can cause the leaves to rot. Greens can be purchased at grocery stores and may be grown in most regions of North America.

White peony (*Paeonia lactiflora* Pall.), aka *bai shao* in Mandarin, is mostly known in the West for the lush, full and abundant flowers that bloom in early spring. The peony was named after Paeon, the Greek physician of the gods, indicating the high regard in which it is held. In Chinese herbal medicine, it is the root that is dried and used in medicinal teas, soups and tinctures. It is always used in conjunction with other herbs; along with licorice, white peony is the other ingredient in the well-known Chinese herbal formula *shao yao gan cao tang*, used to relieve muscle cramping and spasm. Store in a sealed glass jar in a cool dark place for 6 months and no longer than 1 year. Dried white peony root is available through reliable suppliers of Chinese herbs. Look for roots that have not been treated with sulphites.

FOODS THAT HEAL: Their Nature, Flavor and Therapeutic Value According to Chinese Medicine

The following chart offers a quick reference on the properties and therapeutic actions of foods to improve overall health or the state of minor health issues according to Chinese medicine principles. You can use the chart to look up ingredients or learn ways to eat and prepare foods. It includes a number of common foods, many of which are included in the recipes starting on page 206. These foods are described according to their thermal nature (capacity to warm or cool the body), flavor and therapeutic health actions on the body, as well as the typical ways to eat and prepare each food. (See Chapter 3 for more information on the thermal nature and flavor of foods, Chapter 4 for more insight on food groups, and Chapter 6 for additional information on the preparation and therapeutic impact of foods on the body.)

Notes on terms:

- **Decoct** indicates that the essence — and therefore the therapeutic value of this food — has been extracted through boiling in water and consumed as a tea or a soup.

- **Infused** indicates that an herb or food has been soaked in water, juice or alcohol.

- **Steeped** indicates that an herb, fruit or tea has been immersed in liquid, usually water, that has been boiled.

- **Drains or removes damp** indicates a food is being used to increase urination (diuretic) and strengthen the function of the stomach and spleen, the organs responsible for digestion and transformation. "Dampness" is a Chinese medicine term indicating a failure to metabolize and transform moisture in the body. The stomach and spleen act as the central distribution hub for *qi* (energy) in the body. When this organ system is deficient, metabolism suffers and it is easier to retain water and weight. Foods that cause dampness in the body include dairy products, wheat and refined flours, sugar, refined starch, excess raw foods, cold beverages and fatty, greasy and deep-fried food.

- **Middle or central burner** relates to the digestive network: stomach, spleen, liver, gallbladder and small intestine.

Whole Grains

Food	Thermal Nature	Flavor	Organ Network	Therapeutic Action and Benefit	Ways to Eat and Prepare
Barley	Cool	Sweet	Spleen, stomach, bladder	Induces urination; reinforces spleen and stomach; relieves thirst	Boil, steam, bake, decoct as a tea or in soups
Brown rice – short-grain, long grain, jasmine or basmati	Neutral	Sweet	Stomach, spleen	Nourishes; fortifies stomach and spleen; promotes digestion; calming; quenches thirst; treats loss of appetite, diarrhea	Boil, bake, steam, roast, congee
Brown rice – sweet (glutinous)	Warming	Sweet	Stomach, spleen, lung	Calms central nervous system; reinforces and nourishes stomach and spleen; reinforces lung *qi*; counters fatigue, benefits those who feel cold	Boil, bake, steam, roast, congee, ground into a powder to drink as a tea. Sweet rice is often pounded to make a sticky rice paste known as *mochi*, a Japanese treat.
Buckwheat	Cool	Sweet	Stomach, spleen, large intestine	Strengthens spleen; moves *qi* and undigested food; disperses heat; treats food stagnation, diarrhea	Steam, boil, ground into a powder to drink as a tea
Cornmeal – stone-ground, coarse, non-GMO	Neutral	Sweet	Kidneys, large intestine, stomach	Strengthens overall energy; lowers blood sugar; promotes urination	Use in baked goods
Millet	Slightly cold	Sweet, salty	Spleen, stomach, kidneys	Nourishes spleen and kidneys; relieves thirst	Boil, steam, make into a porridge, congee or gruel
Oats	Warming	Sweet	Stomach, spleen, kidneys, heart, lung, large intestine	Builds stamina and warmth; *qi* and blood tonic; stabilizes blood sugar; soothes the digestive and nervous systems	Boil, steam, bake, roast, make into a porridge
Wheat (If you have a sensitivity to gluten, avoid wheat.)	Cool	Sweet	Heart, spleen, kidneys	Nourishes the heart; calming; relieves thirst; induces urination; calms nerves	Boil, steam, bake, decoct as a tea

Beans, Pulses and Other Legumes

Food	Thermal Nature	Flavor	Organ Network	Therapeutic Action and Benefit	Ways to Eat and Prepare
Adzuki beans	Neutral	Sweet/sour	Kidneys	Detoxifies the body; clears heat; disperses stagnant blood; reduces swelling; mildly diuretic; counters edema	Juice is prepared by simmering 1 cup (250 mL) of adzuki beans in 5 cups (1.25 L) of water for 1 hour. Strain before drinking ½ cup (125 mL) juice 30 minutes before meals. Boil, bake, use in soups, grain dishes and desserts
Anasazi beans	Neutral	Sweet	Spleen, kidneys	Induces urination; reduces blood cholesterol; lowers blood pressure	Boil, slow cook, bake
Black-eyed peas	Warming	Sweet	Spleen, stomach	Energizes the lungs and colon; counteracts water retention; reduces blood cholesterol; lowers blood pressure	Boil, slow cook, bake
Black soybeans	Neutral	Sweet	Spleen, kidneys	Reinforces stomach and spleen; nourishes kidney yin; counters water retention and constipation as well as diarrhea; regulates hot flashes; treats sore throat, headache, fevers; relieves muscle cramps, rheumatism, pain in knees	Boil, bake, decoct as a tea. Fermented beans are used in herbal medicine, fermented and salted beans in food preparation.
Bolita beans	Neutral	Sweet	Spleen, kidneys	Mildly diuretic; reduces blood cholesterol; lowers blood pressure	Boil, bake
Chickpeas	Neutral	Sweet	Pancreas, stomach, heart	Induces urination; reduces blood cholesterol; lowers blood pressure	Boil, bake
Fava beans	Neutral	Sweet	Spleen, stomach	Reinforces the spleen; induces urination to relieve edema	Boil, bake, braise, steam
Green peas, fresh (also dried split peas – green and yellow)	Neutral	Sweet	Spleen, stomach	Reinforces spleen; relieves edema; promotes production of body fluids; eases thirst; mildly laxative; clears skin	Boil, steam, decoct as a tea. Fresh peas can be eaten raw; use dried peas in soup.

Beans, Pulses and Other Legumes (continued)

Food	Thermal Nature	Flavor	Organ Network	Therapeutic Action and Benefit	Ways to Eat and Prepare
Kidney beans	Neutral	Sweet	Spleen, large intestine, small intestine	Reinforces spleen; reduces edema; increases blood circulation	Boil, bake
Lentils	Neutral	Sweet	Heart, kidneys	Benefits circulation; stimulates adrenal system; increases vitality	Boil, bake
Lima beans	Cool	Sweet	Liver, lung	Promotes healthy skin; increases yin fluids	Boil or steam
Mung beans	Cool	Sweet	Heart, stomach	Clears summer heat; induces urination; binds and clears toxic residues; reduces heat symptoms that may include skin rashes, blemishes, ulcers, headaches, sore muscles or joints; reduces swelling; helps lower high blood pressure; reduces thirst	Sprout and eat raw, steam, boil, decoct as a tea with lonicera buds to clear heat. Drink liquid from mung bean soup to help reduce mild food poisoning symptoms.
Soybeans (fresh — edamame — and dried)	Neutral	Sweet	Stomach, spleen	Reduces damp; alkalizing action helps eliminate toxins from the body; reinforces spleen; improves circulation; restores pancreatic function	Steam fresh beans (edamame), boil or bake dried beans. Best digested if fermented in forms such as tempeh, natto, miso, tamari. Otherwise, soak for more than 8 hours and then boil. Also made into soy milk and tofu.
Tofu (* If you have sensitivity to soybeans, do not eat tofu. If you have thyroid issues, consult your practitioner. Because of its cooling nature, eat only once a week.)	Cool	Sweet, bland	Spleen	Adds lubrication to body; benefits and moisturizes hair and skin; mildly diuretic; reinforces stomach and spleen; supports milk production in nursing mothers	Steam, bake, stir-fry, mash, boil. Absorbs flavor and adds protein to cooked dishes.

Nuts and Seeds

Food	Thermal Nature	Flavor	Organ Network	Therapeutic Action and Benefit	Ways to Eat and Prepare
Almonds	Neutral	Sweet	Lung, spleen, large intestine	Moistens lungs; relieves difficult breathing	Eat raw, decoct as a tea or infuse in alcohol, blanch, roast, toast, grind into flour. Also made into milk.
Brazil nuts	Neutral	Sweet, slightly bitter	Lung, spleen	Strengthens spleen and lungs	Eat raw, roast, grind into coarse powder
Cashews	Neutral	Sweet	Stomach, large intestine	Replenishes energy; strengthens stomach and large intestine; balances yin	Blanch, roast, toast, soak and blend
Chestnuts	Warming	Sweet	Kidneys, stomach, spleen	Invigorates the *qi*; tonic for stomach, spleen and kidneys; strengthens muscles; promotes circulation; counters weakness, diarrhea	Steam, bake, roast, add to soups and long-cooked stews. Also dried, ground and made into flour.
Chia seeds	Warming	Sweet, bland	Large intestine, kidneys	Moistens; relieves constipation; reduces nervousness; treats insomnia; improves mental focus	Soak for puddings and juices, toast, add raw to almost any dish
Flax seeds	Warming	Sweet	Stomach, spleen, large intestine	Protects mucous membranes; counters dryness and benefits the skin; reduces cholesterol; lowers blood pressure, benefits the bowels; anti-inflammatory	Grind just before use and add to smoothies, dressings, baked goods. Note that cooking at high heat alters the omega-3s.
Gingko nuts	Neutral	Sweet, slightly bitter	Lung, spleen, kidneys	Used in asthma herbal formulas to relieve difficult breathing; nourishes spleen; treats diarrhea and leucorrhea	Boil and add to soups, decoct as a tea. Also dried and ground to a powder. Decoct and drink as a tea.
Hemp seeds	Neutral	Sweet	Large intestine, spleen, stomach	Moistens large intestines and frees the bowels; clears heat (internally or used topically); benefits older people who suffer constipation	Decoct as a tea. Can grind and add to cereals, condiments, dressings. Do not cook at high heat, which destroys omega-3s.
Lotus seeds	Neutral	Sweet, slightly sour	Spleen, kidneys, heart	Nourishes heart; tranquilizes mind; astringes and relieves diarrhea	Eat fresh seeds raw, boil, decoct as a tea, add to soups, grain dishes, stews. Also dried and ground to a fine powder.

Nuts and Seeds (continued)

Food	Thermal Nature	Flavor	Organ Network	Therapeutic Action and Benefit	Ways to Eat and Prepare
Peanuts	Neutral	Sweet	Spleen, lung	Increases spleen *qi*; moistens lungs; clears phlegm	Eat raw, boil, roast, grind into a fine powder or nut butter, decoct as a tea
Pecans	Warming	Sweet	Heart, stomach, spleen	Counters cold; supports the nervous system; promotes heart health	Blanch, roast, toast, grind into powder or nut butter
Pine nuts	Warming	Sweet	Lung, large intestine	Moistens lungs and large intestine; eases constipation	Eat raw, roast, ground into a powder, add to salads, vegetable dishes
Pistachios	Neutral	Sweet	Liver, kidneys	Balances yin and yang; *qi* tonic; eases constipation; reduces blood cholesterol	Eat raw, roast, mix into vegetable dishes, grind into nut butter
Poppy seeds (*Use in moderation. If pregnant or nursing, or a child, avoid due to the seed's addictive nature.)	Neutral	Sour	Large intestine, lung, kidneys	Relieves cough; sedates and calms the nervous system; eases chronic cough and diarrhea	Add to baked goods, salads and salad dressings
Sesame seeds – black	Neutral	Sweet	Kidneys, liver, large intestine	Strengthens liver and kidneys; sesame oil moistens skin and large intestine; counters constipation; yin tonic	Roast, grind. Also made into oil.
Sesame seeds – unhulled brown	Cool	Sweet	Kidneys, liver, large intestine	Supplements blood and body fluids; sesame oil moistens skin and counters constipation	Roast, grind. Also made into oil.
Sunflower seeds	Neutral	Sweet	Spleen, large intestine	Nourishes yin; moistens large intestine; counters constipation	Eat raw, roast, grind, decoct as a tea
Tahini (ground sesame paste)	Cool	Sweet	Kidneys, liver, large intestine	Supplements blood and body fluids	Use in sauces, dressings, spreads
Walnuts	Warming	Sweet, bitter	Kidneys, lung	Strengthens kidneys and lungs; lubricates large intestine; reduces inflammation; alleviates asthma and pain	Eat raw, roast, grind. Also made into milk.

Vegetables

Food	Thermal Nature	Flavor	Organ Network	Therapeutic Action and Benefit	Ways to Eat and Prepare
Beets	Neutral	Sweet, slightly bitter	Heart, liver, large intestine	Balances spleen *qi*; balances stomach *qi*; supports blood circulation	Boil, roast, steam, grate, pickle, add to soups, stir-fries, salads, ferment into kvass
Bitter melon	Cold	Bitter	Stomach, heart, liver	Clears heat; relieves summer heat; improves vision; stabilizes blood sugar	Sauté, juice, ferment, add to stir-fries, soups
Broccoli	Cool	Sweet, slightly bitter	Liver, spleen, stomach	Cools liver; cools blood	Boil, roast, steam, grate, add to soups, stir-fries, salads
Burdock root	Cooling	Bitter, sweet	Liver, kidneys	Stimulates bile secretion; cleanses and purifies blood via liver detoxification pathways; supports digestion; eliminates toxins	Boil, roast, steam, grate, pickle, decoct as a tea, add to soups, stir-fries, salads
Cabbage	Neutral	Sweet	Spleen, stomach	Nourishes and relieves spasms; benefits digestion; clears heat; stimulates liver metabolism	Steam, blanch, roast, sauté, braise, ferment into sauerkraut or kimchi
Carrots	Neutral	Sweet	Spleen, liver, lung	Aids digestion; clears heat; reinforces liver; benefits the eyes; clears coughs	Eat raw, juice, grate, steam, boil, roast, add to soups or cook with sugar to aid food stagnation
Celery	Cool	Pungent, sweet, slightly bitter	Liver, stomach, bladder	Clears heat; calms liver; reinforces stomach; eases urination; lowers blood pressure; resolves headache and dizziness due to hypertension	Eat raw, juice, steam, sauté. Be careful not to overcook.
Chayotes	Neutral to cooling	Sweet, bland	Lung	Helps soften and dissolve kidney stones; treats arteriosclerosis and hypertension; lubricates lungs; clears phlegm	Add to soups and stews. Must be peeled to eat raw.
Chile pepper	Hot	Pungent	Spleen, stomach, heart	Warms middle burner (digestion) to dissolve food stagnation; disperses cold; dries dampness; induces perspiration	Add to beans and other dishes to add spice and warmth

Vegetables (continued)					
Food	Thermal Nature	Flavor	Organ Network	Therapeutic Action and Benefit	Ways to Eat and Prepare
Chinese chives	Warming	Sweet, acrid	Kidneys, stomach, liver	Reinforces kidneys; assists yang; warms and stimulates digestion (middle burner); aids appetite; improves blood circulation	Sauté, use as a garnish, add to soups
Chinese spring onions, also known as green onions or scallions	Warming	Pungent; slightly bitter	Heart, large intestine, lung, stomach	Induces perspiration and sweating; disperses exterior cold; activates yang; expels parasites; eliminates toxins; supports blood circulation; induces urination	Eat raw; use as a garnish; stir-fry; steam, blanch, add to soups, stews; decoct as medicinal tea
Cilantro (fresh coriander)	Warming	Pungent, sweet	Spleen, stomach, lung	Induces perspiration; stimulates the appetite; aids digestion; calms stomach spasms	Use as garnish, add to dressings, condiments, salads, soups
Corn, fresh	Neutral	Sweet	Stomach, bladder	Regulates digestion; acts as a diuretic; treats loss of appetite, edema	Boil, roast, bake, steam
Cucumbers	Cool	Sweet	Stomach, bladder	Clears heat; quenches thirst; relieves edema	Eat raw, add to salads, boil, sauté, pickle or ferment
Daikon	Neutral, cool	Pungent	Lung, stomach	Loosens phlegm in lungs; quenches thirst; diuretic; relieves indigestion	Eat raw, pickle or ferment, steam, boil, decoct as a tea, add to soups
Dandelion greens	Cool	Bitter	Spleen, stomach, kidneys	Cools liver heat; acts as a laxative; reduces swelling and inflammation	Eat raw, steam, blanch, boil
Eggplant	Slightly cold	Sweet	Large intestine, stomach	Clears heat; cools blood; assists bowels; treats dysentery, diarrhea	Steam, roast, grill, stew
Endive	Cooling	Bitter, sweet	Liver	Cools liver heat	Eat raw, add to salads, blanch, roast, steam
Fennel	Slightly warming	Pungent, sweet	Liver, spleen, stomach	Regulates *qi*; relieves pain; reinforces stomach; harmonizes middle burner (digestion)	Eat raw in salads, juice, steam, roast
Garlic	Warming	Pungent, sweet	Spleen, stomach, lung	Warms middle burner (digestion); promotes circulation; antiviral and antibacterial; kills parasites; aids digestion	Eat raw, juice, roast, add to soups, stews and a variety of dishes

Vegetables (continued)

Food	Thermal Nature	Flavor	Organ Network	Therapeutic Action and Benefit	Ways to Eat and Prepare
Leeks	Warming	Pungent, sweet	Lung, liver, kidneys, stomach	Moves *qi*; warms middle burner (digestion); moves blood stasis; dissipates cold; counters bleeding and diarrhea	Steam, blanch, roast, add to soups, stir-fries, stews
Lettuce	Cool, cold	Sweet, slightly bitter	Large intestine, stomach	Cools heat; induces urination; stimulates milk flow in nursing mothers	Eat raw, boil, blanch, grill, roast, stir-fry
Lotus root	Cool (raw), slightly warming (cooked)	Sweet	Spleen, stomach, heart	Clears heat; staunches nosebleeds	Juice, ferment, decoct as a tea, add to soups, stews, stir-fries, salads
Mustard greens	Warming	Pungent	Lung, stomach	Expels phlegm; warms middle burner (digestion); reinforces stomach; dispels cold	Sauté, steam, blanch, ferment with salt, add to soups
Onions	Warming	Bitter, pungent	Lung, stomach, large intestine	Activates yang; descends *qi*; aids bowel movements; lowers blood pressure; reduces cholesterol	Steam, juice, add to soups, stews
Parsnips	Neutral, warming	Sweet, pungent, bitter	Liver, lung, stomach	Balances stomach, lubricates intestines; mildly diuretic; promotes perspiration; clears damp	Steam, boil, bake, roast
Plantain	Cold	Bitter	Large intestine, liver, stomach, spleen	Mildly astringent; anti-inflammatory	Sauté, steam, fry, boil, dried and baked or fried as a chip
Potatoes	Neutral	Sweet	Spleen, stomach	Reinforces stomach and spleen; relieves spasms and pain	Eat raw, juice, sauté, boil, bake, steam
Pumpkin	Warming	Sweet	Spleen, stomach	Reinforces spleen and stomach; warms middle burner (digestion); nourishes *qi*; dissolves phlegm	Steam, bake, roast boil, purée
Radishes	Cool	Pungent	Lung, stomach	Clears mucus and phlegm; treats indigestion; helps with digestion of fatty foods; clears blood heat	Eat raw, juice, steam, stir-fry pickle or ferment

Vegetables (continued)

Food	Thermal Nature	Flavor	Organ Network	Therapeutic Action and Benefit	Ways to Eat and Prepare
Spinach	Cool	Sweet	Large intestine, stomach, liver	Moistens dryness internally; eases bowels; nurtures liver; quenches thirst	Eat raw in salads, sauté, boil, steam, add to soups
Shallots	Warming	Pungent	Lung, stomach, liver, large intestine	Improves blood and *qi* circulation; disperses cold	Eat raw, sauté, add to cooked dishes
Squash – summer	Cooling	Sweet, bitter	Stomach, liver	Reduces inflammation; cools stomach and liver heat	Eat raw, steam, bake, roast
Sweet potatoes	Neutral; cooling if eaten raw	Sweet	Spleen, stomach, large intestine	Supplements middle burner (digestion); supplements *qi*; promotes bowel movements; promotes body fluids; quenches thirst when used raw	Eat raw, boil, bake, roast, steam
Taro root	Neutral	Pungent, sweet	Spleen, stomach	Strengthens stomach and spleen; reduces swelling	Boil, add to soups and stews
Turnips	Cool	Pungent, sweet	Stomach, lung	Clears heat; promotes production of body fluids; dissolves phlegm; cools blood; promotes urination	Eat raw, steam, boil

Wild Vegetables

Food	Thermal Nature	Flavor	Organ Network	Therapeutic Action and Benefit	Ways to Eat and Prepare
Bamboo shoots	Cold	Sweet, slightly bitter	Lung, stomach, large intestine	Cooling; quenches thirst; assists bowel movements; clears stomach heat	Eat raw in salads, sauté, stir-fry
Daylily, buds, fresh or dried	Slightly cold	Sweet	Heart, liver	Tranquilizes mind; cools blood, improves vision	Sauté, boil
Purslane	Slightly cold	Sour, sweet	Large intestine, bladder, liver	Clears heat; improves detoxification process in the body; useful in cases of dysentery; can stop bleeding; as a juice to ease dry cough; treats diarrhea	Eat raw in salads, add to soups, congee, juices; dried as a tea; topically as a poultice for fevers, cuts, inflammation

Wild Vegetables (continued)

Food	Thermal Nature	Flavor	Organ Network	Therapeutic Action and Benefit	Ways to Eat and Prepare
Shepherd's purse (*Capsella bursa-pastoris*)	Cool	Sweet, pungent, a bit bitter	Liver, stomach, bladder, small intestine	Cools the blood; stops bleeding; reduces infection; induces urination; clears heat; minimizes post-partum bleeding and difficult, excessive menstruation; relieves headache; benefits lactation	Eat raw in salads, juice, steam, decoct as a tea

Mushrooms and Fungi

Food	Thermal Nature	Flavor	Organ Network	Therapeutic Action and Benefit	Ways to Eat and Prepare
Cordyceps	Warming	Mild and sweet, slightly pungent and mildly bitter	Lung, kidneys	Rejuvenates and restores *qi*; strengthens the essence (*jing*); strengthens immune system; eliminates phlegm; builds blood; addresses fatigue; treats viral hepatitis, erectile dysfunction due to kidney deficiency, infertility	Add to soups, vegetable dishes, decoct as a tea
Cremini, button and white mushrooms	Neutral to slightly cold	Sweet	Spleen, stomach, lung	Reinforces spleen; replenishes *qi*; moistens dryness; dissolves phlegm	Sauté, add to soups, stir-fries, stews, steep as tea
Oyster mushrooms	Slightly warming	Sweet	Spleen, stomach, lung	Reinforces the spleen; improves appetite; removes damp; relieves spasms; treats loss of appetite, soreness or pain in joints	Add to soups, stir-fries, steep as tea
Shiitake mushrooms	Neutral	Sweet	Spleen, liver, stomach	Reinforces the spleen; builds *qi*; strengthens immune system; resolves phlegm	Add to soups, stews, steep as tea. For stronger flavor, use dried.
Wood ears, dried,	Neutral	Sweet	Lung, stomach, liver	Moistens lungs; nourishes yin; stops bleeding	Boil, add to soups and other dishes. Needs to be soaked.

Seaweeds

Food	Thermal Nature	Flavor	Organ Network	Therapeutic Action and Benefit	Ways to Eat and Prepare
Agar-agar	Cold	Sweet, salty	Lung, large intestine	Moistens internal dryness; dissolves phlegm; clears heat; promotes bowel movements; can chelate heavy metals	Soaked until soft and torn into shreds to add to salads; dissolve in liquid to make vegan gelatin

Seaweeds (continued)					
Food	Thermal Nature	Flavor	Organ Network	Therapeutic Action and Benefit	Ways to Eat and Prepare
Dulse	Cool	Salty	Kidneys	Increases levels of iodine; rich in magnesium; activates enzymes	Roast, soak and add to salads and soups
Hijiki and arame	Cool	Salty	Kidneys	Induces urination; resolves phlegm; detoxifies the body; benefits thyroid; helps normalize blood sugar levels; supports hormone function; soothes nerves	Steam, sauté, soak and add to salads, soups and other cooked dishes
Kombu (aka kelp)	Cold	Salty	Liver, stomach, kidneys	Used to mineralize food; moistens dryness; iodine content benefits the thyroid; dissolves phlegm; relieves edema	Soak and add to broths, soups and cooked dishes, decoct as a tea
Nori	Cold	Sweet, salty	Liver, lung, stomach, kidneys	Highest, most easily digested protein content found in sea vegetables; increases yin; induces urination; lowers cholesterol; aids digestion of fried foods; dissolves phlegm and treats cough with yellow mucus	Toast and add to salads, stews, dressings, soups
Wakame	Cool	Salty	Liver, stomach, kidneys	Rich in calcium and niacin; used in Japanese culture to purify the mother's blood after childbirth; promotes healthy hair and skin	Soak and add to salads and soups

Fruit					
Apples	Cool	Sweet, slightly sour	Spleen, stomach	Quenches thirst; reinforces the spleen; promotes hydration of body tissues; reduces fever	Eat raw, juice, bake, steam, braise
Apricots	Neutral	Sweet, sour	Stomach, lung	Hydrates, eases thirst; moistens lungs; relieves difficult breathing	Used to make jams and preserves, steam, bake, boil, juice, dried
Avocados	Cool	Sweet	Large intestine, liver, lung	Blood and yin tonic; harmonizes liver; lubricates lungs and large intestine	Eat raw. Also pressed into oil.

Food	Thermal Nature	Flavor	Organ Network	Therapeutic Action and Benefit	Ways to Eat and Prepare
Fruit (continued)					
Bananas	Cold	Sweet	Stomach, lung	Nourishes yin; moistens dryness; eases constipation; eases dry throat	Eat raw, steam, boil, bake, roast, sauté
Cherries, sweet	Warming	Sweet, slightly sour	Spleen, liver	Astringes premature ejaculation; used in treatment of gout, arthritis, rheumatism; increases *qi*	Eat raw, juice, bake, decoct as a tea or in alcohol
Coconut	Warming	Sweet	Heart, spleen, stomach, large intestine	Tonifies *qi* and blood; stops bleeding; used for nosebleeds; nourishes whole body; coconut milk clears effects of summer heat	Made into milk used in curries, soups, beverages, sap made into coconut sugar for baking
Cranberries	Cool, neutral	Sweet, sour	Bladder, kidneys, large intestine	Increases appetite; dispels heat and damp	Fresh: juice, boil, bake, preserve; dried: add to baked goods and various dishes
Dates – red (jujubes)	Neutral	Sweet	Stomach, spleen	Supplements *qi* and blood; improves poor appetite; calms spirit	Add to soups, stews, congee, decoct as a tea
Fig	Neutral	Sweet	Spleen, lung, large intestine	Moistens lungs; eases sore throat; moistens large intestine; assists bowel movement	Eat raw; dried: boil, decoct as a tea
Grape	Neutral	Sweet, slightly sour	Kidneys, liver, stomach	Strengthens the liver and kidney; nourishes *qi* and blood; promotes internal hydration; induces urination	Eat raw, juice, decoct for medicinal wines
Grapefruit	Cold	Sweet, sour Peel is sweet, bitter & warming	Stomach, lung	Hydrates; eases thirst; restores appetite, redirects the flow of *qi* downward (nausea or vomiting); eases coughs and clears phlegm	Eat raw, juice, decoct peel as a tea
Kiwifruit	Cold	Sweet, sour	Stomach, bladder	Clears heat; hydrates; harmonizes and settles the stomach; induces urination	Eat raw, juice
Kumquats	Slightly warming	Sweet, sour	Lung, stomach, liver	Clears phlegm with a cough; regulates *qi*; relieves stagnation	Eat raw, candy with honey, decoct as a tea

Food	Thermal Nature	Flavor	Organ Network	Therapeutic Action and Benefit	Ways to Eat and Prepare
				Fruit (continued)	
Lemon	Slightly cold	Sour	Stomach, liver, lung	Relieves summer heat; quenches thirst; relieves coughs and clears phlegm; calms nausea	Eat raw, juice, pickle
Lychee	Slightly warming	Sweet, slightly sour	Spleen, stomach, liver	Nourishes blood; eases thirst; strengthens spleen *qi*; promotes hydration	Raw, decoct as a tea
Longan	Warming	Sweet	Spleen, heart, kidneys, lung	Enriches blood; eases tension; calms nerves; aids sleep; removes damp	Eat raw; dried: decoct as a tea, add to soups or infuse dried longan in alcohol
Oranges	Cool	Sweet, sour	Stomach, gall-bladder	Induces urination; quenches thirst; resolves mucous	Eat raw, juice, add dried orange peel and decoct as tea; add fresh twist of peel and steep as tea
Peaches	Neutral	Sweet, sour	Stomach, large intestine	Reinforces the stomach; promotes production of body fluids; moistens dryness	Eat raw, steam, boil. Also available dried.
Pears	Cool	Sweet, slightly sour	Stomach, lung	Promotes hydration of body tissues; moistens dryness; dissolves phlegm; clears heat	Eat raw, juice, steam, poach, decoct as a tea
Persimmon	Cold	Sweet	Lung, stomach, large intestine	Moistens the lungs; dissolves phlegm; eases thirst; treats dry cough	Eat raw or dried, steam
Pineapple	Slightly cold	Sweet, slightly sour	Stomach, bladder	Quenches thirst; induces urination; promotes digestion	Eat raw, juice, bake, grill
Plums	Cold	Sweet, sour	Liver, stomach	Clears liver heat; relieves dehydration and quenches thirst; benefits constipation	Eat raw, juice, steam, boil, bake, juice. Also available dried.
Pomegranates	Neutral	Sweet, slightly sour, astringent	Stomach, large intestine	Eases thirst; moistens body tissues; relieves diarrhea; can kill worms in intestinal tract	Eat raw, juice, steep as tea
Prunes	Cold	Sweet, sour	Liver, large intestine	Relieves constipation; reduces blood cholesterol	Stew, juice, use in baking
Quince	Cool	Slightly sweet, sour, slightly bitter	Large intestine, stomach	Relieves diarrhea; reduces inflammation in intestinal tract; reduces blood cholesterol	Stew, bake, braise, use to make jams. Quince needs to be cooked.

Fruit (continued)

Food	Thermal Nature	Flavor	Organ Network	Therapeutic Action and Benefit	Ways to Eat and Prepare
Tamarind	Cool	Sweet, sour	Stomach, large intestine	Clears heat; relieves summer heat; stimulates digestion; promotes bowel movements	Decoct to flavor dishes and sauces
Tangerines	Neutral	Sweet, sour	Lung, stomach	Relieves nausea and vomiting; stimulates appetite; clears phlegm	Fresh, juice, peel is dried and used in teas and soups
Tomatoes	Cool	Sweet, sour	Liver, stomach	Clears heat; quenches thirst; cools blood	Eat raw, juice, roast, steam, braise
Umeboshi (aka pickled Japanese plums)	Cold	Sweet, sour	Large intestine, stomach	Enhances digestion; nourishes blood; relieves indigestion and constipation	Add to teas, ingredient in salad dressings and sauces; as a vinegar
Watermelon	Cold	Sweet	Stomach, heart, bladder	Clears excessive heat; quenches thirst; induces urination	Eat raw, juice, add to salads

Meats

Food	Thermal Nature	Flavor	Organ Network	Therapeutic Action and Benefit	Ways to Eat and Prepare
Beef	Warming	Sweet	Spleen, stomach	Nourishes *qi* and blood	Roast, bake, stir-fry, use in soups, stews
Chicken	Warming	Sweet	Stomach, spleen	Nourishes *qi* and blood; tonic for kidneys and *jing*; used for weakness after childbirth	Roast, bake, stir-fry, use in soups, stews
Chicken – Silkie (black-boned)	Neutral	Sweet	Liver, spleen, kidneys	Nourishes liver and kidneys; clears heat; nourishes spleen and stomach	Roast, bake, stir-fry, use in soups, stews
Duck	Neutral	Sweet, salty	Lung, spleen, kidneys	Strong tonic for kidney yin and yang; induces urination	Roast, bake, stir-fry, use in soups, stews
Egg whites (chicken)	Cool to neutral	Sweet	Spleen, stomach	Nourishes blood, yin and *qi*; beneficial after illness; benefits the fetus	Boil, poach, fry, bake
Egg yolks (chicken)	Warming	Sweet	Spleen, stomach	Nourishes blood, yin and *qi*; beneficial after illness	Boil, poach, fry, bake
Eggs (duck)	Cool	Sweet	Lung	Nourishes yin; treats coughs with little mucus, dry mouth; eases thirst	Boil, poach, fry, bake
Lamb	Warming	Sweet	Spleen, kidneys	Benefits digestion; enriches *qi* and blood; dispels cold; aids lactation; treats weakness; promotes appetite	Roast, bake, stir-fry, use in soups, stews

Meats (continued)

Food	Thermal Nature	Flavor	Organ Network	Therapeutic Action and Benefit	Ways to Eat and Prepare
Pork	Neutral	Sweet, salty	Lung, spleen, liver	Nourishes yin; moistens dryness; enriches blood	Roast, bake, stir-fry, use in soups, stews
Rabbit	Cool	Sweet	Spleen	Reinforces spleen; enriches *qi*	Roast, bake, stir-fry, use in soups, stews

Seafood

Food	Thermal Nature	Flavor	Organ Network	Therapeutic Action and Benefit	Ways to Eat and Prepare
Anchovies	Neutral to warming	Sweet, salty	Spleen, stomach	Enriches *qi*; reinforces and warms stomach and spleen; dispels cold	Boil, sauté; marinated, brined or salted form used in salad dressings and sauces
Catfish	Neutral	Sweet	Spleen, stomach	Reinforces spleen; enriches *qi*; promotes production of milk if due to *qi* deficiency; induces urination if due to weak spleen	Steam, poach, fry
Clams	Cold	Sweet, salty	Liver, kidneys	Nourishes yin; improves vision; nurtures the liver; clears internal feelings of heat	Eat raw, steam, boil, in soups, stews
Crabs	Cold	Salty	Liver	Activates blood circulation	Steam, boil
Eels	Neutral	Sweet	Liver, spleen, kidneys	Nourishing; builds *qi*; counters pain; enriches blood; expels parasites and painful obstructions	Boil, sauté, fry
Mussels	Warming	Salty	Liver, kidneys	Nourishes liver and kidneys; enriches *jing* and blood	Boil, steam
Oysters	Neutral	Sweet, salty	Liver	Nourishes yin; enriches blood; clears heat; removes damp	Eat raw, boil, fry
Prawns	Warming	Sweet, salty	Liver, kidneys	Tones kidneys; reinforces yang; nourishes *qi* and blood; dispels blood stasis; clears phlegm	Boil, stir-fry steam, grill
Salmon	Warming	Sweet	Stomach, spleen	Enriches *qi* and blood	Steam, bake, grill, braise, poach
Shrimp	Warming	Salty	Liver, kidneys	Tones kidneys; reinforces yang	Boil, stir-fry, steam, grill

Seafood (continued)

Food	Thermal Nature	Flavor	Organ Network	Therapeutic Action and Benefit	Ways to Eat and Prepare
Squid	Cold	Sweet, salty	Kidney, bladder, liver	Nourishes yin, blood and *qi*; clears heat	Boil, grill, fry
Trout	Warming	Sweet	Stomach, spleen	Builds yang and *qi*; moves *qi*; warms digestion	Braise, grill, bake

Dairy

Food	Thermal Nature	Flavor	Organ Network	Therapeutic Action and Benefit	Ways to Eat and Prepare
Ghee	Neutral	Sweet, fatty	Stomach, spleen	Supplements yin, blood and *jing*; moistens body tissues; anti-inflammatory	Use as cooking oil in frying and baking; as spread
Milk – cow's	Neutral, cooling	Sweet	Lung, heart, stomach	Reinforces lungs; moistens intestinal tract; treats weakness	Boil, fermented to make yogurt, kefir, sour cream, cultured butter or curdled to make some cheeses
Milk – sheep's and goat's	Neutral to warming	Sweet, sour	Lung, stomach	Enriches yin; moistens dryness; reinforces *qi*	Boil, fermented to make yogurt, kefir, sour cream, cultured butter or curdled to make some cheeses

Condiments, Teas and Alcohol

Food	Thermal Nature	Flavor	Organ Network	Therapeutic Action and Benefit	Ways to Eat and Prepare
Cocoa powder, unsweetened	Neutral to warming	Bitter, sweet	Unknown	Induces urination; stimulates energy; can support reduction of cholesterol levels and lower blood pressure	Beverage, sweetened to make candy, desserts
Gardenia flowers	Cool	Pungent, slightly bitter	Lung, liver	Clears heat and phlegm in lungs; cools blood; clears liver	Steep as tea
Honey	Neutral	Sweet	Stomach, spleen, lung	Energizes stomach, spleen and lungs; helpful for fluid retention	Add to beverages such as tea, use as sweetener
Hot peppers (such as, cayenne, jalapeno, habanero, ghost pepper)	Warming to hot	Pungent	Lung, stomach, spleen, heart	Enhances blood and *qi* circulation; aids in digestion; invigorates stomach; activates sweating	Add to cooked dishes
Jasmine flowers	Slightly warming	Pungent	Spleen, stomach	Clears bloating; regulates *qi*; relieves depression	Steep in teas

Food	Thermal Nature	Flavor	Organ Network	Therapeutic Action and Benefit	Ways to Eat and Prepare
Miso	Neutral to warming	Sweet, salty	Spleen, stomach, kidneys	Reinforces and benefits digestion; nourishes blood; detoxifies environmental toxins	Add to soups, broths, cooked dishes, use as a condiment
Molasses, unsulphured	Warming	Slightly sweet, bitter	Kidneys, liver, stomach, spleen, lung	Eases coughs	Adds flavor and moisture to baked goods
Rose, buds or petals, red	Slightly warm	Pungent, sweet	Spleen, liver	Activates *qi* and blood circulation; disperses blood stasis; benefits digestion; calms mind	Use as a condiment, steep in teas, infuse in beverages and liquor
Salt	Neutral	Salty	Kidneys, spleen	Adds flavor; enhances digestion; replaces important mineral	Use as a condiment in cooking but not at the table
Sugar	Neutral	Sweet	Spleen, stomach	Eases muscle spasms; relieves pain; calming; boosts blood sugar quickly	Use as a sweetener
Tea – oolong, black	Neutral to warming	Slightly bitter, sweet	Heart, lung, liver, large intestine, stomach, bladder	Stimulates digestion and aids bowel movement; relieves thirst; its stimulating nature acts to refresh the mind	Infuse, steep, boil
Tea – green and white	Cool	Slightly bitter, sweet	Heart, lung, liver, large intestine, stomach, bladder	Benefits the heart; induces urination; relieves thirst; its stimulating nature acts to refresh the mind; high in anti-oxidants; strengthens the immune system	Infuse, steep, boil
Tea – rooibos	Cool	Slightly bitter, sweet	Heart, lung, liver, large intestine, stomach, bladder	Soothes tension; supports digestion; calms infantile colic	Infuse, steep, boil
Vinegar	Warming	Sour, bitter	Stomach, liver	Assists and activates digestion; disperses blood stasis; activates blood circulation; stops bleeding; eliminates toxins; detoxifies	Drink on its own, add to tea, soups, beans, broths, dressings, use topically to relieve sunburn, contusions and pain

Condiments, Teas and Alcohol (continued)

Food	Thermal Nature	Flavor	Organ Network	Therapeutic Action and Benefit	Ways to Eat and Prepare
Alcohol	Warming	Pungent, sweet	Heart, liver, lung, stomach	Activates blood circulation; disperses cold; stimulates digestion	Drink on its own or infuse with herbs, nuts, flowers or other plant-based foods

Medicinal Herbs

Food	Thermal Nature	Flavor	Organ Network	Therapeutic Action and Benefit	Ways to Eat and Prepare
Astragalus root	Warming	Sweet	Spleen, lungs	Builds and replenishes vitality, especially when feeling weak; strengthens immune system	Decoct as a tea, add to soups; cook with rice and other foods, infuse in alcohol
Barberries – dried	Warming	Sour, sweet	Lung, liver, gall-bladder, urinary bladder, stomach, spleen	Clears heat and toxins; calms stomach; clears fever; treats diarrhea; eases inflammation; treats urinary infections	Use in grain dishes, jams
Cinnamon – dried sticks and twigs	Warming	Pungent, sweet	Heart, lungs, bladder	Warms digestion; disperses cold; promotes blood circulation; used for common colds and joint pain	Decoct in tea formulas
Codonopsis – dried	Neutral	Sweet	Spleen, lung	Invigorates spleen and stomach; builds *qi*; eases shortness of breath, weakness in limbs, loss of appetite, thirst	Add to soups, stews, decoct as a tea, infuse in alcohol
Dang gui – dried	Warming	Sweet, neutral	Liver, heart, spleen	Nourishes blood and invigorates circulation; relieves menstrual problems; benefits anemia	Add to soups, stews, decoct as a tea, infuse in alcohol
Ginger	Slightly warming	Pungent	Lung, spleen, stomach	Increases and benefits digestion; induces perspiration to treat common colds; stops vomiting; warms lungs	Use raw, dried and/or ground, decoct as a tea, infuse in alcohol
Goji berries – dried	Neutral	Sweet	Kidneys, liver	Nourishes blood; improves eyesight, enhances immunity; treats dry cough	Eat on their own, steep as tea, cook in dishes; infuse in alcohol
Hawthorn fruit (crataegus) – dried	Slightly warming	Sweet, sour	Spleen, stomach, liver	Improves digestion; eases food stagnation; invigorates blood circulation; treats post-partum abdominal pain; can aid in lowering blood pressure	Candy, jam, add to soups, decoct as a tea

Medicinal Herbs (continued)					
Food	Thermal Nature	Flavor	Organ Network	Therapeutic Action and Benefit	Ways to Eat and Prepare
Hibiscus flowers – dried	Cool	Sour	Heart, liver	Aids in lowering mild hypertension and cholesterol; supports heart health; eases mild constipation	Juice, desserts, steep as tea
Chinese yam – dried	Neutral	Sweet	Lung, spleen, kidneys	Invigorates spleen and stomach; builds appetite, astringes and helps stop diarrhea	Add to cooked dishes, decoct as a tea, infuse in alcohol
Lily bulbs	Slightly cold	Sweet	Heart, lung	Nourishes and moistens lungs; relieves cough; calms the mind	Simmer with fruit or vegetables, add to soups, stews, cook with rice, decoct as a tea
Lotus seeds – dried	Neutral	Sweet	Lung, heart, kidneys	Nourishes heart; benefits those with poor appetite; arrests diarrhea; treats insomnia; calms the mind	Cook with grains and in dishes, candy, decoct as a tea
Mulberries – dried	Slightly cold	Sweet	Liver, heart, kidneys	Nourishes blood; softens skin; nourishes yin; treats constipation	Eat on their own, add to cooked dishes, infuse in wine, teas
Nettles	Cool	Sweet, mildly salty	Bladder, spleen, liver	Yin and blood tonic; dispels toxins; induces urination; anti-inflammatory; promotes lactation; increases estrogen; strengthens hair	Juice, steam; sauté, stir-fry, add to soups, rice dishes, steep as tea
Rose hips	Neutral	Sour, sweet	Kidneys, large intestine, bladder	Mild immune stimulant; relieves diarrhea; eases constipation; induces urination; acts as a laxative; benefits skin	Use fresh or dried in jams, syrups, infuse in alcohol, decocts as a tea
Schisandra berries – dried	Warming	Sour	Lung, heart, kidney	Replenishes vital energy; can ease chronic diarrhea and insomnia; treats dry coughs	Use in jams, syrups, decoct as a tea, infuse in alcohol
Shiso (perilla) leaves	Warm	Pungent	Lung, spleen	Induces sweat in common cold; eases vomiting and abdominal pain	Add fresh or dried to salads or dressings; decocted as tea; used in pickling umeboshi plums
Solomon's seal (*Polygonatum*) – dried	Slightly cold	Sweet	Lung, stomach	Strengthens heart; nourishes yin; eases thirst and dry throat; promotes production of body fluids; used for dizziness and muscle spasms; eases dry coughs	Add to cooked dishes, decoct as a tea, infuse in alcohol

Medicinal Herbs (continued)

Food	Thermal Nature	Flavor	Organ Network	Therapeutic Action and Benefit	Ways to Eat and Prepare
Tangerine peels	Warming	Sour, bitter	Lung, spleen	Activates *qi* and digestive *qi*; relieves indigestion; eases coughs with phlegm, hiccups and vomiting	Use fresh or dried peels in cooked dishes, steep in teas
Umeboshi plums	Neutral	Salty, sour	Lung, liver, stomach, large intestine	Relieves coughs; treats diarrhea; antibacterial, antifungal; anti-parasitic	Add to hot water and decoct with ginger

Culinary Herbs and Spices

Food	Thermal Nature	Flavor	Organ Network	Therapeutic Action and Benefit	Ways to Eat and Prepare
Allspice	Hot	Pungent and aromatic	Spleen, stomach, kidneys	Carminative (reduces intestinal gas); treats indigestion; promotes peristalsis; eases diarrhea	Use in pickles, marinades, mulled wine, spice blends
Anise seeds *Not recommended if pregnant	Warming	Pungent and aromatic	Heart, lung, liver, spleen, stomach, kidneys	Yang tonic; builds *qi*; aids digestion; clears asthma and phlegm; aids lactation	Decoct as a tea; used in baked goods; added to fish, meat or vegetable dishes; infused in alcohol
Basil	Warming	Pungent, bitter, slightly sweet	Liver, large intestine, spleen, stomach, kidneys	Stimulates digestion; loosens phlegm; generates warmth; resolves phlegm and mucus; antimicrobial; relieves depression and headache	Add fresh or dried to dressings, sauces, salads, cooked dishes, steep in teas
Bay leaves – dried	Warming	Aromatic	Stomach, spleen	Regulates blood circulation; helps regulate menstruation; anti-inflammatory; relieves insomnia; benefits the stomach and digestion; relieves gas, colic and indigestion	Use to cook beans and in soups, stews
Black peppercorns	Hot	Pungent	Spleen, stomach, large intestine	Aids digestion; restores appetite; stimulates blood circulation; relieves pain	Grind fresh and use to add spice to soups, dishes, dressings and teas
Cardamom – dried	Slightly warming	Sweet, aromatic, pungent	Lung, large intestine, spleen, stomach	Warms and aids digestion; eases coughs; moves digestive *qi*; dissolves damp; strengthens stomach	Use in spice blends, decoct in alcohol, steep or infuse in teas

Culinary Herbs and Spices (continued)

Food	Thermal Nature	Flavor	Organ Network	Therapeutic Action and Benefit	Ways to Eat and Prepare
Caraway seeds	Warming	Aromatic, slightly pungent	Bladder, stomach, kidneys	Stimulates digestion, promotes *qi* and blood circulation; disperses cold; eases menstrual pain	Use raw or toast, grind, add to baked goods, fermented vegetables
Cayenne and hot chile peppers	Hot	Pungent	Spleen, stomach, heart, lung	Expels cold; activates yang and warms internal organs; aids digestion	Use fresh or dried as a condiment
Chinese chives	Warming	Sweet, pungent	Kidney, stomach, liver	Reinforces kidneys; assists yang; warms middle burner (digestion) and relieves stomach aches; aids appetite; disperses blood stasis; helps stop overgrowth of intestinal bacteria	Sauté, use as a garnish, add to soups
Citrus zest, lemon, orange, tangerine	Warming	Sour	Spleen, stomach, kidneys	Activates *qi* circulation and digestion; clears phlegm; eases bloating; eases cough with profuse phlegm	Use fresh or dried in cooked dishes or steep in teas
Cloves	Warming	Pungent and aromatic, slightly bitter	Spleen, stomach, kidneys	Expels damp cold; strengthens stomach, spleen and kidneys; aids digestion; moves *qi*; calms nausea and hiccups	Add to meat dishes, grain dishes, baked goods
Coriander seeds	Warming	Pungent	Spleen, stomach, lung	Reinforces stomach; regulates *qi*; induces perspiration	Use raw or toast, grind
Cumin seeds	Warming	Pungent, bitter	Spleen, liver	Stimulates digestion; relieves gas and spasms	Toast and grind, use in spice mixes and as a condiment
Dill	Warming	Pungent, slightly bitter	Stomach, spleen, kidneys	Stimulates appetite; calming; relieves hiccups and intestinal gas	Use fresh or dried (and seeds) in soups, pickles, sauces
Juniper berries – dried	Warming	Bitter	Spleen, stomach, kidneys	Improves digestion; treats urinary infections; relieves arthritic pain	Use in condiments, marinades, infuse in alcohol
Nutmeg – dried and grated	Warming	Pungent and aromatic	Large intestine, stomach, spleen	Moves blood and *qi*; dispels cold; improves digestion	Use in baked goods, spice mixes

Food	Thermal Nature	Flavor	Organ Network	Therapeutic Action and Benefit	Ways to Eat and Prepare
Culinary Herbs and Spices (continued)					
Parsley	Warming	Slightly pungent, bitter	Bladder, kidneys, stomach	Stimulates digestion; induces urination	Eat raw, juice, use as a garnish, add to salads, soups and various cooked dishes
Rosemary	Warming	Pungent, sweet	Spleen, heart, lung, kidneys, liver	Aids digestion; improves circulation; used as a tonic for older people; eases headache; dispels cold and mucus; increases *qi*; potent antioxidant	Use fresh or dried in cooked dishes, decoct in alcohol, vinegar or as a tea
Sage	Warming	Astringent	Lung, liver, heart, kidneys	Relieves spasm; relieves stomach aches and excessive perspiration; potent decongestant	Use fresh or dried in cooked dishes, decoct in alcohol or as a tea, use as a gargle for sore throat, steam for congestion
Sichuan peppercorns	Hot	Pungent	Spleen, stomach, kidneys	Circulates blood and *qi*; soothes pain due to cold; eases stomach ache; kills tapeworms; eases toothache	Add to cooked dishes
Smoked paprika	Warming	Bitter, slightly sweet	Spleen, stomach, kidneys	Stimulates digestion; increases circulation; warms the body	Finishing herb for color and flavor
Thyme	Warming	Pungent and aromatic, bitter	Spleen, lung, bladder, heart, kidneys, uterus	Clears phlegm and mucus; relieves cold and damp; relieves intestinal gas; improves digestion; increases *qi*; antiseptic	Use fresh or dried in herbal teas, vinegars, soups and other cooked dishes
Turmeric	Warming	Bitter, pungent	Spleen, liver	Dries phlegm and cold; relieves pain; anti-inflammatory and antibacterial	Use fresh or dried in spice mixes, soups, cooked dishes
Vanilla	Warming	Sweet	Spleen, stomach, kidneys	Mildly stimulating; aids digestion; antiseptic	Use fresh bean or extract in baked goods, desserts, fruit dishes

Recipes for Every Season

Recipe Assumptions

The quality of the food you cook and eat is key to building vitality. Be sure to source the best-quality foods you can. Seek out your local farmers' markets and food suppliers. Get to know the people and sources of your food. This will strengthen your health and your connection to what you eat.

Unless otherwise noted in the ingredients list, recipes in this book follow these assumptions:

- Produce is organic.
- Produce is washed, peeled and trimmed as appropriate, unless otherwise noted.
- Nuts, seeds and oils are organic.
- Eggs are sourced from sustainably raised organic chickens.
- Meat is sustainably raised; beef and lamb are grass-fed.
- Poultry is sustainably and pasture raised.
- Fish is sustainably fished.
- Dried herbs are organic and food-grade.

Recipes for the Seasons

The recipes in this book are divided by seasons, for the most part, with the exception of the Blood Tonics and Condiments sections. Adjusting the foods we eat from season to season helps the body attune to the energy of the changing cycles of life during the year. Seasonal eating actually helps us to practice making changes from one season to the next. The subtle changes in foods and cooking help optimize our physical participation in a number of natural processes, including the renewing energy of spring, the abundance of summer, the harmony of transitional times, the containing energy of autumn and the regenerative focus needed in winter.

The recipes here are crafted to combine specific whole foods, herbs and spices — each of which provides certain flavors as well as warming and cooling properties — and prepared using a particular method to nurture the body and activate a certain response. When you begin to experiment with seasonal eating, pay attention to how the food makes you feel, and hopefully you will start to notice when you feel satisfied, at ease and in sync.

Let's take a quick look at how eating within the framework of seasons can benefit your health.

Spring

Spring's energy is all about growth, rebirth and renewal. We could say that the energy of spring is up and out as new greens shoot up and out of the earth. Indeed, our energy begins to move up and out into the beauty of nature in spring. Therefore, how we eat should support this upward, renewing activity of the season. The foods and flavors we introduce during spring — for example, pungent (an upward, dispersing flavor) and sweet (a calming and harmonizing flavor) — encourage the breakup of internal energy stored by the body to stay warm through the winter. The pungent and sweet flavors, along with certain cooking styles, will help protect us from the changeable weather and promote a sense of ease and flow.

Summer

As we move into summer, our pores are open to receive the season's abundance, to soak up all its warmth and vibrant energy. This is an active, outward time of year and the foods we eat need to support this activity while providing balance internally. Pungent flavors (both cooling and warming) help open the pores of the body to encourage sweating, helping us to cool off, while bitter flavors (which are cold and detoxifying) balance and drain the summer heat we absorb. Finally, the sour flavor so prevalent in summer fruits helps to keep us hydrated.

Seasonal Transition

Every season has a period of transition. A notable one is when summer begins to wane, with cooler mornings and evenings. In some parts of the world, the end of summer brings a period of harmony and harvest referred to as late summer. In Chinese medicine, this time of the waning season also happens during the last 18 days of each season, affording us a time to transition, to recalibrate our internal balance before we move into the next phase. These transitional times are supported by eating more simply, with naturally sweet bland foods (think of carrots, squashes and cabbages).

Autumn

Autumn is the beginning of a time when we begin to contain our energy to move inward and indoors. We begin to wear more layers of clothing to protect us from the cooling temperatures. The air dries and the leaves begin to drop. It is a time to begin protecting our bodies from cold winds, dryness, and the colds and flu that always seem to come around during this time of year. Adding foods that are more sour (a flavor found naturally in the autumnal fruits) stimulates the body's natural hydration system.

Winter

Finally, winter, the seemingly most barren time of the year, is an important time for focusing inward. It is a time to become more reflective, putting our energy toward regenerating so that we are ready to burst forth in spring with new vigor and vitality. It is also a time for us to, in a sense, hibernate. Rest is tantamount, going to bed earlier and, if possible, awakening later to be in tune with the cycles of light and darkness. This is when we cook with foods that help warm and revitalize our physical and mental energy. The flavors of winter encourage this descent into ourselves through the kidney energy, which according to Chinese medicine is the source of all yin and yang in the body (see Chapter 2 for more information). One such flavor is salty (found in celery, seaweeds, salt, soy and miso), which has a downward movement in the body. As much as it is important to store heat and warmth in the body, however, too much heat can dry us out and interfere with the balance of dryness and hydration. The bitter flavor (as in chicory, escarole, bitter greens, olives, grapefruit) drains and clears out internal heat buildup and acts to regulate internal warming and cooling.

Spring Seasonal Menus

Menu 1
Auntie Katherine's Chicken Adobo
Sautéed Broccoli with Tangy Ginger Dressing
Brown Basmati Rice

Menu 2
Catfish with Pungent Spiced Oil
Spring Greens and Lotus Root Sauté

Menu 3
Qi-Moving Rose Game Hens
Steamed Artichokes with Cashew Sauce
Garlicky Wild Spring Greens

Menu 4
Herbed Nettle and Asparagus Risotto
Fava Beans with Anchovy, Lemon and Mint Dressing

Spring Recipes

Spring Tonic Congee

Congee is a traditional Chinese breakfast dish that can be varied in so many delicious ways. This simple version has a nice blend of textures; a delightfully sweet, mild flavor; and earthiness, thanks to the adzuki beans. You can customize it by adding a furikake-style sprinkle or any of the other tasty toppers in the Condiment Recipes chapter (pages 422 to 465).

MAKES 4 SERVINGS

Tip

Adzuki beans originated in Japan and their name translates as "small beans."

Variation

To nourish the stomach and spleen specifically — and to add a sweeter taste — cook 1 cup (250 mL) chopped peeled seeded winter squash (such as kabocha, acorn or butternut) in the congee.

---

2 tbsp	dried adzuki beans	30 mL
1½ tbsp	hato mugi (Job's tears)	22 mL
½ cup	sweet (glutinous) brown rice (or brown Arborio rice)	125 mL
2 tbsp	dried Chinese yam (dioscorea)	30 mL
1 tbsp	grated gingerroot	15 mL

1. Place adzuki beans in a medium bowl and cover with water. Let stand overnight. Drain well.

2. Meanwhile, place hato mugi in another medium bowl and cover with water. Let stand for 1 hour or overnight if you plan to cook it in the morning. Drain well.

3. In a medium saucepan, combine 6 cups (1.5 L) water, adzuki beans, hato mugi, rice and Chinese yam. Bring to a boil. Reduce heat to low, cover and simmer, stirring occasionally, for 2 hours. The congee should have a souplike consistency; if there is not enough liquid left in the pan, add up to ½ cup (125 mL) water. Stir in ginger. Cover and let cool for 10 minutes.

4. Serve immediately or transfer to an airtight container and refrigerate for up to 3 days. Warm in a small saucepan over low heat before serving.

Health Tips

Congee is light and easy to digest, so it is great for anyone who is recovering from an illness. The food-grade herbs — hato mugi and dried Chinese yam — in this recipe are especially useful for building qi, or vitality. This congee is beneficial for people suffering from low appetite, fatigue or loose stools.

Adzuki beans help control blood sugar and promote urination.

Essential Seed and Nut Porridge with Strawberries and Honey

In this book, we're offering an essential seed and nut porridge for each season, and each contains a different combination. Spring is the time for pecans, because they are warming and perfect for the changeable spring weather. Making the porridge mix the night or several days before is a convenient way to get a head start on breakfast — it's as easy as instant oatmeal but much tastier and more nutritious. The fresh strawberries in this recipe brighten up the porridge's simple, toasty taste.

MAKES 4 SERVINGS

Tips

You can add up to 1 cup (250 mL) more boiling water to the porridge mix if you prefer a thinner consistency.

Health Tips

This porridge provides some of your daily dose of omega-3 essential fatty acids, which nourish the yin and essence (*jing*) of the body. If you are overweight and have digestive issues, eat this dish in moderation. It is important to resolve and clear the yin excess that causes these health issues.

Pecans are warming and counter the cold, changeable winds of spring. Pecans support and balance the nervous system as well.

Honey is sweet, lubricating and nourishing to the stomach and spleen.

- **Blender**

2 cups	boiling water	500 mL
1 cup	thickly sliced hulled strawberries, at room temperature	250 mL
4 tsp	liquid honey or pure maple syrup	20 mL

Porridge Mix

3 tbsp	sunflower seeds	45 mL
3 tbsp	flax seeds	45 mL
2 tbsp	chia seeds	30 mL
½ cup	pecan halves	125 mL
½ cup	unsalted raw cashews	125 mL
1 cup	unsweetened roasted plantain chips	250 mL
½ tsp	salt	2 mL

1. *Porridge Mix:* In a large dry skillet, toast sunflower, flax and chia seeds over medium-low heat, stirring often, for 5 minutes or until fragrant. Transfer to a heatproof bowl. Return skillet to heat and add pecans and cashews. Toast over medium-low heat, stirring often, for 10 minutes or until fragrant. Transfer to another heatproof bowl. Let cool completely.

2. In blender, combine seed mixture and plantain chips and grind until the texture of brown sugar. Add nut mixture and salt and grind to texture of brown sugar.

3. In a medium bowl, stir porridge mix with boiling water. Cover and let stand for 5 minutes.

4. Spoon porridge into serving bowls. Top with strawberries and honey. Serve immediately.

Health Tip

Strawberries are one of the first spring fruits to appear. They are cooling, sweet and sour, nourish the blood and also soothe a sore throat.

Tofu and Snow Pea Breakfast Fried Rice

Around the world, people often eat savory, dinner-style dishes for breakfast. This quick, and simple fried rice is a perfect example that will get you going first thing in the morning! Mild, nourishing tofu and sweet snow peas lighten up this fried rice, making it a delightful spring dish. The star anise gives it an aromatic quality and rounds out the flavors nicely.

> **MAKES**
> **4 TO 6 SERVINGS**

Variation

Substitute an equal weight of cooked drained beans for the tofu. Marinate them as you would the tofu.

Health Tips

Tofu, a product of soybeans, is a semi-raw food and can be an allergen for some people. Eat it only occasionally if you suffer from hypothyroid or have trouble digesting soy products (tofu made from semi-raw soybeans inhibits the digestive enzyme trypsin).

Green peas are sweet and cooling, and nourish the spleen.

Tofu is rich in protein, isoflavones (an estrogen-like plant compound) and omega-3 fatty acids. It is moistening. It is beneficial for people with high blood pressure.

This cooling fried rice is especially good for people who often feel overheated.

1	package (14 oz to 1 lb/420 to 500 g) extra-firm tofu, drained	1
½ cup	tamari or soy sauce	125 mL
1 tbsp	coconut sugar	15 mL
4	whole star anise	4
1 cup	red cargo rice or brown jasmine rice	250 mL
2 tbsp	avocado oil	30 mL
8 oz	snow peas, trimmed and halved	250 g
½ cup	packed chopped fresh Chinese chives or green onions	125 mL

1. Cut tofu into ½-inch (1 cm) cubes. In a bowl, combine tofu, tamari, sugar and star anise. Gently toss to coat. Cover and refrigerate, gently stirring occasionally, for 4 hours or for up to 24 hours.

2. In a medium saucepan, combine 2½ cups (625 mL) water and rice. Bring to a boil. Reduce heat to low, cover and simmer for 30 to 40 minutes or until almost tender. Turn off heat and let pan stand, covered, on burner for 15 minutes. Let cool. Refrigerate for 2 hours.

3. Reserving marinade, drain tofu. Set tofu and marinade aside separately. Remove and discard star anise.

4. In a large skillet, heat oil over medium-high heat. Add snow peas and cook, stirring often, for 2 minutes. Push snow peas to 1 side of the pan. Using a spatula, spread rice over bottom of pan. Cook, without stirring, for 1 minute or until bottom is lightly browned. Turn rice and cook for 1 minute or until lightly browned.

5. Scatter tofu and Chinese chives over rice. Pour reserved marinade around edge of pan and cook for 1 minute or until no liquid remains. Gently fold in tofu and chives. (Avoid stirring the rice, as that will make it gummy.)

6. Spoon into serving bowls. Serve immediately.

Mixed Herb Omelet

This omelet is deliciously simple and fresh tasting, thanks to the addition of delicate spring herbs. The cooking time is minimal, so use a blend of tender herb leaves, which wilt quickly over the heat.

MAKES 2 SERVINGS

Tip

You can easily halve the recipe to make a tasty breakfast for one. Use a medium skillet to keep the omelet from getting too thin.

2 tbsp	avocado oil or ghee	30 mL
1 cup	packed chopped mixed herbs, such as fresh dill, green onions, chervil and/or parsley (about 3 oz/90 g total)	250 mL
4	large eggs, beaten	4
½ tsp	salt, or to taste	2 mL

1. In a large skillet, heat oil over medium-high heat, swirling to coat bottom of pan. Add herbs and cook, without stirring, for 30 seconds or until wilted.

2. Starting in center and spiraling out to edge of pan, pour eggs over herbs. Reduce heat to low and cook, without stirring, until eggs are almost set. Sprinkle with ½ tsp (2 mL) salt.

3. Using a spatula, cut omelet in half. For each half, fold each point into center to make a rectangle. Transfer to serving plates. Serve immediately and season with more salt to taste, if desired.

Health Tips

Green onions, also known as scallions or *cong bai* in Mandarin, are used as an herb in Chinese medicine. They are warming and pungent, so they are often served to people who are just beginning to get the common cold. At the beginning of a cold, when you experience chills, chop up some green onions, stir them into boiling water and drink for a soothing remedy.

Rich in protein, eggs nourish *qi* and the blood. Eat the whole egg, not just the white and you will get the full benefit. Be sure to choose organic eggs (see page 292).

Aromatic fresh herbs embody the positive, upward energy of spring. In this dish, the sweet eggs nourish the body while the warming and pungent herbs increase their effectiveness.

A tendency to get skin rashes can indicate that you have an underlying internal hot condition. In that case, you might want to avoid this recipe, as it is quite warming.

Scallop and Snow Pea Savory Steamed Egg Custard

This dish is simply wonderful and elegant. The scallops and snow peas are a delightful treasure to find hidden at the bottom of the creamy custard.

MAKES 6 SERVINGS

Tips

If your pot is too small to hold all of the ramekins at once, steam the custards in batches.

Rubber-tipped tongs are great for transferring the ramekins to the steamer pot. If you don't have them, you can wrap thick rubber bands around the tips of regular metal tongs.

Health Tips

Scallops are sweet, salty and slightly cold. They act as a kidney tonic.

Eggs nourish both yin and yang. The yolk is warming in nature, while the white is cooling. Eggs are a beneficial food for people who are recovering from illness. Steaming hydrates any food and, in this case, makes the eggs highly digestible. Cooked in this way, this dish can help ease constipation.

- **Six $\frac{1}{2}$- or $\frac{3}{4}$-cup (125 or 175 mL) ramekins or custard cups**
- **Large pot with steamer rack (about 1 inch/2.5 cm above bottom of pot)**

12	snow peas, trimmed and halved crosswise	12
12	medium (or 18 small) scallops (8 to 12 oz/250 to 375 g total)	12
4	large eggs, beaten	4
3 cups	Traditional Dashi (page 297), at room temperature	750 mL
1 tbsp	tamari or soy sauce	15 mL
$\frac{1}{2}$ tsp	salt	2 mL

1. In a medium saucepan, combine snow peas with $\frac{1}{2}$ cup (125 mL) water and bring to a simmer over medium-high heat. Cover, reduce heat and cook for 2 minutes or until tender. Uncover and cook, stirring often, until no liquid remains. Transfer to a plate and let cool. Divide among ramekins.

2. In a small saucepan, combine scallops with $\frac{1}{4}$ cup (60 mL) water and bring to a simmer over medium-high heat. Cook, stirring often, for about 1 minute or until scallops are just opaque. Using a slotted spoon, divide scallops among ramekins and let cool.

3. In a 4-cup (1 L) glass measuring cup, whisk together eggs, dashi, tamari and salt. Strain and gently pour into ramekins.

4. Pour enough water into pot to come scant 1 inch (2.5 cm) up side. Place steamer rack in pan over water. Bring to a boil.

5. Arrange ramekins on rack, cover tightly and steam for 15 to 20 minutes or until custard is barely set in the center (it will be jiggly but not liquid).

6. Serve warm or at room temperature. Or cover and refrigerate for up to 3 days; let come to room temperature for an hour before serving.

Fresh Fish Ball Soup with Napa Cabbage

These tasty fish balls are delicate, tender and easy to make. The delicate shreds of napa cabbage add a subtle sweetness to this soup.

MAKES 4 SERVINGS

Tips

If you don't have a food processor, chop the fish very finely by hand. In a medium bowl, using a fork, mix together fish, $\frac{1}{2}$ tsp (2 mL) of the salt, the ginger and egg. Continue with recipe.

If fish mixture is very sticky, moisten your hands with water before forming it into balls.

- **Food processor (see tips, at left)**

1 lb	boneless mild white fish fillets (such as sole or tilapia), cut into pieces	500 g
1½ tsp	salt, divided	7 mL
1 tsp	grated gingerroot	5 mL
1	large egg, beaten	1
4	green onions, minced	4
3 cups	finely shredded napa cabbage (about ½ small head)	750 mL

1. In bowl of food processor fitted with the metal blade, combine fish, $\frac{1}{2}$ tsp (2 mL) of the salt, the ginger and egg. Pulse until fish is finely ground but not puréed. Stir in green onions. Form into 16 balls and place on a large plate. Cover and refrigerate for 2 hours.

2. In a medium saucepan, bring 4 cups (1 L) water to a simmer. Add fish balls, cabbage and remaining salt. Reduce heat to low and simmer, stirring gently once or twice, for 5 to 10 minutes or until fish balls are opaque in center. (To test, cut one open.)

3. Ladle into serving bowls. Serve immediately.

> ## Health Tips
>
> The benefits you get from the fish in this recipe depend on which variety you choose. Freshwater fish has a sweet-salty flavor and is easy to digest. Ocean fish has a salty flavor; it strengthens *qi*, blood, yin and yang, and benefits liver and kidney yin.
>
> Napa cabbage is neutral and sweet, with a tendency toward cooling. It clears out excessive heat in the stomach and lungs.
>
> Napa cabbage is also the base for a traditional remedy for fevers and colds that include a cough. Grate raw napa cabbage and squeeze out the juice. Mix the juice with grated radish, warm water and honey for a healing drink.

Springtime Chive and Clam Soup with Pea Shoots

Clams have a deep, vibrant and satisfying mineral-rich flavor. The heat from the soup is enough to cook them lightly without simmering (which would make the meat tough). Delicately sweet pea shoots brighten the taste of the savory clear broth.

MAKES 4 SERVINGS

Tips

Only buy live clams that are firmly closed; open clams are dead and can cause food poisoning. Store live clams for up to 3 days in the refrigerator in a bowl covered with a wet towel.

You can skip Steps 1 through 3 and substitute 2 cans (each 6½ oz/184 g) minced or whole clams, with juices, in Step 4. The can sizes are slightly different, so just use the same total weight.

Pea shoots are the delicate, growing tips of garden pea (not sweet pea) plants. They are available in the spring in Asian grocery stores and health food stores. If you are growing peas, you can harvest the top 6 inches (15 cm) of the plant for this dish.

Health Tip

Clams clear internal heat and mucous, and reduce water retention (mild edema). When cooked with pungent chives and sweet pea shoots, as in this soup, they make an excellent dish for combatting night sweats.

4 lbs	small cherrystone or Manila clams (see tips, at left)	2 kg
	Cold water	
⅓ cup	salt	75 mL
4 cups	Traditional Dashi (page 297)	1 L
1 cup	packed coarsely chopped pea shoots (3 oz/90 g)	250 mL
½ cup	minced fresh chives	125 mL
2 tbsp	rice wine, such as sake	30 mL

1. Using a stiff vegetable brush, rinse and scrub each clam to remove any grit. Pour enough cold water into a large stockpot to come about halfway up side. Stir in salt until dissolved. Rinse clams again and add to pot. Pour in more cold water to cover, if necessary. Discard any clams that float. Let stand for 30 minutes or until clams purge any remaining grit.

2. In a colander, drain clams and rinse well. Discard any that are open. Rinse out pot and add clams and 1 cup (250 mL) water. Cover and bring to a boil over high heat. Steam for 2 to 3 minutes or until clams open. Immediately remove from heat and transfer clams and their cooking juices to a large heatproof bowl. Let cool enough to handle.

3. Discard any clams that have not opened. Using a sharp knife, cut clams from shells and place in a medium bowl. Strain cooking juices through a fine-mesh sieve over clams.

4. In a medium saucepan, bring dashi to a boil over medium-high heat. Stir in pea shoots and cook for about 30 seconds or just until wilted. Remove from heat. Stir in chives, clams and their juices, and rice wine.

5. Ladle into serving bowls. Serve immediately.

Two-Pea Soup with Spicy Fennel-Pepper Oil

This gently sweet and aromatic soup, made with dried split peas and sweet green peas, is a lovely dish to welcome spring. The sweet green peas lighten up the hearty base created by the split peas. If you like, try the soup with a complementary dry condiment (see pages 440 to 453) sprinkled over top instead of the spiced oil.

MAKES 4 SERVINGS

Tip

The shiny black seeds in Sichuan peppercorns are hard and gritty, so it's best to remove them before adding this spice to recipes.

Health Tips

Split and green peas are both sweet — neither warming nor cooling — and offer vitalizing nourishment. Legumes are considered drying, so in Chinese nutritional therapy they are used to relieve edema and promote the circulation of fluids throughout the body.

The pungent, slightly spicy Sichuan peppercorns are warming and activate digestion.

- **Immersion blender or countertop blender**

1 cup	dried green split peas	250 mL
1	leek	1
2 cups	shelled fresh or thawed frozen green peas (about 9 oz/275 g)	500 mL
2 tsp	salt	10 mL
2 tbsp	fresh cilantro leaves	30 mL

Spicy Fennel-Pepper Oil

1/4 cup	avocado oil	60 mL
1 tsp	Sichuan peppercorns, shiny black seeds removed (see tip, at left)	5 mL
1 tsp	fennel seeds	5 mL
1/2 tsp	hot pepper flakes	2 mL

1. *Spicy Fennel-Pepper Oil:* In a small saucepan, combine oil, Sichuan peppercorns, fennel seeds and hot pepper flakes. Warm over medium-high heat for about 5 minutes or until spices are sizzling and oil is fragrant. Remove from heat and let cool completely. Pour into an airtight container and set aside. (Oil can be refrigerated for up to 2 months.)

2. In a medium saucepan, combine split peas with enough water to cover. Bring to a boil. Remove from heat, cover and let stand for 1 hour.

3. Trim roots and all but 1 inch (2.5 cm) of the dark green leaves off leek and discard. Cut leek in half lengthwise, then cut crosswise into 1/2-inch (1 cm) wide pieces. Rinse very well in 2 changes of water to remove grit. Set aside.

4. Drain split peas well. Rinse, drain and return to pan. Add 4 cups (1 L) water and leeks. Bring to a boil. Reduce heat, cover and simmer for 1 hour.

5. Stir in green peas and simmer for 30 minutes or until split peas are completely soft and broken down. Stir in salt. Using immersion blender, purée soup. (Let cool slightly if using countertop blender.)

6. Ladle into serving bowls. Drizzle with spicy fennel-pepper oil and sprinkle with cilantro. Serve immediately.

Spring Greens Tonic Soup

This refreshing soup is chock-full of sweet, aromatic greens and nourishing medicinal herbs. It's perfect for renewing your body's energy in the spring.

MAKES 4 SERVINGS

Tip

If you would like a garnish but don't care for chives, try one of the dry condiments on pages 440 to 453.

Health Tips

Dried white peony root (called *bai shao* in Mandarin) is a perfect spring herb. It has a bitter, sour flavor and is cooling in nature. It is beneficial to the liver, *qi* and blood. The herb astragalus (called *huang qi* in Mandarin) is sweet and warming. It lifts the *qi* and acts as a tonic. Together, these two herbs help balance and support vital energy and blood circulation.

The aromatic and pungent greens in this soup stimulate digestion, help reduce water retention and provide warmth against the gusty winds of spring.

- **Cheesecloth and kitchen string**

2	leeks	2
1 oz	dried white peony root	30 g
1 oz	dried astragalus root	30 g
1 tsp	avocado oil	5 mL
3	stalks celery, chopped	3
2	cloves garlic, smashed	2
1	piece (3 inches/7.5 cm square) dried kombu	1
1 cup	shelled fresh or thawed frozen green peas	250 mL
1 cup	coarsely chopped watercress	250 mL
1 cup	coarsely chopped fresh parsley	250 mL
1 tsp	sea salt	5 mL
	Chopped fresh chives (optional)	

1. Trim roots and all but 1 inch (2.5 cm) of the dark green leaves off leeks and discard. Cut leeks in half lengthwise, then cut crosswise into ½-inch (1 cm) wide pieces. Rinse very well in 2 changes of water to remove grit. Set aside.

2. On a square of cheesecloth, arrange white peony and astragalus roots. Bring corners up over herbs and tie with kitchen string to form a bundle. Set aside.

3. In a large saucepan, heat oil over medium heat. Add leeks and cook, stirring, for 1 to 2 minutes. Add celery and garlic and cook, stirring, for 1 to 2 minutes. Add 5 cups (1.25 L) water, kombu and herb bundle. Bring to a boil. Reduce heat and simmer for 25 minutes.

4. Remove and discard herb bundle and kombu. Stir in peas, watercress, parsley and salt. Simmer for 5 minutes or just until watercress is wilted.

5. Ladle into serving bowls. Sprinkle with chives (if using). Serve immediately.

Brothy White Bean and Greens Minestra

This variation on a traditional Italian-style minestra (soup) is a hearty and satisfying one-pot dinner. This recipe is an homage to the wonderful brothy minestras made in northern Italy.

Tips

This soup should be brothy. If it's too thick, add more water, a bit at a time, until you reach the desired consistency.

Lacinato kale goes by a number of different names, including dinosaur kale, Tuscan kale (or cabbage) and *cavolo nero*.

Health Tips

This soup can help reduce mild water retention, especially for women who are in the premenstrual phase of their cycle.

Beans are nourishing and help lower blood pressure and prevent constipation. Beans are drying, so they can also reduce water retention. However, if you often feel dry or have dry skin, don't consume too much of this soup.

1 cup	dried cannellini (white kidney) or navy beans	250 mL
2	bay leaves	2
1	piece (3 inches/7.5 cm square) dried kombu	1
1 tbsp	dried thyme	15 mL
1 tsp	salt, or to taste	5 mL
2	carrots, cut in half lengthwise, then crosswise into 1-inch (2.5 cm) chunks	2
2	stalks celery, cut in half	2
1	onion, cut into quarters	1
1	bunch tender leafy greens or lacinato kale, stemmed and thinly sliced	1
1 tsp	unfiltered cider vinegar	5 mL
1/4 tsp	freshly ground black pepper	1 mL

1. Place cannellini beans in a large bowl and pour in enough water to cover. Let stand overnight. Drain and rinse well. Drain again.

2. In a large saucepan, combine 5 cups (1.25 L) water, beans, bay leaves, kombu and thyme. Bring to a boil. Reduce heat to medium-low and simmer for 1 hour. Stir in salt, after 30 minutes, adding up to 1 tsp (5 mL) more to taste, if desired.

3. Reserving cooking liquid, drain beans and set aside. Return cooking liquid to saucepan and add carrots, celery and onion, adding additional water if necessary (see tips, at left). Bring to a boil. Reduce heat and simmer for about 20 minutes or until carrots are tender. Remove celery.

4. Return beans to soup. Stir in greens and vinegar and cook for 8 to 10 minutes or until greens are tender. Stir in pepper. Discard bay leaves.

5. Ladle into serving bowls. Serve immediately.

Herbed Nettle and Asparagus Risotto

Nettles have a lovely, fresh vegetal taste with mineral notes. They make a wonderful partner to the grassy asparagus in this risotto.

Tips

When risotto is cooking, it should bubble very gently. If you use up all the broth before the rice is tender, you can add hot water for the last few additions.

To make the chicken broth, see the recipe variation on page 418. Omit the ginger.

Health Tips

Traditionally, nettles have been eaten and steeped to make teas to calm allergy and hay fever symptoms. They are cooling and a diuretic (astringent), with a sweet flavor. Nettles are used in the West to nourish and build the blood; for example, in cases of anemia.

Asparagus is slightly warm and bitter. It can help to clear internal heat buildup (common with allergies) through urination.

The combination of nettles and asparagus in this soup will nourish the blood and yin.

3 cups	chicken broth or vegetable broth (see tips, at left)	750 mL
2 tbsp	avocado oil	30 mL
¼ cup	finely chopped onion	60 mL
2 cups	short-grain brown rice	500 mL
¼ cup	dried nettles (or 2 cups/500 mL chopped fresh nettle leaves)	60 mL
8 oz	asparagus, trimmed and cut into 1-inch (2.5 cm) pieces	250 g
½ cup	minced mixed fresh herbs, such as basil, chives and/or parsley	125 mL
	Salt to taste	

1. In a medium saucepan, combine broth and 3 cups (750 mL) water. Bring to a simmer over low heat. Turn off heat, cover and keep warm.

2. In another medium saucepan, heat oil over medium-high heat. Add onion and cook, stirring often, for 3 to 5 minutes or until translucent.

3. Stir in rice and cook, stirring, for 1 or 2 minutes or until coated and translucent. Reduce heat to medium-low and, using a heatproof spatula, stir in about 1 cup (250 mL) of the warm broth. Cook, stirring almost constantly and scraping bottom of pan to prevent sticking, for 5 to 10 minutes or until no liquid remains.

4. Stir in 1 cup (250 mL) of the remaining broth and nettles (if using dried). Cook, stirring almost constantly and scraping bottom of pan to prevent sticking, for 5 to 7 minutes or until no liquid remains.

5. Continue cooking, stirring and adding remaining broth, 1 cup (250 mL) at a time, as directed for 20 to 25 minutes total or until rice is just tender to the bite and has absorbed enough of the broth to be creamy but not soupy (see tips, at left).

6. Add asparagus and nettles (if using fresh). Cook, stirring often, for 5 minutes or just until asparagus is tender. Stir in herbs and salt to taste.

7. Spoon into serving bowls. Serve immediately.

Catfish with Pungent Spiced Oil

This nourishing fish is frequently served fried in the United States. Steaming catfish, however, brings out its sweet flavor and tender texture. Serve with Simple Sautéed Greens (page 263) and water-sautéed Asian sweet potatoes.

MAKES 4 SERVINGS

Tip

The shiny black seeds in Sichuan peppercorns are hard and gritty. It's best to remove them so that you don't bite into them.

Health Tip

Catfish is warming, sweet and very nourishing. Steaming the fish preserves its light, fresh texture and its moistening effect on the body. The pungent spiced oil invigorates the digestion.

- **Large pot with steamer rack (about 1 inch/2.5 cm above bottom of pot)**
- **6-cup (1.5 L) glass or ceramic baking dish that fits in steamer pot**

1 lb	boneless skinless catfish fillets	500 g
½ tsp	salt	2 mL
¼ cup	minced green onions	60 mL

Pungent Spiced Oil

¼ cup	avocado oil	60 mL
1 tsp	Sichuan peppercorns, shiny black seeds removed	5 mL
1 tsp	grated lemon zest	5 mL
1 tsp	minced gingerroot	5 mL
1 tsp	salt	5 mL
½ tsp	hot pepper flakes (optional)	2 mL

1. *Pungent Spiced Oil:* In a small saucepan, combine oil, Sichuan peppercorns, lemon zest, ginger, salt and hot pepper flakes (if using). Warm over medium heat for about 5 minutes or until spices are sizzling and oil is fragrant. Remove from heat and set aside. (To make ahead, let cool completely. Pour into an airtight container and set aside. Oil can be refrigerated for up to 2 months.)

2. Pour enough water into pot to come scant 1 inch (2.5 cm) up side. Place steamer rack in pan over water. Bring to a boil. Arrange catfish fillets in baking dish, cutting in half crosswise if necessary to fit. Sprinkle with salt. Place on rack, cover tightly and steam for 10 to 15 minutes or until fish is barely opaque.

3. Transfer fish to a serving platter and sprinkle with green onions. Keep warm. Reheat spiced oil until sizzling and immediately pour over fish and green onions. Serve immediately.

Auntie Katherine's Chicken Adobo

This recipe comes from Ellen's sister-in-law Katherine, whose mother passed it down to her and makes it for special family dinners. Adobo is known as the national dish of the Philippines, and is served often in homes across the country. This chicken version is a perfect comfort food and builds qi in the spring. It is an easy dish to make and a family favorite, served with steamed rice and freshly cooked greens.

	MAKES 4 SERVINGS	

Tips

We prefer organic chicken in all of our recipes. Conventionally raised chickens are given antibiotics and genetically modified feeds, and are subject to overcrowding and unhealthy conditions. This all runs counter to building your personal health, so choose organic whenever possible.

Cut the chicken into serving-size portions: thighs, drumsticks, wings, breasts, back and neck.

1	whole chicken (about 3 lbs/1.5 kg), cut into pieces	1
1 cup	unfiltered cider vinegar	250 mL
½ cup	tamari or soy sauce	125 mL
6	cloves garlic, smashed	6
1 tbsp	black peppercorns	15 mL
6 or 7	bay leaves	6 or 7

1. In a stockpot, combine 3 cups (750 mL) water, chicken, vinegar, tamari, garlic, peppercorns and bay leaves. Bring to a boil. Immediately reduce heat, cover and simmer, skimming surface occasionally to remove excess fat, for 40 minutes or until chicken is falling off the bones.

2. Spoon chicken and sauce into a deep serving platter. Serve immediately.

Health Tips

This dish — made from warming, sweet, *qi*-building chicken and warming vinegar — will help you perk up if you feel run-down after a cold (once all the symptoms are gone). It is also great for rebuilding the *qi* and blood in postpartum women.

The warming and pungent herbs boost digestion.

Do not eat this adobo if you have a cold, or experience symptoms related to excessive heat in the body.

Sweet Potato Noodles with Spring Greens and Shredded Lamb

Glistening, slippery sweet potato noodles balance the deep, rich flavor of lamb and the surprising freshness of wild spring greens. Tempeh is earthy like lamb, and a delicious alternative to it if you want to make this a vegetarian dish (see variation, below).

MAKES 4 SERVINGS

Tips

If you cannot find sweet potato noodles, substitute with mung bean noodles and cook them the same way. The latter are finer and softer.

To toast sesame seeds, place them in a small dry skillet. Toast over low heat, stirring or shaking pan constantly, for 3 minutes or until fragrant.

Variation

Substitute the same weight of plain tempeh for the lamb and cut into cubes. Follow the recipe through Step 3. Add ½ cup (125 mL) water. Reduce heat to low, cover and simmer for 10 minutes. Uncover and cook until water is evaporated, and then continue with Step 4.

Health Tip

Lamb is sweet, warming and nourishes the *qi*, yang and blood. It is good for women who often feel cold and those who experience irregular periods.

8 oz	sweet potato noodles (see tips, at left)	250 g
2 tbsp	avocado oil, divided	30 mL
1 lb	lamb shoulder	500 g
¼ cup	tamari or soy sauce	60 mL
¼ cup	rice wine, such as sake	60 mL
4 oz	trimmed mixed spring greens, such as arugula, purslane, baby kale or shepherd's purse	125 g
¼ cup	sesame seeds, toasted (see tips, at left)	60 mL
4	green onions, minced	4

1. In a large saucepan, bring 8 cups (2 L) water to a boil. Add noodles and cook, stirring once or twice, for 10 minutes or until tender. Drain well and return to pan. Stir in 1 tbsp (15 mL) of the oil and set aside.

2. Cut the lamb across the grain into ¼-inch (0.5 cm) thick slices. Stacking a few slices at a time, cut into ¼-inch (0.5 cm) strips.

3. In a large skillet, heat remaining oil over medium-high heat, swirling to coat bottom of pan. Add lamb and cook, stirring often, for 2 to 3 minutes or until edges are browned.

4. Stir in tamari, rice wine and greens and cook, stirring often, for 2 to 3 minutes or until greens are wilted and lamb is no longer pink in center.

5. Remove from heat. Add noodles and sesame seeds and toss to coat.

6. Divide noodle mixture among serving bowls. Sprinkle with green onions. Serve immediately.

Health Tip

Sweet potato noodles are neutral and pick up the seasonings and flavors from the other ingredients around them.

Qi-Moving Rose Game Hens

These fragrant game hens are a unique and special dish to serve to company with rice or a simple pilaf. They get their wonderful aromas, flavors and qi-moving properties from a delicious homemade spice blend (see recipe, opposite page).

> **MAKES**
> **4 LARGE SERVINGS**

Tips

If your game hens are smaller, turn after 35 minutes.

It's important to buy food-grade dried rose petals for cooking (not the ones used in potpourri). Choose organic ones, which don't contain any pesticide or other chemical residues.

- **Preheat oven to 400°F (200°C).**
- **Rimmed baking sheet, lined with lightly oiled foil**

2 tbsp	Ras el Hanout (see recipe, opposite)	30 mL
2 tsp	salt, divided	10 mL
2	Cornish game hens (each 1½ lbs/ 750 g), giblets removed	2
1	apple (such as Pacific Rose or Pink Lady), cored and coarsely chopped	1
1 tbsp	food-grade dried rose petals (see tips, at left)	15 mL

1. In a small bowl, stir ras el hanout with 1 tsp (5 mL) of the salt. Rub all over game hens.

2. In another small bowl, stir together apple, rose petals and remaining salt. Stuff apple mixture into hens. Using 6-inch (15 cm) bamboo skewers, skewer cavities, making an X over each opening.

3. Arrange hens, breast sides down, on prepared pan. Roast in preheated oven for 45 minutes.

4. Turn hens breast side up. Roast for 5 to 10 minutes or until juices run clear when thickest part of thigh is pierced.

5. Remove from oven and cover pan loosely with foil. Let stand for 15 minutes.

6. Cut each hen in half lengthwise. Arrange on serving plates and spoon stuffing alongside. Serve immediately.

> ## Health Tip
>
> Chicken is sweet, warming and builds the *qi*. Every time we emphasize augmenting or nourishing the *qi*, it is important to move it as well — this helps prevent stagnation. The combination of chicken and the fragrant and aromatic ras el hanout does just that.

Ras el Hanout

The name of this North African spice mixture translates as "top of the shop," indicating the high quality of the spices that go into it. It may contain as many as 20 different spices, and the recipe varies from cook to cook.

MAKES GENEROUS ½ CUP (125 ML)

Tip

See page 175 for more information on this spice mixture.

- Spice grinder, or mortar and pestle

1 tbsp	food-grade dried rose petals (see tips, opposite page)	15 mL
1 tsp	cumin seeds	5 mL
1 tsp	black peppercorns	5 mL
1 tsp	whole allspice	5 mL
1 tsp	green cardamom pods	5 mL
1 tsp	crumbled cinnamon stick	5 mL
½ tsp	coriander seeds	2 mL
1 tbsp	ground ginger	15 mL
1½ tsp	freshly grated nutmeg	7 mL
1 tsp	ground turmeric	5 mL
Pinch	ground cloves	Pinch
Pinch	cayenne pepper	Pinch

1. In spice grinder, combine rose petals, cumin seeds, peppercorns, allspice, cardamom pods, cinnamon stick and coriander seeds. Grind until powdery. Strain through a fine-mesh sieve into a small bowl. Discard any solids in sieve.

2. Stir in ginger, nutmeg, turmeric, cloves and cayenne.

3. Store in an airtight container in a cool, dark, dry place for up to 3 months.

Health Tips

Ras el hanout is a unique mixture of anti-inflammatory, digestive, balancing and *qi*-moving herbs and spices. Cardamom and nutmeg warm and activate digestion. Allspice is a carminative (meaning it relieves gas). Turmeric is a warming aromatic herb known as the "golden spice"; it has powerful anti-inflammatory effects, thanks to its active component, curcumin. It has been shown to reduce arthritis pain, lower cholesterol and protect liver function. Ginger soothes and protects the stomach. Rose petals ease liver *qi* and promote *qi* flow. Spring is the time for activating movement internally and externally, which the *qi*-moving herbs and spices in this blend do.

Quick-Pickled Radish Tops over Steamed Red Radishes and Cauliflower

Steaming makes simple red radishes beautifully translucent and almost sweet. This side is a delightful way to eat a range of fresh spring ingredients in a single dish.

MAKES 4 SERVINGS

Tips

If your bunch of radishes doesn't include enough tops to make 1 cup (250 mL) minced, supplement with trimmed arugula or chopped mustard greens.

You can substitute an equal amount of another type of radish, cut into 1-inch (2.5 cm) chunks.

Unpasteurized sauerkraut contains live bacteria, which are beneficial to gut health. Here, it is used to soften the greens and aid digestion.

- **2-cup (500 mL) canning jar**

1	bunch red radishes (8 oz/250 g)	1
1 tbsp	sauerkraut juice (from store-bought unpasteurized sauerkraut)	15 mL
½ tsp	kosher or non-iodized sea salt	2 mL
1	small head cauliflower (1 lb/500 g)	1

1. Remove tops (leaves and tender stems) from radishes. Mince and measure to make 1 cup (250 mL). (If not enough, see tips, at left.) Trim radishes and set aside.

2. In jar, combine radish tops, sauerkraut juice and salt. Seal lid and gently shake jar to make sure radish tops are evenly coated with juice and salt. Open jar. Using the back of a spoon, pack mixture down, making sure liquid covers radish tops. Cover loosely and let stand at room temperature for 24 hours. Seal jar and refrigerate for up to 2 days if not completing recipe immediately.

3. Cut cauliflower into bite-size florets. Halve radishes (or quarter if large).

4. In a large saucepan, bring 2 cups (500 mL) water to a boil. Add radishes and cauliflower. Reduce heat to medium-low, cover and cook for 5 minutes or until radishes are tender-crisp. Uncover pan and cook, shaking pan often, for 3 to 5 minutes or until no liquid remains.

5. Spoon radishes and cauliflower into a serving bowl. Scatter radish top mixture and its juices over top. Serve immediately.

Health Tips

Pungent greens, like these spicy radish tops, activate circulation and digestion and enhance fat digestion. Their spicy bite disperses internal stagnation — if you are looking to lose weight, add these greens to your diet.

This tasty side dish is excellent if you are getting over a spring cough with congestion.

Shredded Carrot and Dulse Salad

This chewy seaweed-and-veggie mixture is bursting with perfectly balanced flavors. The sweet carrots are complemented by the salty dulse, sour lemon and aromatic fresh parsley.

Tip

To toast sunflower seeds, place them in a small dry skillet. Toast over low heat, stirring or shaking pan often, for 3 to 4 minutes or until golden and fragrant.

½ cup	firmly packed dried dulse	125 mL
1 lb	carrots, grated	500 g
½ tsp	sea salt	2 mL
	Freshly squeezed juice of ½ lemon, or to taste	
¼ cup	minced fresh parsley	60 mL
2 tbsp	hulled raw sunflower or pumpkin seeds (optional), toasted	30 mL

1. Rinse dulse under cold running water until soft. Chop coarsely and set aside.

2. In a medium bowl, combine carrots and salt. Toss until carrots have a slight sheen and begin to release liquid. Stir in dulse.

3. Add lemon juice to taste, and parsley. Toss to coat. Sprinkle with sunflower seeds (if using). Serve immediately.

Health Tips

Dulse is a sea vegetable that is very high in minerals, including calcium, iron and magnesium. Sea vegetables are a traditional food consumed in coastal cultures throughout the world. They detoxify the body and strengthen the endocrine system. Small, regular servings of them make a delicious addition to your diet.

Carrots are sweet, encourage healthy digestion and elimination, and benefit the stomach. Lemons are sour and cooling. They support the production of saliva and other vital bodily fluids that lubricate the internal organs. Parsley is pungent, slightly bitter and salty. It moderates the strong flavors of fish and meat, helping the body to digest them.

Fava Beans with Anchovy, Lemon and Mint Dressing

Fava beans have a mildly earthy taste that's perfect for spring. Adding a zesty, tangy and highly aromatic dressing complements their flavor. Look for them in the spring at your local farmers' market, Asian grocery store or, if you are lucky, your favorite supermarket.

MAKES 4 SERVINGS

Tips

Fava beans are generally considered a nutritious food. But some people of African, Mediterranean or Southeast Asian descent have a genetic condition called favism, in which contact with fava flowers or beans can cause life-threatening anemia.

Fava beans are a quintessential spring bean. They are often planted in the autumn as a cover crop, and sprout and grow in the spring. If you have a garden, try your hand at planting them — you will harvest plenty, and your soil will be happy!

4 lbs	fava bean pods (or 1 lb/500 g shelled fava beans)	2 kg
2 tbsp	minced fresh spearmint	30 mL
½ tsp	grated lemon zest	2 mL
1 tbsp	freshly squeezed lemon juice, or to taste	15 mL
1	can (2 oz/56 g) anchovy fillets	1
	Salt (optional)	

1. Shell fava beans, discarding pods. Pour enough water into a large saucepan to come 1 inch (2.5 cm) up side. Bring to a boil. Add beans and cook, stirring occasionally, for 5 minutes or until tender. (To test, remove a bean and peel it; the center should be tender).

2. Drain well. Let stand until cool enough to handle. Peel skins off beans and discard. Place beans in a medium bowl and set aside.

3. In a small bowl, stir together mint, lemon zest and juice. Add anchovies and oil from can to mint mixture. Mash until chunky and well combined. Taste and add more lemon juice if desired. Season to taste with salt (if using).

4. Drizzle dressing over beans and toss to coat. Serve immediately.

Health Tips

Fava beans are sweet and neutral. They improve circulation and reduce water retention, which helps relieve edema.

The anchovy, lemon and mint dressing stimulates digestion and builds strength.

If you have a skin condition such as acne, decrease the lemon juice to 1 tsp (5 mL) and omit the anchovies (they are too warming).

Garlicky Wild Spring Greens

This simple, traditional way of cooking wild greens mellows their bitterness. It doesn't, however, reduce their value to your health. And they taste delicious!

MAKES 4 SERVINGS

Tip

If you pick wild greens yourself, make sure to avoid any areas that may have been sprayed with chemical pesticides, herbicides or fertilizers. Wild greens are often available in the spring at health food stores and farmers' markets.

1 lb	coarsely chopped dandelion or other wild greens (such as purslane or shepherd's purse)	500 g
4	cloves garlic	4
2 tbsp	extra virgin olive oil	30 mL
½ tsp	salt	2 mL

1. Pour enough water into a large saucepan to come 1 inch (2.5 cm) up side. Bring to a boil.

2. Add greens and garlic. Reduce heat and simmer for 5 to 8 minutes or until greens are very tender. Drain well and discard garlic.

3. Spoon into a serving bowl. Drizzle oil over top and sprinkle with salt. Serve immediately.

Health Tips

Wild spring greens are usually bitter or pungent. That makes them very powerful at clearing and draining excessive heat from the body. It is important to include these greens in your spring diet to eliminate the yang and heat you've built up over the winter.

Wild greens are packed with chlorophyll, which brings renewed energy to the body. They are proven blood cleansers and tonics.

Reduce the number of garlic cloves if you have a cold, fever or feel agitated. Garlic is very warming.

Steamed Artichokes with Cashew Sauce

The magnificent yet humble artichoke is much easier to cook than it looks. It's also delicious and fun to eat with this savory dipping sauce.

MAKES 4 SERVINGS

Tips

To eat artichokes, pull off a single leaf and dip it into the sauce. Pull it between your upper and lower teeth to scrape off the tender base of the leaf and the sauce. Discard the woody portion of the leaf. Repeat with the remaining leaves until you reach the fuzzy center (called the choke). Using a spoon, scrape out and discard the choke. Cut the heart and stem into bite-size pieces and dip into the sauce.

Artichokes are one of the oldest cultivated vegetables. They are actually the flower buds of a type of thistle — and cousins to cardoons.

- **Blender or food processor**

1	lemon		1
4	fresh artichokes		4
1	clove garlic		1
1 cup	warm water		250 mL
¾ cup	salted cashew butter		175 mL
1 tbsp	tamari or soy sauce		15 mL
	Salt		

1. Cut lemon in half. Squeeze 2 tbsp (30 mL) of the juice into a small bowl. Set juice and both lemon halves aside.

2. Trim artichokes and rub cut edges with lemon.

3. Pour enough water into a large saucepan to come 3 inches (7.5 cm) up side. Bring to a boil. Add garlic. Reduce heat and simmer for 5 minutes. Using a slotted spoon, remove garlic and discard.

4. Add artichokes, stem ends up, to pan. Cover and simmer for 15 to 20 minutes or until bases are very tender when tested with a fork.

5. Meanwhile, in blender, combine warm water, cashew butter and tamari. Blend until smooth. Taste and add some of the reserved lemon juice to taste. Season to taste with salt.

6. Drain artichokes well. Place on serving plates and serve immediately with sauce for dipping.

Health Tips

Artichokes are cooling, bitter and slightly sweet. They are an age-old remedy that stimulates bile flow in the liver, an organ that is particularly active in the spring. A tincture made from this wonderfully bitter food is high in antioxidants and is often used to help lower cholesterol, promote liver function and encourage fat digestion.

Cashews are sweet and add a nourishing component to this liver-stimulating food.

Braised Taro and Baby Vegetables with Citrus Oil

Taro is a starchy root vegetable with a mild, earthy, nutty flavor. It is typically eaten as part of Chinese New Year celebrations. In this simple braised spring side dish, fresh baby vegetables and a citrus oil drizzle brighten it up and make it even tastier. The vegetables are good warm or at room temperature; just drizzle with oil and sprinkle with cilantro right before serving.

MAKES 4 SERVINGS

Tip

Raw taro root peel contains compounds that can irritate the skin. To avoid that, we cook the root before peeling it.

Health Tip

Taro is pungent, sweet and neutral. Its high carbohydrate content is nourishing and reinforcing. The cooked root is easily digested. It is a beneficial food to eat if you have loss of appetite and fatigue due to weak digestion.

1 lb	taro roots (unpeeled)	500 g
1 lb	mixed baby vegetables, such as radishes, carrots and turnips	500 g
1 tbsp	avocado oil	15 mL
1 tsp	salt	5 mL
2 tbsp	minced fresh cilantro or parsley	30 mL
Citrus Oil		
1/4 cup	avocado oil	60 mL
1 tsp	grated grapefruit zest (preferably white grapefruit)	5 mL
1 tsp	grated lemon zest	5 mL
1/2 tsp	hot pepper flakes	2 mL

1. *Citrus Oil:* In a small saucepan, combine oil, grapefruit zest, lemon zest and hot pepper flakes. Warm over medium-high heat for about 3 minutes or until oil is fragrant. Remove from heat and set aside. (To make ahead, let cool completely. Pour into an airtight container and set aside. Oil can refrigerated for up to 2 months.)

2. Place taro in a medium saucepan and pour in enough water to cover. Bring to a boil. Reduce heat and simmer for 20 minutes or until taro is almost tender when tested with a fork. Drain well and peel.

3. Cut taro and baby vegetables into 3/4-inch (2 cm) chunks. In a large skillet, heat oil over medium-high heat. Add baby vegetables and stir to coat. Cook, stirring often, for 5 minutes or until edges of vegetables are starting to brown.

4. Add taro, 1 cup (250 mL) water and salt. Cover and steam for 5 minutes or until vegetables are tender.

5. Spoon into serving bowls. Drizzle with citrus oil and sprinkle with cilantro. Serve immediately.

Sautéed Broccoli with Tangy Ginger Dressing

Simple, familiar broccoli is more delightful with the addition of a zippy, tangy-sweet dressing — and kids will often enjoy it prepared this way. Serve it as a side dish with simply steamed fish, roasted chicken or tofu.

MAKES 4 SERVINGS

Tips

If you're preparing this dish ahead, add the dressing and nuts just before serving.

To toast pecans, place them in a small dry skillet. Toast over low heat, stirring or shaking pan frequently, for about 5 minutes or until fragrant.

- **2-cup (500 mL) canning jar**

2	green onions, finely chopped	2
3 tbsp	avocado oil, divided	45 mL
2 tbsp	unfiltered cider vinegar	30 mL
2 tbsp	slivered dried apricots	30 mL
2 tsp	grated gingerroot	10 mL
1 tsp	salt	5 mL
1	bunch (1½ lbs/750 g) broccoli, cut into small florets	1
½ cup	coarsely chopped pecans, toasted	125 mL

1. In jar, combine green onions, 2 tbsp (30 mL) of the oil, the vinegar, apricots, ginger and salt. Shake to combine and set aside.

2. In a large skillet, heat remaining oil over medium-high heat, swirling to coat bottom of pan. Add broccoli and ½ cup (125 mL) water. Cover and steam for 2 minutes. Uncover and sauté for 5 minutes or until broccoli is bright green and tender.

3. Spoon broccoli into a serving bowl. Shake dressing well to recombine and drizzle over broccoli. Sprinkle with pecans. Serve immediately.

Health Tips

Broccoli is cooling and clears out excess liver heat, counters eye inflammation and acts as a diuretic.

The warming pungency of green onions will disperse cold. Warming ginger supports digestion.

Be sure to eat broccoli cooked. It contains compounds called goitrogens, which can interfere with the thyroid's capacity to absorb iodine, causing goiters. Avoid raw broccoli altogether if you have hypothyroidism.

Spring Greens and Lotus Root Sauté

The vivid freshness of young spring greens is enlivening. They're even more delightful paired with crunchy, mild lotus root. If you like, garnish this dish with Citrus Oil (page 233) or Umeboshi with Jasmine Tea Leaves (page 435).

MAKES 4 SERVINGS

Tip

For more information how to purchase the best-quality lotus root and pea shoots, turn to pages 173 and 218, respectively.

8 oz	lotus root	250 g
2 tbsp	avocado oil	30 mL
8 oz	mixed baby greens, such as spinach, kale or pea shoots, coarsely chopped	250 g
½ tsp	salt	2 mL

1. Pour enough water into a medium saucepan to come 2 inches (5 cm) up side. Bring to a simmer.

2. Trim ends off lotus root and peel. Immediately place in simmering water and cook for 15 to 20 minutes or until tender-crisp. Drain and let cool to room temperature.

3. Cut lotus root into ⅛-inch (3 mm) thick slices. Set aside.

4. In a large skillet, heat oil over medium-high heat, swirling to coat bottom of pan. Add greens and salt and cook, stirring often, for 2 to 3 minutes or until wilted. Add lotus root and cook, stirring often, for 1 minute or just until heated through.

5. Spoon into a serving bowl. Serve immediately.

Health Tips

Uncooked lotus root is sweet and cooling, whereas cooked is more warming. It can be beneficial for people with hypertension and high cholesterol. In traditional Chinese medicine, lotus root juice mixed with honey is used to treat thirst during fevers.

Spring greens are usually pungent, sweet or slightly bitter. They are filled with chlorophyll, which brings renewed cleansing energy back to the body after a long winter.

Simple Roasted Asparagus

Asparagus is a tender spring vegetable and one of the first treats of the season. The good news is that it's incredibly easy to cook and is so delicious when roasted with a little oil and salt.

MAKES 4 SERVINGS

Tip

Thin asparagus is more intensely flavorful. But because it takes fewer large spears to make 2 lbs (1 kg), you'll have them trimmed and peeled in less time — and they're still very tasty.

- **Preheat oven to 400°F (200°C)**
- **Large rimmed baking sheet**

2 lbs	asparagus	1 kg
2 tbsp	avocado oil	30 mL
1 tsp	salt	5 mL

1. Trim off cut ends of asparagus and discard. Using a vegetable peeler, peel off tough skin from bottoms of spears.

2. Arrange asparagus on prepared pan. Drizzle with oil and sprinkle with salt. Roll spears to coat with oil.

3. Roast in preheated oven, stirring 2 or 3 times, for about 20 minutes or until tender.

4. Transfer to a serving platter. Serve immediately.

Health Tip

Asparagus is a wonderful natural diuretic. This vegetable is mildly cooling, so it is also good for people with hypertension and those who tend to feel hot and irritable. Asparagus can also be a good treatment for a cough, as it moistens the lungs.

Spring Nettle and Fragrant Flowers Tea

This beautifully aromatic, clean-tasting tea will leave you refreshed and feeling calm. We recommend dried rose buds for their concentrated flavor and fragrance in this tea.

MAKES 4 SERVINGS

Tip

If you like, you can leave out the flowers and make a nettle-only tea. Some people find the grassy, almost bitter aftertaste of nettles takes a little getting used to. Feel free to add a squeeze of lemon or a spoonful of honey to soften the flavor.

4 tsp	dried nettles	20 mL
4 tsp	food-grade dried red rose buds	20 mL
2 tsp	dried chrysanthemum flowers	10 mL

1. In a small saucepan, bring 4 cups (1 L) water to a boil. Remove from heat.

2. Stir in nettles, rose buds and chrysanthemum flowers. Let stand for 5 minutes.

3. Strain into teacups. Serve immediately.

Health Tips

This tea is great for anyone who suffers from spring allergies with itchy eyes. It soothes, clears out excess heat and gets the *qi* moving.

Nettles are well known for their capacity to enrich liver yin, nourish the blood, regulate metabolism, promote detoxification and fight allergies. They are also beneficial during pregnancy and afterwards to boost breast-milk production. Add steamed fresh nettle leaves to soups, or quickly braise or sauté them as a side dish.

Fragrant dried red rose buds are slightly warming and gently pungent, so they move the liver *qi* — which is just what you want in springtime. They open the body and mind up, stimulating the senses and stirring the heart.

Ginger and Tangerine Peel Tea

As the famous jazz song goes, "Spring can really hang you up the most." This season is so fickle: one day it's warm, the next, blustery; you really have to keep your jacket buttoned up. This tea helps with that, thanks to the warming essences of ginger and dried tangerine peel. Its spicy, lightly bitter citrus flavor will warm you and help fight off spring colds.

| | MAKES 2 SERVINGS | |

Tips

You can buy dried tangerine peel from a Chinese herb supplier or any acupuncturist who stocks medicinal herbs. But it's also easy to dry your own. Peel a tangerine and rip into 1-inch (2.5 cm) long strips. Lay the strips on a piece of parchment paper and let dry in a cool, dark, dry place for 2 days or up to 1 week or until completely dried. Store in a glass jar at room temperature for up to 3 months.

You can use raw tangerine peel instead of dried to make this tea, but you will not get as strong a warming effect from it.

3	slices (quarter-size) gingerroot, lightly crushed	3
2	strips dried tangerine peel (see tips, at left)	2
	Liquid honey (optional)	

1. In a small saucepan, bring 2 cups (500 mL) water to a boil. Remove from heat.

2. Stir in ginger and tangerine peel. Cover and let stand for 10 minutes.

3. Strain into teacups. Stir in honey (if using) to taste. Serve immediately.

Health Tips

The tangerine peel and ginger are both warming and soothe stomach upsets. Use this tea to help boost digestion, warm the stomach and clear out phlegm.

If you are just coming down with a cold, add 1 tsp (5 mL) dried mint along with the tangerine peel. It will help the tea clear your head and throat.

Qi-Moving Rose Liquor

Spring is a time to relax and appreciate the beautiful growth happening all around in nature. This spring beverage stimulates the senses with a light floral fragrance as it warms your body and lifts your spirits. It makes a delicious, soothing aperitif and is a terrific stress buster.

> **MAKES ABOUT 3 CUPS (750 ML)**

Tip

A little bit of this liquor goes a long way. Enjoy a very small amount — about a shot glass worth, or 3 tbsp (45 mL) — once a day.

This liquor is best drunk straight up, without ice.

- **1-quart (1 L) canning jar**
- **1-quart (1 L) glass bottle**

4 oz	food-grade dried rose buds or rose petals	125 g
3 cups	vodka	750 mL
¼ cup	liquid honey	60 mL

1. Place rose buds in jar and pour in vodka. Add honey and shake gently to combine. Seal with lid and let stand at room temperature, gently shaking jar occasionally, for 3 to 4 weeks.

2. Strain liquid through a fine-mesh sieve into bottle. Discard solids. Store at room temperature for up to 6 months.

> ### Health Tip
>
> Alcohol warms the body and invigorates the circulation. Roses awaken and move the liver *qi* and are most useful for relaxing the body and mind.

Strawberry-Rose Fruit Salad

This delectable, aromatic and ultra-fresh salad is infused with the heart-opening fragrance of roses. It makes a refreshing finish to a spring dinner and is lovely with Ginger and Tangerine Peel Tea (page 238).

---

2 tbsp	orange juice	30 mL
1 tbsp	liquid honey	15 mL
¼ tsp	rose water	1 mL
4 cups	strawberries, hulled and halved	1 L
2 tsp	thinly sliced fresh spearmint (optional)	10 mL

MAKES 4 TO 6 SERVINGS

Tip

The acid in the orange juice stabilizes the color compounds in the strawberries, so the salad stays beautifully red.

Rose water is easy to find in supermarkets, Middle Eastern grocery stores and online shops.

1. In a small bowl, whisk together orange juice, honey and rose water.

2. Place strawberries in a serving bowl and drizzle with orange juice mixture. Toss gently to coat. Sprinkle with mint (if using). Serve immediately.

Health Tips

This delicious dessert quenches thirst, lubricates tissues and soothes a dry throat and a dry cough.

In Chinese medicine, wind is one of the five external climate factors (known as pathogens) that can activate illness. Wind, cold and damp are common springtime climate elements. Strawberries are cooling and can help to eliminate the effects of wind and heat.

Baked Spiced Rhubarb

Vibrant rhubarb stalks are one of the first plants to emerge from the ground in the spring. Rhubarb is a vegetable that is mostly treated like a fruit; it's a star in pies and cobblers. This warm, comforting, easy-to-make dessert is nice on a windy spring day. The shape and texture of the rhubarb holds up nicely when it's baked — you will be pleasantly surprised!

MAKES 6 SERVINGS

Tip

To make ginger juice, grate gingerroot and press through a fine-mesh sieve into a small bowl. Discard fibers.

- **Preheat oven to 350°F (180°C)**
- **13- by 9-inch (33 by 23 cm) glass baking dish**

1 cup	unsweetened white grape juice	250 mL
2 tsp	ground cinnamon	30 mL
2 lbs	fresh rhubarb stalks, trimmed and cut diagonally into 1-inch (2.5 cm) pieces	1 kg
½ cup	liquid honey	125 mL
2 tsp	ginger juice (see tip, at left)	10 mL

1. In baking dish, whisk grape juice with cinnamon. Add rhubarb. Drizzle with honey and ginger juice.

2. Cover tightly with foil and bake in preheated oven for 15 minutes or until liquid is bubbling vigorously. Uncover and bake, stirring gently once or twice, for 15 minutes or until almost no liquid remains. Serve warm. (To make ahead, let cool completely. Cover and refrigerate for up to 1 week. Reheat before serving.)

3. Spoon into serving bowls. Serve immediately.

Health Tips

Rhubarb's sour flavor, astringency and cold nature make it an excellent food for clearing out excess internal heat that builds up over the winter. It is also beneficial for people who suffer from constipation.

While rhubarb stalks are safe to eat, they do contain some oxalic acid. Eat them sparingly if you suffer from any inflammatory joint conditions, which can be exacerbated by this compound.

Do not eat rhubarb leaves — they contain dangerously high levels of oxalic acid.

Summer Seasonal Menus

Menu 1
Braised Tomatoes and Sweet Potatoes with Eggs
Simple Sautéed Greens

Menu 2
Roasted Eggplant and Tomato with Peanut Sauce
Five-Flavor Sautéed Cucumbers

Menu 3
Herb-Grilled Chicken
Arame Salad with Lemon and Chives
Vibrant Summer Vegetables with Tofu Dressing

Summer Recipes

Breakfasts

Soups

Meats, Fish and Other Mains

Mostly Vegetables

Snack

Teas and Tonic Beverages

Desserts

Clear-the-Heat Mung Bean Congee

Warm mung bean congee is a typical Chinese breakfast on a summer morning. Mung beans are known for their cooling nature. Cooking the beans in green tea gives them a light astringency, which contrasts nicely with the sweet, mellow rice.

> **MAKES 4 SERVINGS**

Tip

Pure coconut milk is used in this recipe, not coconut milk beverage. Look for a brand that is preservative-free — it will have better flavor.

1 cup	sweet (glutinous) brown rice (or brown Arborio rice)	250 mL
1 cup	coconut milk (see tip, at left)	250 mL
½ cup	chopped pitted dates	125 mL
2 cups	Mung Beans Cooked in Green Tea (see recipe, opposite)	500 mL
½ cup	hulled hemp seeds	125 mL

1. In a medium saucepan, combine 2 cups (500 mL) water, rice and coconut milk. Bring to a boil. Reduce heat, cover and simmer for 45 minutes to 1 hour or until very tender. The congee should have a souplike consistency; if there is not enough liquid left in the pan, add up to ½ cup (125 mL) water.

2. Stir in dates. Cover and let cool for 30 minutes. Serve immediately or transfer to an airtight container and refrigerate for up to 5 days. Warm in a small saucepan over low heat before serving.

3. In a small saucepan, warm mung beans over low heat, stirring occasionally, for 2 to 3 minutes or until heated through. Meanwhile, in a small dry skillet, toast hemp seeds over low heat, stirring or shaking pan often, for about 5 minutes or until fragrant.

4. Spoon warm congee into serving bowls. Divide mung beans and hemp seeds among bowls. Serve immediately.

> ## Health Tip
>
> Mung beans are sweet and cooling. They are a classic remedy for clearing heat from the surface of the body during the hot, humid summer months. They are also beneficial for people with diabetes, high cholesterol, or skin issues that cause redness (heat) and itching.

Mung Beans Cooked in Green Tea

These lightly astringent, cooling beans are also delicious in Thai-Style Textured Salad (page 255). They are very easy to make, so keep them on hand for cooling down in the hot weather.

MAKES ABOUT 2 CUPS (500 ML)

½ cup	dried green mung beans	125 mL
2	green tea bags (or 2 tsp/10 mL loose green tea)	2

1. In a medium saucepan, combine 4 cups (1 L) water and mung beans. Bring to a boil. Remove from heat, cover and soak for 1 hour. Drain and rinse well.

2. In another medium saucepan, bring 4 cups (1 L) water to a boil. Add tea bags or loose tea. Remove from heat, cover and let stand for 5 minutes.

3. Discard tea bags or strain out leaves and discard. Stir mung beans into tea. Return to a simmer over medium-high heat. Reduce heat to low, cover and simmer for 30 to 40 minutes or until mung beans are tender. Drain before adding to recipes. (Drained cooked beans can be refrigerated in an airtight container for up to 3 days.)

White Fish and Celery Congee

Seafood, paired with delicately aromatic celery and fennel seeds, makes this congee a pleasing option to eat any time of day — though it is an especially satisfying breakfast. It's fresh, savory and light enough to enjoy on a sunny summer day.

MAKES 4 SERVINGS

Tip

Make sure the congee is simmering before you stir in the fish. The residual heat will cook it through but won't overcook it and make it fall apart. If the fish still looks underdone for your taste, gently simmer for a minute or two more until it's cooked to your liking.

1	piece (3 inches/7.5 cm square) dried kombu	1
2 cups	thinly sliced celery (about 4 stalks)	500 mL
½ cup	sweet (glutinous) brown rice (or brown Arborio rice)	125 mL
1 tsp	fennel seeds	5 mL
1 tsp	salt, or to taste	5 mL
1 lb	boneless mild white fish fillets, such as snapper	500 g

1. In a medium saucepan, combine 5 cups (1.25 L) water, kombu, celery, rice and fennel seeds. Bring to a boil. Reduce heat to low, cover and simmer for 10 minutes. Discard kombu.

2. Simmer, stirring occasionally, for 2 hours. The congee should have a souplike consistency; if there is not enough liquid left in the pan, add up to ½ cup (125 mL) water. Stir in 1 tsp (5 mL) salt; taste and season with more salt, if desired.

3. Cut fish into 1-inch (2.5 cm) chunks and stir into congee. Remove from heat, cover and let stand for 10 minutes or until fish is opaque.

4. Serve immediately or transfer to an airtight container and refrigerate for up to 3 days. Warm in a small saucepan over low heat before serving.

Health Tip

People either love or avoid celery. If you fall into the latter camp, give it another chance, because it offers so many wonderful health benefits. Cooling, slightly pungent, slightly salty, slightly bitter and sweet celery stalks are most beneficial for people who run hot or have high blood pressure. It is known for its calming action. Celery helps clear heat out of the body, calms agitation, eases headaches and encourages detoxification.

Essential Seed and Nut Porridge with Feta and Fresh Fruit

The combination of salty, creamy feta cheese and sweet-tart fruit gives this porridge a nice balance of tastes. Sheep's milk feta is the traditional favorite for its earthier flavor profile.

MAKES 4 SERVINGS

Tips

You can add up to 1 cup (250 mL) more boiling water to the porridge mix if you prefer a thinner consistency.

If you can only find salted roasted pistachios, shake them in a colander to remove excess salt and skip the toasting step. Do, however, toast the almonds as directed.

Make sure the plantain chips you purchase are cooked in a healthy oil and don't contain added sugar.

Health Tips

This porridge provides some of your daily dose of omega-3 essential fatty acids. If you are overweight and have digestive issues, eat this dish in moderation. It is important to resolve and clear the yin excess that causes these health issues.

Honey is sweet, lubricating and nourishing to the stomach and spleen.

* **Blender**

2 cups	boiling water	500 mL
1 cup	cubed pitted fresh apricots or peaches, at room temperature	250 mL
4 oz	drained sheep's milk feta cheese, crumbled	125 g
¼ cup	liquid honey (optional)	60 mL

Porridge Mix

3 tbsp	hulled hemp seeds	45 mL
3 tbsp	flax seeds	45 mL
2 tbsp	chia seeds	30 mL
½ cup	unsalted raw pistachios	125 mL
½ cup	unsalted raw almonds	125 mL
1 cup	unsweetened roasted plantain chips	250 mL
½ tsp	salt	2 mL

1. *Porridge Mix:* In a large dry skillet, toast hemp, flax and chia seeds over medium-low heat, stirring often, for 5 minutes or until fragrant. Transfer to a heatproof bowl. Return skillet to heat and add pistachios and almonds. Toast over medium-low heat, stirring often, for 8 to 10 minutes or until fragrant. Transfer to another heatproof bowl. Let cool completely.

2. In blender, combine seed mixture and plantain chips and grind until the texture of brown sugar. Add nut mixture and salt and grind until the texture of brown sugar.

3. In a medium bowl, stir porridge mix with boiling water. Cover and let stand for 5 minutes.

4. Spoon porridge into serving bowls. Top with apricots and feta cheese. Drizzle with honey (if using). Serve immediately.

Mushroom, Buckwheat and Egg Bowl

This toothsome assortment of mushrooms complements and echoes the earthiness of the creamy buckwheat. This robust, savory bowl could become a go-to comfort food for starting your day.

Tip

Remove and discard the stems from shiitake mushrooms, as they are often quite tough.

Health Tip

Buckwheat looks and cooks up like a grain, but it is not one. Buckwheat has a nutty, earthy flavor and is rich in B vitamins. It helps regulate blood sugar, and disperses heat and dampness in the body, so it is great for people who have a difficult time losing weight.

3 tbsp	ghee, divided	45 mL
6 cups	thinly sliced mixed mushrooms, such as shiitake, button, cremini or oyster	1.5 L
1 tsp	salt	5 mL
4 to 8	large eggs	4 to 8
1	batch Creamy Buckwheat (recipe, below), warmed	1

1. In a large skillet, heat 2 tbsp (30 mL) of the ghee over medium heat. Add mushrooms and cook, stirring often, for 5 to 7 minutes or until softened and almost no liquid remains. Sprinkle with salt and transfer to a plate. Keep warm.

2. Wipe out skillet. Add remaining ghee and heat over medium heat. Break eggs into pan and fry to desired doneness.

3. Spoon warm buckwheat into serving bowls. Top with eggs and mushrooms. Serve immediately.

Creamy Buckwheat

Cooking the buckwheat with plenty of water yields the same creamy texture as corn grits, making them into an earthy porridge-style breakfast cereal. Garnish this porridge with a condiment or chopped nuts, or with your favorite toppings.

Tip

Whole, unprocessed buckwheat seeds are called groats.

1 cup	buckwheat groats	250 mL

1. In a medium saucepan over medium heat, toast buckwheat, stirring often, for 5 minutes or until fragrant.

2. Stir in 5 cups (1.25 L) water and bring to a simmer. Reduce heat to low and simmer, stirring often, for 30 minutes. Remove from heat, cover and let stand for 30 minutes before serving.

Pungent-Herb Breakfast Fried Rice

Fresh summer herbs enliven this simple fried rice, which you can vary according to whatever is in season and appeals to you most. Keep in mind that herbs with tender (not woody) leaves work best in this dish.

MAKES 4 SERVINGS

Tip

Green onions (also known as scallions) are not usually considered an herb, but their potent pungency and heat-clearing attributes make them a perfect crossover into herbal terrain. In winter, pair them with ginger to warm the body; in summer, eat them if you experience a fever, as their pungency will induce sweating and help you cool down.

1 cup	brown jasmine rice or brown basmati rice	250 mL
2 tbsp	avocado oil	30 mL
1 cup	packed chopped mixed fresh herbs, such as green onions, dill, cilantro or parsley (3 oz/90 g total)	250 mL
1 tsp	salt	5 mL
4	large eggs, beaten	4

1. In a medium saucepan, combine $2\frac{1}{2}$ cups (625 mL) water and rice. Bring to a boil. Reduce heat to low, cover and simmer for 30 to 40 minutes or until almost tender. Turn off heat and let pan stand, covered, on burner for 15 minutes. Let cool. Refrigerate for 2 hours or up to 2 days.

2. In a large skillet, heat oil over medium-high heat. Using a spatula, spread rice over bottom of pan. Cook, without stirring, for 1 minute or until bottom is lightly browned.

3. Sprinkle herbs and salt over rice and turn. Cook, without stirring, for 1 minute or until lightly browned.

4. Push rice to 1 side of the pan and pour eggs into open space. Cook, without stirring, for 2 minutes or until eggs are set on bottom. Turn eggs and cook, without stirring, for 1 minute or until set on bottom. (Avoid stirring the rice, as that will make it gummy.)

5. Remove from heat. Using spatula, roughly chop eggs and fold into rice. Spoon into serving bowls. Serve immediately.

Health Tip

Strongly flavored fresh herbs — such as dill, parsley, cilantro, chives and green onions — stimulate and support digestion in this nourishing dish. Parsley also acts as a mild diuretic.

Okra, Corn and Basil Savory Steamed Egg Custard

A steamed egg custard, resplendent with summer vegetables, has a multidimensional flavor and texture. This might just be the perfect height-of-summer dish. It is also very nourishing and ultra-digestible.

MAKES 6 SERVINGS

Tips

If your pot is too small to hold all of the ramekins at once, steam the custards in batches.

Rubber-tipped tongs are great for transferring the ramekins to the steamer pot. If you don't have them, you can wrap thick rubber bands around the tips of regular metal tongs.

Health Tip

Cooked okra has a slippery texture that people either love or hate. Even if you haven't liked it before, try it in this custard — it's so good. Okra aids digestion and can ease constipation. Basil, another summer food, is pungent and warming, and promotes good digestion. Corn, the third summery ingredient in this custard, is cooling.

- **Six ½- or ¾-cup (125 or 175 mL) ramekins or custard cups**
- **Large pot with steamer rack (about 1 inch/2.5 cm above bottom of pot)**

6	okra pods	6
6 tbsp	fresh or thawed frozen corn kernels	90 mL
6	fresh basil leaves	6
4	large eggs, beaten	4
3 cups	Traditional or Vegetarian Dashi (page 297), at room temperature	750 mL
1 tbsp	tamari or soy sauce	15 mL
½ tsp	salt	2 mL

1. In a medium saucepan, bring 1 cup (250 mL) water to a boil. Add okra and cook for 2 to 3 minutes or just until tender. Using a slotted spoon, transfer to a small bowl and let cool.

2. Add corn to boiling water and cook for about 1 minute or until color brightens. Drain and let cool.

3. Cut okra into ½-inch (1 cm) pieces. Divide okra and corn among ramekins. Add 1 basil leaf to each. Set aside.

4. In a 4-cup (1 L) glass measuring cup, whisk together eggs, dashi, tamari and salt. Strain and gently pour into ramekins.

5. Pour enough water into pot to come scant 1 inch (2.5 cm) up side. Place steamer rack in pan over water. Bring to a boil.

6. Arrange ramekins on rack, cover tightly and steam for 15 to 20 minutes or until custard is barely set in the center (it will be jiggly but not liquid).

7. Serve warm or at room temperature. Or cover and refrigerate for up to 3 days; let come to room temperature for an hour before serving.

Tilapia and Arugula Soup

This light soup celebrates the subtle flavors of good homemade dashi, a savory Japanese broth — made with dried bonito flakes and/or kombu seaweed, it gives the soup a foundation of umami. You only need the cobs from the corn to make the broth; save the kernels to use in another recipe, such as Quick-Pickled Summer Salad with Squash and Corn (page 264).

**MAKES
2 TO 4 SERVINGS**

Tip

Katsuobushi are flakes of shaved dried bonito, a product commonly used in Japanese cuisine. Look for packages of them in Asian grocery stores and well-stocked supermarkets. They're sold by weight — you'll only need about $1/6$ ounce (5 g) to make $1/2$ cup (125 mL). Learn more about them in the ingredient profile on page 171.

2	ears corn, husked	2
1	piece (4 inches/10 cm square) dried kombu	1
½ cup	katsuobushi (see tip, at left)	125 mL
1½ tsp	salt	7 mL
2 oz	mixed baby greens, such as baby arugula, baby kale or baby spinach	60 g
8 oz	boneless skinless tilapia or other mild white fish fillets, cut into bite-size pieces	250 g
2 tbsp	finely chopped green onions	30 mL

1. Cut kernels off corn cobs and reserve for another use. Break cobs in half and place in a large saucepan. Add 4 cups (1 L) water and kombu. Bring to a boil.

2. Turn off heat and stir in katsuobushi. Cover and let stand on burner for 10 minutes. Strain broth through a fine-mesh sieve into a bowl, discarding solids.

3. Return broth to pan and bring to a boil. Stir in salt and greens. Reduce heat and simmer for 2 to 3 minutes or just until wilted.

4. Gently stir in fish and turn off heat. Cover and let stand on burner for 5 minutes or until fish is opaque.

5. Ladle soup into serving bowls. Sprinkle with green onions. Serve immediately.

Health Tip

The sweet-salty fish mingled with sweet corn and spicy arugula makes this nourishing summer soup excellent if you tend to feel overheated and can help boost *qi*.

Corn Silk and Chicken Soup

The sweetness of the meat coupled with corn and its silk makes this a nourishing, well-balanced soup for summer that's not too warming. A simple corn silk tea gives a lovely, mellow sweetness to the broth for this soup. Make sure your corn is organic or at least unsprayed before using the silk.

MAKES 4 SERVINGS

Tip

Corn silk is a pretty name for the tassels that appear at the top of an ear of corn. You can use fresh or dried in recipes.

2	ears corn (unhusked)	2
1	large egg, beaten	1
1 lb	ground chicken (preferably thighs)	500 g
2 tsp	salt, divided	10 mL
4	green onions, minced	4
¼	napa cabbage (about 2-lb/1 kg cabbage), cored and thinly sliced	¼

1. Reserving silk, remove husks from corn. Set silk aside and discard husks. Cut off corn kernels, discarding cobs.

2. In a medium bowl, combine corn kernels, egg, chicken, ½ tsp (2 mL) of the salt and green onions. Mix until well combined. Shape into 16 meatballs and place on a large plate. Cover and refrigerate for 2 hours or for up to 24 hours.

3. In a medium saucepan, combine 4 cups (1 L) water and corn silk. Bring to a simmer. Immediately remove from heat, cover and let stand for 10 minutes. Strain through a fine-mesh sieve into a bowl, discarding solids. Return liquid to pan.

4. Bring liquid to a simmer. Add meatballs and remaining salt. Reduce heat to low and simmer, gently stirring once or twice, for 10 minutes.

5. Stir in cabbage and cook, gently stirring occasionally, for 2 to 3 minutes or until cabbage is wilted and meatballs are no longer pink inside.

6. Ladle into serving bowls. Serve immediately.

Health Tip

Corn silk is used by Western herbalists to soothe the inflammation of the urinary system, ease edema and reduce hypertension. It is also administered to help with kidney stones. Corn silk is sweet, cooling, and it balances the warming aspect of the sweet chicken.

Borscht

This tasty beet soup is a variation on the wonderful vegan borscht that was served at Nosmo King, a now-defunct New York City vegan restaurant. The sweetness of the beets is heightened by a small amount of lemon juice. For a creamy finish, top it with a spoonful of Greek, sheep's milk or goat's milk yogurt.

MAKES 6 SERVINGS

Tip

This soup is best served at room temperature or slightly chilled. Of course, you can also eat the soup hot.

- **Blender or immersion blender**

3	beets, cut into small chunks	3
1	large onion, coarsely chopped	1
1	large carrot, coarsely chopped	1
1	piece (3 inches/7.5 cm square) dried kombu (optional)	1
1	bay leaf	1
1 tsp	salt	5 mL
1½ tsp	freshly squeezed lemon juice	7 mL
	Black pepper	
	Fresh dill sprigs	

1. In a stockpot, combine 6 cups (1.5 L) water, beets, onion, carrot, kombu (if using), bay leaf and salt. Bring to a boil. Reduce heat and simmer for 30 minutes or until beets are tender.

2. Remove from heat. Discard kombu and bay leaf. Stir in lemon juice.

3. In blender, in batches if necessary, purée soup until smooth. Let cool to room temperature. (To make ahead, let cool completely, cover and refrigerate for up to 3 days.)

4. Ladle into serving bowls. Sprinkle with pepper to taste and garnish with dill sprigs. Serve immediately.

Health Tip

Beets are the original blood-building vegetable, and are especially beneficial for people who are anemic or have lower-than-normal iron levels. If you are vegetarian or vegan, make sure to include them in your diet. Beets also promote healthy liver function, clear phlegm and ease constipation.

Saffron Seafood Soup

An exquisite, subtle spice, saffron is also a medicinal herb (see health tips, below). Just a couple of generous pinches gives this fish-and-shrimp soup depth of flavor and a bright yellow hue that evokes a sunny day at the beach.

MAKES 4 SERVINGS

Tips

This soup is terrific for a picnic! Pack it in a vacuum flask to keep it warm, and bring along the parsley and lemon wedges in separate airtight containers.

This soup does not reheat well, so plan to eat it all right away.

Saffron is the most expensive spice in the world. By some counts, it can take upwards of 75,000 *Crocus sativus* flowers to extract a single pound (500 g) of saffron!

Caution

Do not use saffron if you are pregnant, as it can induce contractions.

---

2 tbsp	avocado oil	30 mL
4	cloves garlic, chopped	4
½	large onion, chopped	½
1	can (14 oz/398 mL) diced tomatoes, with juices	1
½ tsp	saffron threads	2 mL
¼ tsp	fennel seeds	1 mL
2 cups	Traditional Dashi (page 297)	500 mL
8 oz	boneless skinless mild white fish fillets, such as snapper, cut into 1-inch (2.5 cm) pieces	250 g
8 oz	uncooked peeled deveined shrimp	250 g
¼ cup	finely chopped fresh parsley or basil	60 mL
2	small lemons, cut into wedges	2

1. In a medium saucepan, heat oil over medium heat. Add garlic and onion. Cook, stirring often, for 5 minutes or until onion is translucent and golden.

2. Stir in tomatoes and juices, saffron and fennel seeds. Cook, stirring often, for 15 minutes. Stir in dashi and bring to a simmer.

3. Gently stir in fish and shrimp. Turn off heat, cover and let stand on burner for 5 minutes or until fish and shrimp are just opaque.

4. Ladle soup into serving bowls. Sprinkle with parsley. Serve immediately with lemon wedges.

Health Tips

In traditional Chinese medicine, saffron — also known as Tibetan red flower, or *zang hong hua* in Mandarin — is a powerful herb that invigorates and moves the blood. It is often given to women who suffer from amenorrhea, or in the absence of menstruation. Saffron is also beneficial in reducing flatulence.

Thai-Style Textured Salad

This lightly cooked Southeast Asian salad is great for a potluck because it holds for a while without wilting. The dressing has a zippy, assertive flavor, thanks to the fish sauce, garlic and shallots.

<table>
<tr><td colspan="3">• 2-cup (500 mL) canning jar</td></tr>
<tr><td>1 cup</td><td>unsweetened flaked coconut (preferably large flakes)</td><td>250 mL</td></tr>
<tr><td>¼</td><td>large head green or red cabbage (3-lb/1.5 kg cabbage), cored and cut into 2-inch (5 cm) chunks</td><td>¼</td></tr>
<tr><td>¼ cup</td><td>fish sauce</td><td>60 mL</td></tr>
<tr><td>¼ cup</td><td>freshly squeezed lime juice</td><td>60 mL</td></tr>
<tr><td>1</td><td>disc (1 oz/30 g) palm sugar</td><td>1</td></tr>
<tr><td>2</td><td>cloves garlic, thinly sliced</td><td>2</td></tr>
<tr><td>½</td><td>jalapeño pepper (optional), thinly sliced</td><td>½</td></tr>
<tr><td>1</td><td>large shallot, thinly sliced</td><td>1</td></tr>
<tr><td>2 cups</td><td>Mung Beans Cooked in Green Tea (page 245)</td><td>500 mL</td></tr>
<tr><td>1</td><td>large tomato, cored and cut in 1-inch (2.5 cm) chunks</td><td>1</td></tr>
<tr><td>½</td><td>English cucumber, cut into 1-inch (2.5 cm) chunks</td><td>½</td></tr>
<tr><td>1 tsp</td><td>minced fresh basil or spearmint</td><td>5 mL</td></tr>
<tr><td>1 cup</td><td>chopped toasted cashews</td><td>250 mL</td></tr>
</table>

1. In jar, combine coconut with 1 cup (250 mL) water. Seal with lid and refrigerate overnight, shaking jar once or twice, or for up to 2 days. Drain and set aside.

2. In a medium saucepan, bring 4 cups (1 L) water to a boil. Add cabbage and cook for 1 to 2 minutes or until translucent. Drain and set aside.

3. In a large skillet, combine fish sauce, lime juice, sugar, garlic and jalapeño. Warm over low heat, stirring often, for 5 minutes or until sugar is dissolved. Remove from heat and stir in shallot.

4. In a serving bowl, combine coconut, cabbage and mung beans. Drizzle with dressing and toss gently to coat. Gently stir in tomato, cucumber and basil. Sprinkle with cashews and serve immediately or let cool to room temperature.

**MAKES
4 TO 6 SERVINGS**

Tip

To toast cashews, place them in a medium dry skillet over low heat. Toast, stirring or shaking pan often, for about 5 minutes or until fragrant and golden.

Health Tips

Coconut is a rich, versatile nut. Its water is well known for its cooling and refreshing powers. The meat, on the other hand, is warming and nourishing to the blood — it is rich in fat, which builds energy and strength, counters dryness and nourishes yin. Coconut oil is an excellent source of fat for vegetarians and vegans.

If you have a tendency to feel hot, agitated or irritable, leave out the jalapeño pepper and reduce (or omit) the garlic. The warm pungency from the shallots will bring enough of a bite to the dish without those other elements.

Roasted Eggplant and Tomato with Peanut Sauce

Here, fragrant, punchy herbs and greens enliven and contrast well with the sweet-and-sour flavors of roasted tomato and eggplant. A luscious Asian-inspired peanut sauce enriches and completes this hearty dish.

MAKES 4 SERVINGS

Tip

To make the chopped mixed herbs and greens, use a combination of fresh spearmint, fresh cilantro and tender greens, such as arugula or baby kale. You can customize the mix to your tastes; add more cilantro or mint if you love them, or more greens if you like a less-herbaceous dish.

- **Preheat oven to 400°F (200°C)**
- **Rimmed baking sheet**

1	large eggplant (about 2 lbs/1 kg)	1
2	large plum (Roma) tomatoes	2
2 tbsp	avocado oil	30 mL
½ cup	chopped mixed herbs and greens (see tip, at left)	125 mL
1 cup	Peanut Sauce (see recipe, opposite)	250 mL

1. Trim ends off eggplant and core tomatoes. Cut each into ¾-inch (2 cm) cubes and place on baking sheet. Drizzle with oil and gently toss to coat.

2. Roast in preheated oven, stirring 2 or 3 times, for about 20 minutes or until eggplant is softened and browned. Let cool slightly.

3. Spoon eggplant mixture into a serving bowl. Add mixed herbs and greens and drizzle with peanut sauce. Gently toss to combine. Serve immediately.

> ### Health Tips
>
> Tomato and eggplant clear excessive heat, and hydrate and moisten the body tissues. Eggplant is also considered a blood mover that soothes skin irritations and rashes. A traditional remedy for both hypertension and bloodshot eyes is to eat one or two raw tomatoes on an empty stomach right after waking up in the morning.
>
> Peanuts are nourishing, benefiting the stomach and spleen *qi*. They also strengthen the body and counter generalized weakness.
>
> This dish is quite beneficial for elderly people — it's nutritious, and easy to chew and digest.

Peanut Sauce

This rich sauce is delicious on all sorts of simple dishes, from steamed vegetables to grilled chicken.

MAKES ABOUT 1 CUP (250 ML)

Tip

To make ginger juice, grate gingerroot and press it through a fine-mesh sieve into a small bowl. Discard fibers.

6 tbsp	smooth or chunky peanut butter	90 mL
¼ cup	unseasoned rice vinegar	60 mL
2 tbsp	coconut sugar	30 mL
2 tbsp	tamari or soy sauce	30 mL
1 tbsp	toasted sesame oil	15 mL
1 tsp	ginger juice (see tip, at left)	5 mL

1. In a medium bowl, whisk together peanut butter, vinegar, sugar, tamari, sesame oil and ginger juice until as smooth as possible.

Rosemary Grilled Fish with Lemony Greens and Pilaf

Fresh grilled fish can be so satisfying — crispy outside, moist and tender inside. The rosemary and citrus harmonize beautifully in this dish, as they both have resin-like flavor notes. The greens and pilaf can be prepared ahead and reheated, but the fish is best cooked just before serving.

MAKES 4 SERVINGS

Tips

If it's not grilling season, you can easily cook the fish under a preheated broiler. Broil it, skin side up, on a lightly oiled foil-lined baking sheet.

You can buy ghee in many grocery stores, but it's easy to make at home. Melt butter in a medium saucepan over low heat. Cook, stirring occasionally, until solids are golden brown and granular. Strain ghee through a paper towel–lined sieve into a heatproof bowl; discard solids. Transfer ghee to a sealed jar and store at room temperature in a cool dark place for up to 3 months or in the refrigerator for up to 6 months.

- **Preheat oven to 350°F (180°C)**
- **Preheat barbecue to medium-high**

1 tsp	coriander seeds	5 mL
1 tsp	mustard seeds	5 mL
¼ cup	ghee or avocado oil, divided	60 mL
1 cup	long-grain brown rice or brown basmati rice	250 mL
1 tbsp	salt, divided	15 mL
1 lb	chopped stemmed mustard greens	500 g
1 tsp	grated lemon zest	5 mL
1 tbsp	freshly squeezed lemon juice	15 mL
1½ lbs	boneless skin-on oily fish fillets, such as mackerel, large sardines or salmon	750 g
4	large sprigs fresh rosemary	4

1. Place coriander and mustards seeds in a medium ovenproof saucepan. Toast over low heat for 2 minutes or until fragrant. Using a large spoon, crush coriander seeds. Stir in 2 tbsp (30 mL) of the ghee. Stir in rice and 1 tsp (5 mL) of the salt. Cook, stirring, for 5 minutes.

2. Stir in 2¼ cups (560 mL) water and bring to a simmer. Cover and transfer to preheated oven. Bake for 45 minutes.

3. Remove from oven and let stand for 15 minutes or up to 1 hour.

Rosemary — a sweet, aromatic and pungent herb — has traveled the world. It originated in Europe and was taken to China by travelers from the Roman Empire in 452 BCE. This herb is very easy to grow in a pot outside in summer or in a sunny window in winter. Adding rosemary to any dish will increase its vitality and flavor.

4. In a large skillet, heat remaining ghee over medium-high heat, swirling to coat bottom of pan. Add mustard greens and cook, stirring often, for 3 to 5 minutes or until wilted and tender. Remove from heat. Toss with lemon zest and juice just before serving.

5. Cut fish into 4 portions and press 1 sprig of the rosemary onto each to adhere. Sprinkle with remaining salt. Place on oiled grill on preheated barbecue, skin side down, and grill for 10 minutes per each 1 inch (2.5 cm) of thickness or until fish is opaque.

6. Serve fish immediately with pilaf and greens.

Health Tip

The herbalist Peter Holmes, in his book *The Energetics of Western Herbs,* describes rosemary as having divergent healing properties that meet at the heart and lungs. It is a *qi* tonic and is beneficial for treating a number of conditions, including low blood pressure, headaches and acute sinusitis. Rosemary also soothes the nervous system, increases reproductive *qi* and clears the mind.

Braised Tomatoes and Sweet Potatoes with Eggs

The smell of tomatoes and basil on the table evokes summer. This unique combination of vegetables, herbs and spices creates an alluring dish, and it only takes small amounts of curry powder and basil to give it a gently aromatic flavor. The egg boosts the protein content and makes it a satisfying vegetarian entrée.

**MAKES
2 TO 4 SERVINGS**

Tips

You can prepare the sauce ahead of time and refrigerate it for up to 3 days. Bring it to a simmer before adding the eggs.

Try different types of heirloom tomatoes for varying textures and flavors.

Health Tip

Tomatoes are full of sweet and sour flavors that help hydrate the body and clear buildup of summer heat. Sweet potatoes are high in carbohydrates and nutrient-dense, and tonify the *qi*, blood and yin. They can ease dryness and constipation. Arugula's spicy bite, basil's fragrance and flavor and curry spices all aid and benefit digestion when used in moderation. The eggs nourish both yin and yang. All together, these ingredients make a wonderfully nutritious and balanced recipe.

2 tbsp	ghee, avocado oil or coconut oil	30 mL
1 tsp	curry powder or garam masala	5 mL
1 cup	chopped trimmed arugula or baby kale	250 mL
1	sweet potato (about 12 oz/375 g), peeled and cubed	1
1 tbsp	chopped fresh basil	15 mL
2	large tomatoes, cored and diced (about 1¼ lbs/625 g)	2
1 tsp	salt	5 mL
2 to 4	large eggs	2 to 4

1. In a large skillet, heat ghee over medium heat. Add curry powder and cook, stirring, for about 30 seconds or until fragrant.

2. Add arugula, sweet potato and basil. Cook, stirring often, for 5 minutes or until sweet potato is just starting to soften.

3. Add tomatoes and salt and bring to a boil. Cook, stirring occasionally, for 5 minutes or until tomatoes break down and form a sauce.

4. Reduce heat to low. Using the back of a spoon, make 2 to 4 depressions in sauce. Crack eggs into depressions. Cover and cook for 2 minutes or until yolks reach desired doneness.

5. Gently spoon 1 egg into each serving bowl. Divide sauce among bowls. Serve immediately.

Herb-Grilled Chicken

For many people, summertime means being outdoors and grilling food. This simple grilled chicken is sweet, flavorful and warming, enhanced by the pungent and aromatic herbs — perfect for this season.

> **MAKES
> 4 TO 6 SERVINGS**

Tip

To broil the chicken, preheat broiler with rack in upper third. Place chicken, skin side down, on a foil-lined baking sheet. Broil, turning once, for 10 minutes or until juices run clear when chicken is pierced.

- **Preheat barbecue to high**
- **Blender or food processor**

1 cup	packed chopped mixed herbs, such as basil, parsley, dill and celery leaves	250 mL
½	large onion, coarsely chopped	½
1½ tsp	salt	7 mL
2 lbs	boneless skin-on chicken thighs (4 to 6)	1 kg

1. In blender, combine herbs, onion and salt. Purée until smooth. Pour into a resealable plastic bag and add chicken, turning to coat. Seal and refrigerate, turning bag once or twice, for 2 hours or up to 24 hours,

2. Place chicken, skin side up, on oiled grill on preheated barbecue. Cover and grill, turning once, for 10 minutes or until juices run clear when chicken is pierced.

3. Transfer to a warmed platter, skin side up, and let stand for 10 minutes. Serve immediately.

Health Tip

If you suffer from a hot condition, such as a fever, high blood pressure, agitation or irritability, avoid grilled meat. Instead, try grilling up some tofu or vegetables such as cooling zucchini, summer squash or eggplant. Marinate them for up to 2 hours, adding ¼ cup (60 mL) avocado oil to the onion mixture when it is blended.

Grits, Greens and Sausage Bowl

The gentle sweetness of dried apples complements the savory, freshly made sausage patties in this nourishing main dish. Both are a nice contrast to the earthy greens and creamy grits.

<table>
<tr><td>¼ cup</td><td>dried apples, cut into ¼-inch (0.5 cm) pieces</td><td>60 mL</td></tr>
<tr><td></td><td>Warm water</td><td></td></tr>
<tr><td>1 lb</td><td>ground pork</td><td>500 g</td></tr>
<tr><td>½ tsp</td><td>fennel seeds</td><td>2 mL</td></tr>
<tr><td>1 tsp</td><td>chopped fresh sage</td><td>5 mL</td></tr>
<tr><td>1 tsp</td><td>salt</td><td>5 mL</td></tr>
<tr><td>1 tbsp</td><td>avocado oil</td><td>15 mL</td></tr>
<tr><td>4 cups</td><td>Simple Sautéed Greens (see recipe, opposite)</td><td>1 L</td></tr>
</table>

Grits

1 cup	coarse cornmeal	250 mL

1. *Grits:* In a medium saucepan, bring 3 cups (750 mL) water to a boil. Mix cornmeal with an additional 1 cup (250 mL) water and stir into boiling water. Reduce heat to low and simmer, stirring often, for 30 minutes or until slightly translucent. Remove from heat, cover and let stand for 30 more minutes.

2. Meanwhile, place dried apples in a small airtight container. Add enough warm water to fill container. Cover and let stand at room temperature, shaking container often, for 1 hour.

3. Drain apples. In a medium bowl, combine apples, pork, fennel seeds, sage and salt. Mix until well combined. Shape into 8 patties, each about ½ inch (1 cm) thick and 3 inches (7.5 cm) in diameter.

4. In a large skillet, heat oil over medium-high heat. Add patties and cook, turning once, for 3 to 4 minutes per side or until no longer pink inside.

5. Spoon grits into serving bowls. Top with sausage patties and greens. Serve immediately.

MAKES 4 SERVINGS

Tip

You can make the grits ahead and let them cool. Reheat them by bringing a little water to a boil in a medium saucepan, then adding the grits and stirring until smooth. Alternatively, you can cut the cold grits into ½-inch (1 cm) thick slices and pan-fry them in a little oil or ghee over high heat until they're browned and crisp at the edges.

Health Tips

Fennel seeds are used in Chinese medicine to ease abdominal pain, stimulate digestion and expel cold in the abdomen.

Pork is a meat that supplements blood and yin. It can be beneficial for women, in small amounts.

Simple Sautéed Greens

These greens are a quick and easy side dish. If you are serving them separately, top with a condiment of your choice.

MAKES 4 CUPS (1 L), ENOUGH FOR 4 SERVINGS

| 2 tbsp | avocado oil | 30 mL |
| 1½ lbs | chopped stemmed greens (see health tips, below) | 750 g |

1. In a large skillet, heat oil over medium-high heat, swirling to coat bottom of pan. Add greens and cook, stirring often, for 3 to 5 minutes or until wilted and tender. Serve immediately.

Health Tips

You can never eat enough greens, it seems. This simple sauté provides a richer way to get your daily dose of chlorophyll to cleanse your liver and blood, while infusing fresh life into your cells.

The recipe works with a wide variety of leafy greens: spinach, beet greens, Swiss chard, dandelion greens, arugula, kale, collards, escarole, chicory, radicchio, mustard greens, bok choy, tatsoi, Chinese broccoli (*gai lan*), amaranth leaves, snow pea shoots, sweet potato vine greens, chrysanthemum greens, shepherd's purse and more.

Quick-Pickled Summer Salad with Squash and Corn

Sweet, tangy and light is the theme of this salad. Preparing the bell pepper in this way can help make it more digestible — it certainly makes it tastier!

Tip

To easily cut the kernels off an ear of corn, stand the ear up on its stem end in a large bowl. Place a chef's knife at the top of the cob and cut straight down the side to release the kernels into the bowl. Repeat all the way around the cob.

Health Tips

The digestive benefits of fermented foods, like sauerkraut, are the healthy highlight of this salad. Red bell peppers are warming, support circulation and can stimulate appetite.

Cilantro boosts the immune system and eases digestion.

If you suffer from any inflammatory condition, such as arthritis, avoid this dish. It contains red bell pepper, a member of the nightshade family, which can exacerbate symptoms.

- **2-cup (500 mL) canning jar**

1	red bell pepper, seeded and thinly sliced	1
½ tsp	kosher or non-iodized sea salt	2 mL
1 cup	unpasteurized sauerkraut (store-bought or homemade), with juices	250 mL
2	ears corn, husked	2
1 lb	yellow summer squash (about 3 small), cubed	500 g
2 tbsp	chopped fresh cilantro	30 mL

1. In jar, combine red pepper and salt, tossing well to combine. Add sauerkraut with juices but do not mix. Using the back of a spoon, pack mixture down, making sure liquid covers peppers. Cover loosely and let stand at room temperature for up to 24 hours. Seal jar and refrigerate for up to 3 days if not completing recipe immediately.

2. Cut kernels off corn cobs, discarding cobs (see tip, at left). In a medium saucepan, combine corn kernels, squash and ½ cup (125 mL) water. Cover and cook over medium-high heat, stirring once or twice, for 4 to 5 minutes or just until squash is barely tender.

3. Uncover and cook, stirring occasionally, for 2 to 3 minutes or until no liquid remains. Watch carefully so vegetables do not brown. Remove from heat and let cool for 20 to 30 minutes, or refrigerate for up to 1 day.

4. Drain pepper mixture and place in a serving bowl. Add corn mixture and toss gently to combine. Sprinkle with cilantro. Serve immediately. (To make ahead, cover and refrigerate for up to 3 days. Serve cold.)

Arame Salad with Lemon and Chives

Arame seaweed is versatile — it has a light, crunchy texture and pleasing neutral flavor. Here, it absorbs the freshness of lively herbs and the tanginess of lemon juice. This dish is easy to make and can be used as a topping on a simple green salad or as a side dish with a meal.

MAKES 4 SERVINGS

Tip

For more information on arame and other seaweeds, see pages 177 and 178.

1 cup	dried arame	250 mL
2 tsp	sesame seeds	10 mL
¼ cup	chopped fresh chives	60 mL
¼ cup	chopped fresh parsley	60 mL
	Freshly squeezed juice of 1 lemon	
1 tsp	extra virgin olive oil	5 mL
¼ tsp	sea salt	1 mL
Pinch	black, white or cayenne pepper	Pinch

1. Place arame in a medium bowl. Pour in enough water to cover by 3 inches (7.5 cm). Let stand for 15 minutes or until plump. Drain and rinse well. Drain again and squeeze out excess water. Transfer to a serving bowl and set aside.

2. Place sesame seeds in small dry skillet. Toast over medium heat, stirring or shaking pan constantly, for 3 minutes or until golden and fragrant. Transfer to a small bowl and set aside.

3. In another small bowl, whisk together chives, parsley, lemon juice, oil, salt and pepper. Pour over arame and toss to coat. Sprinkle with sesame seeds and serve immediately.

Health Tips

Arame is high in calcium, magnesium, phosphorus, iron and iodine. It is good at helping to stabilize blood sugar, regulate hormones, soothe nerves and boost thyroid function. Its saltiness softens phlegm and helps the body expel it.

Different types of seaweed are chelating agents, which mean they bind with environmental toxins and help remove them from the body.

Vibrant Summer Vegetables with Tofu Dressing

This fresh, gently cooked salad is colorful and offers a balance of sweet flavor from the vegetables and rich umami goodness from the tofu and miso. Cooking the vegetables separately preserves their bright hues and textures.

Tips

To toast sesame seeds, place them in a small dry skillet. Toast over low heat, stirring or shaking pan constantly, for 3 minutes or until fragrant. Immediately transfer to a plate and let cool.

If you'd like to prepare the dressing and vegetables ahead of time, let them come to room temperature before serving for the best flavor.

Health Tips

Green beans and beets supplement the blood and *qi*. Carrots benefit those who may suffer from indigestion. Tofu is cooling. This is a beneficial dish to clear heat out of the body, combat dryness and build *qi*. It is an excellent choice for vegetarians or vegans.

If you suffer from soy sensitivity, enjoy this dish without tofu in the dressing.

• **Large rimmed baking sheet**

8 oz	small green beans, trimmed and halved crosswise if large	250 g
8 oz	carrots, cut into matchsticks	250 g
8 oz	beets, cut into matchsticks	250 g
2 tbsp	sesame seeds (preferably black), toasted (see tips, at left)	30 mL

Tofu Dressing

1	package (14 oz to 1 lb/420 to 500 g) soft or medium tofu, drained	1
2 tbsp	white miso	30 mL
1 tbsp	toasted sesame oil	15 mL
1 tbsp	freshly squeezed lemon juice	15 mL

1. *Tofu Dressing:* In a large bowl, whisk together tofu, miso, sesame oil and lemon juice until smooth. Set aside.

2. In a large saucepan of boiling water, cook beans for 3 to 4 minutes or just until tender. Using a slotted spoon, transfer to baking sheet and spread out. Let cool completely.

3. Add carrots to saucepan and cook for 3 to 4 minutes or just until tender. Using a slotted spoon, add to baking sheet and spread out. Let cool completely.

4. Add beets to saucepan and cook for 5 to 7 minutes or just until tender. Using a slotted spoon, add to baking sheet and spread out. Let cool completely. (To make ahead, cover vegetables and refrigerate for up to 2 days.)

5. Transfer vegetable mixture to a serving bowl. Drizzle with dressing and toss to coat. Sprinkle with sesame seeds. Serve immediately.

Millet with Corn, Cauliflower and Fresh Herbs

This light, fluffy vegetable-and-grain dish is a little bit sweet and a really enjoyable way to eat millet. Paired with grilled fish and greens, it makes a complete summer meal.

MAKES 4 SERVINGS

Tip

Millet tends to harden quickly as it cools. You can use leftover millet to make a breakfast congee bowl the next morning (just add more water or broth to loosen it up). Serve with a source of protein and some cooked greens.

- **Preheat oven to 350°F (180°C)**
- **Rimmed baking sheet**

2	ears corn, husked	2
½	head cauliflower	½
1 cup	millet	250 mL
1 tbsp	extra virgin olive oil	15 mL
1	onion, finely diced	1
½ cup	chopped fresh parsley	125 mL
½ cup	chopped fresh basil	125 mL

1. Cut kernels off corn cobs. Discard cobs and set kernels aside.

2. Chop cauliflower into small florets.

3. Place millet in a medium bowl and rinse in several changes of cold water. Drain well and spread on baking sheet. Toast in preheated oven for 15 minutes.

4. Meanwhile, in a medium saucepan, bring 2 cups (500 mL) water to a boil. Cover, reduce heat and keep hot.

5. In another medium saucepan, heat oil over medium-low heat. Add millet and stir to coat. Add onion, cauliflower and corn kernels. Pour reserved hot water over millet mixture and return to a boil. Reduce heat to medium-low and simmer for about 20 minutes or until no liquid remains.

6. Fluff millet mixture with a fork. Stir in parsley and basil. Spoon into serving bowls. Serve immediately.

Health Tips

Millet is slightly cold in its thermal nature, making it a perfect grain for summer. It has the distinction of tasting both sweet and salty. Millet is nourishing, can relieve thirst and is a diuretic. It is rich in iron, phosphorus and B vitamins, and is gluten-free.

Millet congee is beneficial for people who have poor appetites and generally feel weak. It is considered a yin tonic and helps relieve the thirst or difficult urination that results from a fever.

Five-Flavor Sautéed Cucumbers

Cooked cucumbers are firm and pleasantly astringent — and this is a surprisingly delightful way to enjoy these vegetables. In this side dish, they are a cool foil to the aromatic elements: Sichuan peppercorns, vinegar and basil.

Tips

To toast peanuts, place them in a medium dry skillet. Toast over low heat, stirring or shaking pan often, for about 7 minutes or until golden and fragrant.

The shiny black seeds in Sichuan peppercorns are hard and gritty, so it's best to remove them before adding this spice to recipes.

1	English or Persian cucumber, about 12 inches (30 cm) long	1
1 tbsp	avocado oil	15 mL
½ cup	unsalted raw peanuts, toasted	125 mL
2 tbsp	unseasoned rice vinegar	30 mL
1 tsp	Sichuan peppercorns, shiny black seeds removed (see tips, at left), crushed	5 mL
½ tsp	salt	2 mL
½ tsp	hot pepper flakes	2 mL
2 tbsp	chopped fresh basil	30 mL

1. Trim ends off cucumber and partially peel, making alternating lengthwise stripes. Cut cucumber into quarters lengthwise. Cut crosswise into ½-inch (1 cm) thick slices.

2. In a large skillet, heat oil over medium-high heat. Add peanuts, vinegar, Sichuan peppercorns, salt and hot pepper flakes. Cook, stirring, for 1 minute. Add cucumber and cook, stirring often, for 4 to 5 minutes or until translucent.

3. Stir in basil and remove from heat. Spoon into a serving bowl. Serve immediately.

Health Tips

Cucumbers are another quintessentially summer food. Refreshing, cooling and hydrating, they are well-known blood cleansers and act as a diuretic. Cucumbers can also be used to soothe swollen, hot, dry or irritated eyes; cut slices and place them over your lids as a poultice.

If you have a tendency toward diarrhea or poor digestion, avoid raw cucumber. This dish is fine, however — quickly sautéing the cucumbers with warming and pungent spices boosts their digestibility.

Bitter Melon and Ground Pork

Bitter melon is known (and loved) for its strong bitter flavor. It can be an acquired taste, but don't shy away from it — it is worth trying more than once. Bitter melon gives this dish an intense flavor. It's most delicious paired with a bland side, such as steamed rice or water-sautéed vegetables, which will let the bitter melon be the star of the plate.

MAKES 4 SIDE-DISH SERVINGS

Tip

There are two varieties of bitter melon. One is shiny and light green, with smooth, elongated bumps. The other is darker green with sharp, pointy bumps. We prefer the latter for its firmer texture.

Caution

If you are pregnant, nursing or trying to conceive, be moderate in your bitter melon intake. Eating too much can cause digestive issues, such as bloating, diarrhea or abdominal cramping. In pregnancy, the medicinal element, *Momordica charantia*, can cause toxicity in some people. It also can disturb the fetus and cause premature labor.

8 oz	bitter melons (2 or 3 small)	250 g
1 tsp	salt	5 mL
8 oz	ground pork	250 g
2 tbsp	minced fresh basil	30 mL
2 tsp	minced gingerroot	10 mL
1	clove garlic, minced	1
2 tbsp	tamari or soy sauce	30 mL

1. Cut bitter melons in half lengthwise and scrape out seeds and white pulp. Cut crosswise into $1/8$-inch (3 mm) thick slices. In a medium bowl, toss bitter melon slices with salt and let stand for 30 minutes.

2. In a medium saucepan, bring 4 cups (1 L) water to a boil. Drain bitter melon and add to pan. Return to a boil. Remove from heat and drain well.

3. In a large skillet over medium-high heat, cook pork, breaking up with a spoon, until no longer pink. Stir in bitter melon, basil, ginger and garlic and cook, stirring often, for 5 to 7 minutes or just until bitter melon is tender.

4. Stir in tamari and cook for 5 to 7 minutes or until almost no liquid remains.

5. Spoon into serving dishes. Serve immediately.

Health Tips

Bitter melon stabilizes blood sugar levels, improves digestion, reduces inflammation and boosts the immune system so it can fight off infections and viruses. It also helps improve circulation.

The pork helps balance the bitterness of the melon while nourishing the yin and supplementing the qi and blood. For a winter version of this dish, try Bitter Melon with Shrimp (page 385).

Sesame Seed–Crusted Eggplant

Stylish and satisfyingly delicious: what more could you ask for in a side dish? Here, a crunchy crust encloses a savory, creamy-textured eggplant interior. This recipe requires some last-minute preparation, but it quickly pays off with delicious results.

MAKES 4 SERVINGS

Tip

You can find black sesame seeds in Asian markets or online. If you can't find them, use all white sesame seeds.

Caution

If you are pregnant, eat eggplant only occasionally. In Japan, women are advised to avoid it altogether during pregnancy, because it's believed that the vegetable's blood-moving properties can cause miscarriage.

Health Tip

Eggplant is the basis for an age-old canker sore remedy, too. A powder made from charred eggplants is applied to the sores in order to remove the excess heat that causes them.

- **Preheat oven to 400°F (200°C)**
- **Rimmed baking sheet, lined with parchment paper**

¼ cup	tamari or soy sauce	60 mL
¼ cup	rice wine, such as sake	60 mL
¼ cup	pure maple syrup	60 mL
2 tbsp	white miso	30 mL
2 tbsp	avocado oil	30 mL
1 tbsp	toasted sesame oil	15 mL
1	large eggplant (1½ lbs/750 g)	1
½ cup	mixed sesame seeds (black and white)	125 mL

1. In a large bowl, whisk together tamari, wine, maple syrup, miso, avocado oil and sesame oil until smooth. Set aside.

2. Trim ends off eggplant. Cut lengthwise into ½-inch (1 cm) thick slices. Cut slices lengthwise into ½-inch (1 cm) wide strips, then crosswise to make 3-inch (7.5 cm) long pieces.

3. Add eggplant to tamari mixture and stir gently to coat. Cover and refrigerate, stirring once or twice, for 8 hours or up to 24 hours.

4. Spread sesame seeds on a large plate. Drain eggplant and press into sesame seeds, turning to coat all over. Arrange slices on prepared pan.

5. Bake in preheated oven for 15 minutes. Using a long flexible spatula, turn eggplant slices. Bake for 15 minutes or until coating is browned and eggplant is very tender.

6. Transfer to a serving platter. Serve warm or at room temperature.

Health Tip

In Chinese medicine, eggplant is used to clear internal heat, cool down fevers, soothe pain and treat dysentery. Eggplant has an affinity for the uterus and is thought to move stagnant blood, and is often recommended for women who suffer from menstrual cramps.

Savory Summer Nuts

This fragrant, herbal twist on roasted salted nuts makes a delightful snack. The almonds and walnuts are so savory and satisfying when prepared this way.

MAKES ABOUT 3 CUPS (750 ML)

Tip

Make these nuts when the weather is dry — if it is humid, they won't stay crisp.

2 tbsp	packed minced fresh basil	30 mL
2 tbsp	white miso	30 mL
1 tbsp	unseasoned rice vinegar	15 mL
¼ tsp	black pepper	1 mL
1½ cups	unsalted raw almonds	375 mL
1½ cups	walnut halves	375 mL
1 tbsp	avocado oil	15 mL

1. In a medium heatproof bowl, combine basil, miso, vinegar and pepper. Mix until well combined. Using a spatula, spread up and onto side of bowl. Set aside.

2. In a large dry skillet, combine almonds and walnuts. Toast over medium-low heat, stirring often, for 5 to 10 minutes or until golden and fragrant.

3. Immediately add nuts to bowl with basil mixture. Using spatula, stir well to coat, scraping down side of bowl.

4. Add oil to skillet and heat over low heat. Return nut mixture to pan and cook, stirring constantly, for 2 to 3 minutes or until seasoning paste is dry and nuts are crisp.

5. Remove from heat and let cool in pan. Store in an airtight container at room temperature for 1 or 2 days.

Health Tips

The combination of pungent, warming, aromatic basil, miso and vinegar help the body digest the rich almonds and walnuts.

Nuts are rich in beneficial fats and protein, and are vitalizing for the body. Their rich oils can be very stabilizing for people who regularly feel high-strung. If you tend to gain weight easily and have a hard time losing it, eat only moderate amounts of nuts.

Corn Silk Tea

The delicate flaxen silk, or tassels, just inside the husk of a fresh ear of corn are the key to making this light tea. This is a traditional cooling summer drink in Asian countries, such as Korea. Its sweet, delicate flavor is very pleasant.

---

2 tbsp	chopped fresh or dried corn silk	30 mL
	Liquid honey (optional)	

MAKES 2 SERVINGS

Tip

If you can't find fresh ears of corn with the silk attached, dried corn silk makes a fine substitute.

1. In a small saucepan, bring 2 cups (500 mL) water to a boil. Remove from heat.

2. Stir in corn silk. Cover and let stand for 15 minutes.

3. Strain into teacups. Stir in honey (if using) to taste. Serve immediately.

Health Tips

The Latin name for corn is *Zea mays*. Corn silk is a demulcent (which means it's soothing) and has anti-inflammatory and antiseptic powers. It is used by Western herbalists to reduce edema and hypertension. It also soothes acute urinary tract infections and can help dissolve kidney stones.

This tea is not only refreshing but also cooling — which is perfect for hot days.

Basil Tea

In North America, Italian cuisine tends to come to mind when we think of basil. However, the herb has long been used in medicinal teas throughout India, Europe and Mexico. This simple tea is one you can enjoy anytime, and its beautiful, restorative fragrance will lift your spirits.

¼ cup	chopped fresh basil (or 2 tbsp/ 30 mL dried basil)	60 mL
2	strips lemon zest	2

1. In a small saucepan, bring 2 cups (500 mL) water to a boil. Remove from heat.

2. Stir in basil. Cover and let stand for 5 minutes.

3. Strain into teacups. Garnish with lemon zest. Serve immediately.

MAKES 2 SERVINGS

Tips

Heat fresh basil as briefly as possible or it will lose its aromatic potency.

You can also make sun tea: pour water in a glass jar, add basil and let stand in the sun until it is infused. Strain and add the lemon zest just before drinking.

Variation

Try this if you enjoy the zing of fresh ginger: add 1 slice (quarter-size) gingerroot, smashed, along with the basil.

Health Tips

This is a wonderful tea to enjoy after a meal — it helps with digestion. It's also excellent if you are feeling a bit blue and need more energy.

If you often feel cold or have an upper respiratory infection with a cough, make the ginger variation on this tea (see variation, left). It will boost the warming power of the basil.

Green Tea with Rose Hips

This fragrant, cooling green tea makes an excellent summer beverage that hydrates and clears the mind. The tangy rose hips bring color and a bright flavor to it.

MAKES 2 SERVINGS

Tip

Dried rose hips are sold in herbal stores and sometimes in bulk at the grocery store. They are also easy to find as a stand-alone tea, in tea bags.

- **Teapot**

1 tbsp	dried rose hips	15 mL
2 tbsp	loose green tea (or 1 green tea bag)	30 mL

1. In a small saucepan, bring 3 cups (750 mL) water to a boil. Reduce heat and bring to a simmer. Stir in rose hips. Cover and simmer for 5 minutes.

2. Pour into teapot. Cover and let stand for 2 minutes. Stir in green tea, cover and let stand for 2 to 3 minutes.

3. Strain into teacups. Serve immediately.

Health Tips

Green tea is cooling, with a slightly bitter flavor. Drink it to clear out excess heat, quench your thirst and refresh your mind.

Rose hips are sweet and sour, with a cooling nature. They relieve heat in the summer and quench thirst. Paired with green tea, they stimulate digestion and reduce the feeling of abdominal fullness you experience when you have eaten too much.

Chrysanthemum and Goji Berry Wine

Chrysanthemum wine was considered auspicious in ancient Chinese culture. People drank it to bring luck and blessings during the Double Ninth Festival, which normally occurred in autumn — it is also known as the Double Yang Festival in China and the Chrysanthemum Festival in Japan. This lightly floral, sweet beverage is delightfully refreshing.

MAKES 8 SERVINGS

Tips

To make a refreshing, bubbly summer beverage, mix a serving of the wine with sparkling water.

If you don't want to drink alcohol, you can still enjoy the benefits of the herbs in this recipe. Infuse the chrysanthemum flowers and goji berries in boiling water and enjoy the resulting tea with a little bit of honey.

- **4-cup (1 L) canning jar**

2 cups	rice wine, such as sake	500 mL
¼ cup	dried chrysanthemum flowers	60 mL
2 tbsp	dried goji berries	30 mL
1 tsp	liquid honey	5 mL

1. In jar, combine rice wine, chrysanthemum flowers, goji berries and honey. Seal with lid and shake well to combine.

2. Let stand in a cool, dark place, shaking every 2 to 3 days, for up to 1 week.

3. Using a fine-mesh sieve, strain into sake cups. Serve immediately.

Health Tips

All medicinal liquors and wines should be enjoyed in very small amounts. Drink them once or twice daily for a short period of time — and only when you are suffering from the symptoms the herbs in them are designed to treat.

Both of the herbs in this beverage benefit and nourish the liver.

This wine soothes eyes that are dry and tired from the heat. Drink a small sake cup or shot glass of it once daily while symptoms appear.

Plum Drinking Vinegar

Drinking vinegars have a long history in Asian culture, both as satisfying beverages and as health enhancers. In Europe and colonial America, this type of drink was known as a shrub. Here, the spices contribute complex flavors that mix well with the sweet juice and acidic vinegar. This vinegar is a delicious base for an aperitif (see recipes, opposite).

> **MAKES**
> **2½ TO 3 CUPS**
> **(625 TO 750 ML)**

Tips

Any plums will work well in this recipe, so use whatever variety is in season and looks tastiest.

Be aware that acid in vinegar is hard on your teeth. Easy does it with this beverage!

- **4-cup (1 L) canning jar**

1 cup	unseasoned rice vinegar	250 mL
1 cup	unsweetened white grape juice	250 mL
1 tsp	finely chopped gingerroot	5 mL
1	piece (2 inches/5 cm long) cinnamon stick	1
1 lb	plums (about 3 large or 4 medium)	500 g

1. In a small nonreactive saucepan, combine vinegar, grape juice, ginger and cinnamon stick. Bring to a simmer over low heat.

2. Meanwhile, pit plums and cut into ½-inch (1 cm) thick wedges. Place in jar and pour vinegar mixture over top. Seal jar and let cool. Refrigerate for up to 1 week.

3. To serve, strain vinegar mixture through a fine-mesh sieve. Discard solids. Store in refrigerator for up to 2 weeks.

> ### Health Tips
>
> It is best to stir 1 to 2 tbsp (15 to 30 mL) plum vinegar into a glass of room temperature or warm water to enhance and move the liver *qi*. Drink a glass of this mixture to stimulate digestion prior to eating.
>
> Moderation is key with this vinegar. Too much can cause diarrhea and weaken the digestion. Remember, there can be too much of a good thing.

Plum Vinegar Wine Cocktail

Dry rice wine harmonizes beautifully with the plum drinking vinegar, creating a zesty, interesting cocktail.

MAKES 5 COCKTAILS			
2 cups	Plum Drinking Vinegar (see recipe, opposite)	500 mL
2 cups	rice wine, such as sake	500 mL

1. Divide plum vinegar and rice wine among 5 cocktail glasses. Stir well to combine. Serve immediately.

Plum Vinegar Fizzy Cocktail

Sometimes, especially in the summer, people want their drinks to have a little pizzazz. Adding plum drinking vinegar to sparkling water is a bit fancier and fun than normal mocktails.

MAKES 4 COCKTAILS			
1 cup	Plum Drinking Vinegar (see recipe, opposite)	250 mL
2 cups	sparkling water	500 mL

1. Divide plum vinegar among 4 tall glasses. Top with sparkling water. Stir to combine and serve immediately.

Variations

If you want to make this drink more refreshing, add a sprig of fresh mint. If you prefer a spicier flavor, add a cinnamon stick or slice of gingerroot. You can also adjust the amount of drinking vinegar to suit your palate.

Fragrant Rose-Watermelon Cooler

Summer is not summer without magnificent, cooling, sweet watermelon. Here, it's given a gentle floral aroma by rose water and bit of acidity by pomegranate juice. On the hottest of summer days, this beverage is very elegant and cooling.

MAKES 4 SERVINGS

Tip

If you're very fond of rose water, feel free to increase the amount to 1 tsp (5 mL).

- **Blender**
- **4-cup (1 L) canning jar**

3 cups	cubed seedless watermelon	750 mL
2 cups	unsweetened pomegranate juice	500 mL
1	strip (6 inches/15 cm long) lemon zest	1
½ tsp	rose water (see tip, at left)	2 mL

1. In blender, combine watermelon and pomegranate juice. Blend until smooth.

2. Twist lemon zest to release essential oils and place in jar. Add watermelon mixture and rose water. Seal with lid and shake to combine. Refrigerate for up to 3 days if desired and shake to recombine before serving.

3. Pour into glasses, discarding lemon zest. Serve immediately.

Health Tips

Watermelon is cold in nature and, of course, oh-so-sweet. It is beneficial for people who are feeling hot and dried out, or those who sweat profusely in the summer. Watermelon acts like internal air conditioning, quickly cooling you down and quenching your thirst.

Watermelon is extremely cooling, so avoid it in all seasons except summer. Likewise, if you suffer from poor digestion, don't eat large amounts of this fruit, it has a very high sugar content and can cause digestive distress.

Pineapple Chrysanthemum Kanten

Kanten might just become your child's favorite summer treat. It is Ellen's family's go-to summer dessert. This sweet, fruity vegan gelled dessert will quench your thirst and cool you right down on a sweltering summer day.

Tips

Kanten is gelled with agar-agar seaweed and has a similar texture to Western-style gelatin desserts. If you would like a super-smooth, less-firm version, feel free to blend it after it has gelled.

Agar-agar comes in different forms. If you can't find the powdered version, you can substitute 1/2 bar (1/3 oz/10 g bar) dried agar-agar.

- **8-inch (20 cm) square glass baking dish**

2 cups	unsweetened pineapple juice, divided	500 mL
1 tbsp	powdered agar-agar (see tips, at left)	15 mL
2 tbsp	crumbled dried chrysanthemum flowers	30 mL

1. In a medium nonreactive bowl, stir 1 cup (250 mL) of the pineapple juice with agar-agar. Set aside.

2. In a small nonreactive saucepan, bring the remaining pineapple juice to a boil. Stir in agar-agar mixture and return to a simmer.

3. Remove from heat and stir in chrysanthemum flowers. Cover and let stand for 3 minutes. Strain through a fine-mesh sieve into baking dish. Cover and refrigerate for 2 hours or until set.

4. Cut into squares. Serve immediately.

> ## Health Tip
>
> Agar-agar soothes the digestive tract and eases constipation. It's also good for dissolving phlegm.
>
> Chrysanthemum flowers brighten the eyes, soothe tension and clear out excessive heat in the body.

Raspberry Coulis and Peaches with Maple-Spiced Pecans

This is a gorgeous, elegant way to dress up fragrant summer peaches. If you overheat easily, try Hibiscus-Poached Peaches (page 282) instead.

MAKES 4 SERVINGS

Tips

Thawed frozen raspberries will make a thicker sauce than fresh raspberries.

For the best flavor, use whichever variety of peaches is ripest and in season.

• **Blender**

12 oz	thawed frozen raspberries (or 1 pint/500 mL fresh raspberries)	375 g
1 tbsp	freshly squeezed lemon juice	15 mL
2 tbsp	liquid honey	30 mL
4	large ripe peaches	4
1 cup	Maple-Spiced Pecans (see recipe, opposite)	250 mL

1. In blender, combine raspberries and lemon juice. Purée until as smooth as possible. Using a spatula, press purée through a fine-mesh sieve into a small bowl. Discard seeds.

2. Stir honey into purée. Cover and refrigerate until ready to serve.

3. Just before serving, slice peaches and place in serving bowls. Drizzle with coulis and sprinkle with pecans. Serve immediately.

Health Tips

Raspberries are beneficial for the blood. When combined with peaches, they are especially helpful for women suffering from menstrual cramps.

The leaves of the raspberry plant are medicinal and recommended for a number of women's health conditions. Tea made from them, taken regularly, supports a healthy pregnancy and delivery.

Peaches restore bodily fluids, moisten and relieve dry conditions, such as a dry cough. They are also beneficial for the elderly, who often suffer from constipation.

Maple-Spiced Pecans

These are also nice as a nibble. This batch is twice as much as you will need to top the dessert.

**MAKES
2 CUPS (500 ML)**

1 tbsp	ghee	15 mL
2 cups	pecan halves	500 mL
2 tbsp	coconut sugar	30 mL
2 tbsp	pure maple syrup	30 mL
Pinch	salt	Pinch
1/4 tsp	ground cinnamon	1 mL
1/4 tsp	ground nutmeg	1 mL

1. Place a large piece of parchment paper or lightly oiled foil on a heatproof surface.

2. In a large skillet, heat ghee over medium heat. Add pecans and cook, stirring often with a heatproof spatula, for 2 minutes.

3. Stir in coconut sugar, maple syrup and salt. Cook, stirring often, for 2 minutes or until fragrant.

4. Remove from heat. Stir in cinnamon and nutmeg. Immediately scrape nut mixture onto parchment paper and spread in single layer. (Be careful as the nut-and-sugar mixture is very hot.) Let cool to room temperature.

5. Serve immediately or store in an airtight container at room temperature for up to 2 days.

Health Tips

Pecans are a yin tonic and warming food. They strengthen the nervous system and are high in Vitamin B6.

Ghee is nourishing, promotes healing of gastro-intestinal inflammation and is highly digestible, making it a healthy source of fat for elderly people.

Hibiscus-Poached Peaches

Tangy hibiscus flowers have a long history in the food cultures of Asia, Africa and the Middle East. Here, a tea made from them blends with rose water to give simple peaches a floral note. The fragrant nectar of this dessert is a delight that will instantly boost your mood.

MAKES 4 SERVINGS

Tips

You'll often find dried hibiscus flowers in Latin American grocery stores, where they are called *flor de jamaica*. Packages are usually sold by weight; you'll need about $1/3$ oz (10 g) to get the $1/4$ cup (60 mL) for this recipe.

If you'd like your peaches to have a stronger floral flavor, you can increase the rose water to 2 tsp (10 mL)

1 cup	unsweetened white grape juice	250 mL
$1/4$ cup	crushed dried hibiscus flowers (see tips, at left)	60 mL
1 lb	firm ripe yellow peaches (about 2 large or 3 medium)	500 g
2 tbsp	liquid honey	30 mL
1 tsp	rose water	5 mL

1. In a medium nonreactive saucepan, combine grape juice and hibiscus flowers. Bring to a simmer over medium heat. Remove from heat, cover and let stand for 5 minutes.

2. Strain hibiscus mixture through a fine-mesh sieve into a small bowl. Return liquid to pan and discard solids. Return to a simmer.

3. Meanwhile, pit and cut peaches into $1/2$-inch (1 cm) thick wedges. Add to pan along with honey. Simmer, stirring gently once or twice, for 10 minutes or until peaches are tender. Remove from heat, cover and let cool slightly.

4. Stir in rose water. Spoon into serving bowls and serve immediately. Or refrigerate in airtight container for up to 1 week.

Health Tip

Hibiscus is widely used to maintain healthy blood pressure, and to support heart health and the lungs. Rose is also soothing for liver. When combined with the peaches in this dessert, these herbs cool the body and quench summer thirst.

Coconut Tapioca Pudding with Mango

If you need a summer comfort dessert, this cooling coconut tapioca is a luscious choice. The pudding goes well with other types of fresh or water-sautéed tropical fruit, too.

Tip

Canned Asian coconut milk is the right choice for this recipe; don't use a coconut milk beverage.

Variation

To make a sugar-free pudding, omit sugar and increase water to make 3 cups (750 mL) of liquid. Stir in 1/2 cup (125 mL) chopped dried pitted dates along with vanilla.

1	can (14 oz/400 mL) coconut milk (see tip, at left)	1
3 tbsp	small pearl tapioca (not instant)	45 mL
1	disc (1 oz/30 g) palm sugar	1
Pinch	salt	Pinch
1/2 tsp	vanilla extract	2 mL
1	large mango (12 oz/ 375 g), peeled, pitted and sliced	1

1. Pour coconut milk into a measuring cup and add enough water to make 2 1/2 cups (625 mL).

2. In a medium saucepan, combine tapioca, sugar and salt. Slowly add coconut milk mixture, stirring constantly.

3. Place pan over medium heat and bring to a simmer. Simmer, stirring constantly, for 15 to 17 minutes or until tapioca is translucent and tender. Stir in vanilla.

4. Remove from heat, cover and let stand for 15 minutes. Serve immediately or let cool completely and refrigerate for up to 3 days. Serve with mango slices.

Health Tips

Tapioca pudding has a creamy texture that induces a calm, relaxed feeling. Desserts may not offer as many direct health benefits as other dishes, but every time you relax with one, your *qi* moves more smoothly. And that is positive!

Coconut milk is rich in lauric acid, which has antibacterial and antiviral properties. This milk has been found to have good effect on blood cholesterol and contains a rich, healthy and satisfying type of saturated fat. Coconut milk is warming and nourishing to the *qi* and yin.

Cardamom-Roasted Plums with Pistachios

Have a plethora of plums? Then this dessert is for you! It is even delicious if your plums aren't quite ripe. In fact, underripe fruit will hold its shape nicely and make the flavors of the other ingredients pop.

MAKES 4 SERVINGS

Tips

You can toast the pistachios while the plums are baking. Sprinkle them in a small metal baking pan or dish and add to the oven. Toast for 5 to 7 minutes or until fragrant.

Save any leftover syrup from the baking dish. Mix 3 parts syrup with 1 part gin and serve over ice as a delicious cocktail.

- **Preheat oven to 350°F (180°C)**
- **13- by 9-inch (33 by 23 cm) glass baking dish**

2 cups	unsweetened white grape juice	500 mL
2 tbsp	freshly squeezed lemon juice	30 mL
2 tbsp	liquid honey	30 mL
¼ tsp	cardamom seeds (from 2 or 3 green cardamom pods)	1 mL
6	large plums (or 8 medium)	6
½ cup	chopped toasted pistachios	125 mL

1. In baking dish, whisk together white grape juice, lemon juice, honey and cardamom seeds. Set aside.

2. Pit and halve plums. Arrange, cut side down, in baking dish. Bake in preheated oven, turning halfway through, for 1 hour or until juices in baking dish are syrupy.

3. Transfer dish to a wire rack and let cool for 30 minutes. Serve immediately or cover and refrigerate for 3 days.

4. Sprinkle with pistachios just before serving.

Health Tips

Plums are sour and sweet, and cold in thermal nature. They ease thirst, calm irritability and help resolve constipation. Plum juice is beneficial for a sore, dry throat.

If you have a tendency toward diarrhea, don't eat too many plums. In this dessert, they are combined with *qi*-moving and warming cardamom, which enhances digestion. This spice balances the fruit's cooling nature, and protects the stomach and digestion — try a little to see if it agrees with you.

Pistachios are very nutritious. In Ayurvedic medicine, they are considered an important whole-body tonic food and benefit the liver and kidney *qi*. They are beneficial for those with constipation. Pistachios are neutral in thermal nature. They are sweet yet slightly bitter and sour in flavor.

Mixed Berry Crumble

Summer brims with berries! Whichever way you eat them — fresh or cooked — they are packed with nutrients and flavor. Baking the crumble and filling separately ensures a super-crisp topping.

**MAKES
4 TO 6 SERVINGS**

Tips

If you like your crumble a little sweeter, increase the coconut sugar to ½ cup (125 mL).

Thawed frozen berries make a thicker sauce than fresh berries, and the fruit is softer overall.

If you are refrigerating any leftovers, place a paper towel over top before covering with plastic wrap to keep condensation off the crumble.

Health Tips

Berries are sweet, sour and astringent. They are rich in antioxidants and flavonoids, making them an excellent choice for countering inflammation and supporting circulation.

In traditional Chinese medicine, berries nourish the essence, hydrate the body and strengthen the blood.

- **Preheat oven to 400°F (200°C), with racks in upper and lower thirds**
- **Deep 8-cup (2 L) casserole dish**
- **Rimmed baking sheet, lined with parchment paper**

5 cups	thawed frozen or fresh mixed berries, such as blueberries, blackberries, huckleberries or raspberries	1.25 L
3 tbsp	large-flake (old-fashioned) rolled oats	45 mL
2 tbsp	freshly squeezed lemon juice	30 mL
¼ cup	liquid honey	60 mL

Crumble Topping

½ cup	large-flake (old-fashioned) rolled oats	125 mL
½ cup	sliced almonds	125 mL
6 tbsp	almond flour	90 mL
6 tbsp	coconut sugar	90 mL
2 tbsp	ghee	30 mL
¼ tsp	ground cinnamon	1 mL
⅛ tsp	salt	0.5 mL

1. In casserole dish, stir together berries, oats and lemon juice. Drizzle with honey. Bake on lower rack in preheated oven for 15 minutes. Stir well. Bake, stirring 1 or 2 more times, for 30 minutes or until juices are bubbly in center.

2. *Crumble Topping:* Meanwhile, in a large bowl, combine oats, sliced almonds, almond flour, coconut sugar, ghee, cinnamon and salt. Using a fork, stir until crumbly. Spoon onto prepared baking sheet, making a single layer about ½ inch (1 cm) thick. Bake on upper rack in oven for 6 to 8 minutes or until edges are browned. Remove from oven and set aside.

3. Remove berry mixture from oven. Sprinkle crumble over top. Serve warm or at room temperature. Refrigerate leftovers for up to 5 days.

Seasonal Transition Menus

Menu 1
Nourishing Vegetable Treasures
Short-grain Brown Rice

Menu 2
Chunky Vegetable Bean Stew
Mixed Crunchy Lettuce Salad with Tofu Miso Dressing

Menu 3
Mixed Mushroom Sauté
Tangy Carrot, Beet and Potato Salad

Menu 4
Grilled Squid
Sautéed Celery and Cabbage Ribbons

Seasonal Transition Recipes

Chinese Yam Congee with Lotus Seeds and Hato Mugi

The delicate, humble taste of congee on a cool morning is a simple pleasure. In 600 CE, Sun Simiao included congee recipes in his book, Prescriptions Worth a Thousand Pieces of Gold. *Xu Zong-Heng of the Qing Dynasty, in the 700s, wrote, "Cook congee until water and rice are indivisible and eat before dawn. It is sweet and beautiful to the mouth, and entering the abdomen, it is cool and refreshing." The herbs in this recipe add texture and enhance* qi. *If you are seeking a simple and delightful congee, try this one.*

MAKES 4 SERVINGS

Tip

Enjoy the congee as-is or with your favorite condiments, vegetables or protein sources.

¾ oz	dried lotus seeds	20 g
¾ oz	hato mugi (Job's tears)	20 g
	Cold water	
½ cup	sweet (glutinous) brown rice (or brown Arborio rice)	125 mL
¾ oz	dried Chinese yam (dioscorea)	20 g

1. In a medium bowl, combine lotus seeds and hato mugi. Pour in enough cold water to cover. Let soak for 1 hour (or overnight if you plan to cook in the morning). Drain.

2. In a medium saucepan, combine 6 cups (1.5 L) water, lotus seeds, hato mugi, rice and Chinese yam and bring to a simmer. Reduce heat to low, cover and simmer, stirring occasionally, for 2 hours. The congee should have a souplike consistency; if there is not enough liquid left in the pan, add water as needed. Cover and let cool for 10 minutes.

3. Serve immediately or transfer to an airtight container and refrigerate for up to 3 days. Warm in a small saucepan over low heat before serving.

> **Health Tip**
>
> Congee is beneficial for anyone recovering from an illness because it is light and easy to digest. The herbs in this congee are especially good for building *qi* in people who feel weak, have a lingering dry cough or suffer from poor appetite.

Chicken Broth Congee with Aromatic Peanut Condiment

The fragrant seasoned peanuts sprinkled over this simple healing congee brighten its delicate flavor and support good digestion. This condiment is so delicious you might have trouble not eating it all up before your congee is ready!

MAKES 4 SERVINGS

- **Blender, mortar and pestle, or spice grinder**

1	batch Chicken Broth Congee (page 414)	1

Aromatic Peanut Condiment

½ cup	unsalted raw peanuts	125 mL
½	sheet nori	½
½ tsp	dried basil	2 mL
1 tsp	coconut sugar	5 mL
½ tsp	salt	2 mL

1. *Aromatic Peanut Condiment:* In a large dry skillet, toast peanuts over medium heat, stirring often, for 5 to 10 minutes or until browned and fragrant. Transfer to a bowl. Let cool.

2. Meanwhile, place nori in warm skillet and let dry for 5 minutes or until crispy. (Do not place skillet on burner; the residual heat in the skillet is enough.)

3. In blender, combine peanuts, nori and basil. Grind until the texture of brown sugar. Transfer to a small bowl and stir in coconut sugar and salt.

4. Spoon warm congee into serving bowls. Sprinkle with peanut condiment.

Health Tips

Chicken meat is sweet, warming and nourishing. This congee is especially beneficial for women who have menstrual cramps and feel weak during their periods. The *qi*- and blood-nourishing properties of the chicken broth also help boost *qi* after childbirth.

Sweet, neutral peanuts (which become warming when toasted) are a common component in Chinese cooking. They nourish the digestive system and promote milk production in lactating women.

Warming, fragrant basil enhances digestion and eases headaches that come with the common cold, while cooling nori contributes health-enhancing minerals and a lightly salty flavor.

Essential Seed and Nut Porridge with Sautéed Apples and Sheep's Milk Yogurt

If you love porridge in the morning but are avoiding grains such as oats, this quick breakfast is a gentle way to start your day. It's as simple as instant oatmeal but much tastier, more nourishing and truly satisfying. If you prep the porridge mix ahead of time (up to the grinding step), you'll have a quick breakfast that's high in essential fatty acids — and that will keep hunger at bay until lunchtime.

MAKES 4 SERVINGS

Tips

You can add up to 1 cup (250 mL) more boiling water to the porridge mix if you prefer a thinner consistency.

You can make the sautéed apples up to 3 days ahead and refrigerate them. Warm them gently in a saucepan before serving.

Check the package to make sure the plantain chips are cooked in a healthy oil and don't contain added sugar.

Unsweetened plantain chips are available in either the bulk aisle of the grocery store or in packages in the snack section. You can also find them in health food stores and online; see Resources (page 466) for sources. Check the package to make sure the plantain chips are cooked in a healthy oil and don't contain added sugar.

- **Blender**

2 cups	boiling water	500 mL
1 tbsp	ghee	15 mL
2	large sweet apples, such as Fuji or Golden Delicious, peeled, cored and thinly sliced	2
1 tbsp	freshly squeezed lemon juice	15 mL
1 tbsp	liquid honey	15 mL
1 cup	plain sheep's milk or other yogurt	250 mL

Porridge Mix

¼ cup	shelled raw pumpkin seeds (pepitas)	60 mL
2 tbsp	chia seeds	30 mL
2 tbsp	flax seeds	30 mL
½ cup	shelled pistachios (2 oz/60 g)	125 mL
½ cup	Brazil nuts (2 oz/60 g)	125 mL
1 cup	unsweetened roasted plantain chips (3 oz/90 g)	250 mL
½ tsp	salt	2 mL

1. *Porridge Mix:* In a large dry skillet, toast pumpkin, chia and flax seeds over medium-low heat, stirring often, for 5 minutes or until fragrant. Transfer to a heatproof bowl. Return skillet to heat and add pistachios and Brazil nuts. Toast over medium-low heat, stirring often, for 10 minutes or until fragrant. Transfer to another heatproof bowl. Let cool completely.

2. In blender, combine seed mixture and plantain chips and grind until the texture of brown sugar. Add nut mixture and salt and grind to the texture of brown sugar.

Variation

If you don't want cooked fruit in your porridge, try sprinkling chopped fresh apples on top.

3. In a medium bowl, stir porridge mix with boiling water. Cover and set aside.

4. In a large skillet, heat ghee over medium-high heat. Add apples and sauté for 2 to 3 minutes or until almost tender. Stir in lemon juice and honey.

5. Spoon porridge into serving bowls. Top with apples and yogurt. Serve immediately.

Health Tips

Apples are cooling, sweet and sour; cooking them boosts their digestibility. They also make this dish an appetite stimulant, raise the blood sugar and moisten lung tissue. Apples promote hydration in the body by encouraging fluid production in the tissues.

Sheep's milk yogurt is warming, sour and sweet. It helps remedy constipation, nourishes the yin and relaxes the liver. If you suffer from lactose intolerance and experience indigestion and diarrhea when consuming dairy, choose a non-dairy yogurt instead.

Sweet honey is lubricating and nourishing to the stomach and spleen.

Pan-Fried Vegetable Cakes

These tasty, nourishing cakes are delicious at the start your day or as part of another meal. Try them with a pungent pickled condiment, such as Digestive Shiso and Citrus Condiment (page 431) or Parsley and Radish Top Sauerkraut (page 436) to offset their natural richness.

**MAKES ABOUT
12 PIECES**

Tip

Make larger patties from the batter and you have tasty, nutritious veggie burgers for lunch or dinner. Serve them with Tangy Carrot, Beet and Potato Salad (page 306) or Mixed Crunchy Lettuce Salad with Tofu Miso Dressing (page 308).

1½ cups	almond meal	375 mL
2	large eggs	2
1 tsp	salt	5 mL
1 cup	coarsely shredded peeled turnip	250 mL
1 cup	coarsely shredded peeled sweet potato	250 mL
½ cup	finely shredded greens, such as tender mustard greens, napa cabbage or arugula	125 mL
¼ cup	avocado oil, divided	60 mL

1. In a medium bowl, whisk together almond meal, eggs and salt. Stir in turnip, sweet potato, greens and ½ cup (125 mL) water.

2. In a large skillet, heat 1 tbsp (15 mL) of the oil over medium heat, swirling to coat bottom of pan. Using ¼ cup (60 mL) of batter for each, drop 2 patties into pan, pressing gently until about ½ inch (1 cm) thick. Cook, turning once, for 2 minutes per side or until lightly browned all over. Repeat with remaining batter and oil. Serve immediately. (Or let cool, cover and refrigerate for up to 2 days. Warm in a skillet over medium heat for 1 to 2 minutes before serving.)

Health Tips

Sweet potatoes are neutral with a tendency toward warming, and are nourishing. They help people who feel weak or fatigued.

Organic eggs are the perfect yin-yang food. The yolk is warming and nourishes the yang and *qi*. The whites nourish the yin and the blood. Eggs are most beneficial to people recovering from illness, or who suffer from fatigue or weakness. Avoid eggs if you have recurring rashes.

Frying makes the ingredients in these patties more warming and nourishing. If you are a more excessive, hot type of person, they may not be the best dish for you.

Lox Eggs with Winter Vegetable Hash and Pungent Greens

This luxurious fish, egg and vegetable dish is excellent for brunch. The tension between the salty, pungent and sweet flavors — and the contrast of different textures — creates a very satisfying dish.

MAKES
4 TO 6 SERVINGS

Tips

If you want to get a head-start on this dish, prep, simmer and dice the turnip, potato and parsnips ahead of time and refrigerate them until you're ready to cook.

You can adjust the saltiness of this dish by reducing the amount of lox. You can also increase the amount of pungent green onion to offset the richness of the dish.

Health Tip

This is an excellent recipe for supplementing and augmenting physical energy. It is filled with tonic foods, including eggs, salmon, parsnip and potato, which all nourish the yin, yang, *qi* and blood. The cool, moistening spinach eases constipation, while the pungent turnip clears heat and increases digestibility.

1	large turnip (about 8 oz/250 g), halved	1
1	large russet potato or Asian sweet potato (about 8 oz/250 g), halved	1
2	parsnips (about 8 oz/250 g total)	2
6 tbsp	avocado oil, divided	90 mL
½ cup	chopped green onions	125 mL
8 oz	trimmed spinach leaves	250 g
8 oz	lox, cut into large pieces	250 g
8	large eggs, beaten	8

1. In a medium saucepan, bring 8 cups (2 L) water to a boil. Add turnip, potato and parsnips. Reduce heat, cover and simmer for 15 minutes or until barely tender, removing each vegetable with a slotted spoon as it is done. Let cool. Peel and cut each into ¼-inch (0.5 cm) cubes. Set aside.

2. In a large skillet, heat 2 tbsp (30 mL) of the oil over medium-high heat, swirling to coat bottom of pan. Add green onions and spinach. Cook, stirring often, for 3 to 5 minutes or until wilted and tender. Transfer to a small bowl and keep warm. Wipe out skillet.

3. Add 2 tbsp (30 mL) of the remaining oil to skillet and heat over medium-high heat. Add turnip, potato and parsnips and cook, without stirring, for 2 minutes. Turn and cook for 1 minute or until lightly browned on both sides. Transfer to a medium bowl and keep warm.

4. Add remaining oil to skillet and heat over medium-high heat. Add lox and cook, turning once, for 1 minute per side. Push to edge of pan. Pour eggs into center of pan, reduce heat to low and cook, stirring often, for 2 to 3 minutes or until large curds form. When eggs are almost dry, stir in lox and remove from heat.

5. Spoon turnip mixture onto serving plates. Top with egg mixture and spinach mixture.

Steamed Egg Custard with Chopped Greens

Steamed egg custards are an excellent comfort food: they are easy to digest, nourishing and flavorful. If you need to save some time, use leftover cooked greens instead of prepping and simmering the spinach. There's no need to reheat the greens first — just chop and place 1 tbsp (15 mL) in each ramekin before adding the egg mixture.

MAKES 6 SERVINGS

Tips

If your pot is too small to hold all of the ramekins at once, steam the custards in batches.

Rubber-tipped tongs are great for transferring the ramekins to the steamer pot. If you don't have them, you can wrap thick rubber bands around the tips of regular metal tongs.

Variation

If you don't have greens on hand, substitute 2 tbsp (30 mL) minced fresh herbs. Don't cook them; just add 1 tsp (5 mL) to each ramekin before pouring in the egg mixture.

- **Six 1/2- or 3/4-cup (125 or 175 mL) ramekins or custard cups**
- **Large pot with steamer rack (about 1 inch/2.5 cm above bottom of pot)**

2 oz	tender greens, such as baby spinach or baby kale	60 g
4	large eggs, beaten	4
3 cups	Traditional or Vegetarian Dashi (page 297), at room temperature	750 mL
1 tbsp	tamari or soy sauce	15 mL
1/2 tsp	salt	2 mL

1. In a medium saucepan, combine greens with 1/2 cup (125 mL) water and bring to a simmer over medium-high heat. Cover, reduce heat and cook for 2 minutes or until wilted and tender. Uncover and cook, stirring often, until no liquid remains. Transfer greens to a plate and let cool. Chop finely and divide among ramekins.

2. In a 4-cup (1 L) glass measuring cup, whisk together eggs, dashi, tamari and salt. Strain and gently pour into ramekins.

3. Pour enough water into pot to come scant 1 inch (2.5 cm) up side. Place steamer rack in pan over water. Bring to a boil.

4. Arrange ramekins on rack, cover tightly and steam for 15 to 20 minutes or until custard is barely set in the center (it will be jiggly but not liquid).

5. Serve warm or at room temperature. Or cover and refrigerate for up to 3 days; let come to room temperature before serving.

> ## Health Tip
>
> The addition of pungent or sweet dark leafy greens balances the supplementing eggs. Greens will detoxify and clear heat.

Bean and Vegetable Pistou

The marvelous French macrobiotic chef and author Hélène Magariños-Rey's passion for wild, fresh foods is infectious. She taught Ellen how to make this beautiful Provençal soup and multi-textured one-pot meal.

MAKES 4 SERVINGS

Tips

Kombu is dried kelp, a type of seaweed. Look for it in Japanese grocery or health food stores.

Blend a portion of the soup with fresh basil and garlic to give it a vibrant green color and a punch of flavor, and stir it back in to the soup.

Health Tip

The vibrant mixture of warming pungent herbs (garlic and basil), sweet vegetables and beans makes this simple, nourishing soup good for people who have a tendency to gain weight and/ or those who have trouble losing weight. It strengthens the spleen *qi*.

• **Blender or food processor**

1 cup	dried white beans	250 mL
1	piece (1 inch/2.5 cm square) dried kombu	1
1	sprig fresh thyme	1
1	large carrot	1
1	turnip, peeled	1
1	leek	1
1	zucchini	1
1	onion	1
1	stalk celery	1
1 tsp	salt	5 mL
1 cup	halved trimmed green beans	250 mL
1	large bunch fresh basil	1
2	cloves garlic	2
1 tbsp	extra virgin olive oil	15 mL

1. Place white beans in a large bowl and cover with water. Let stand overnight. (Or in a large saucepan, combine 4 cups/1 L water and white beans and bring to a boil. Cook for 2 minutes. Remove from heat, cover and let stand for 1 hour.) Drain well.

2. In a large saucepan, combine white beans, 4 cups (1 L) water, kombu and thyme. Bring to a boil. Reduce heat and simmer for 30 minutes. Remove kombu.

3. Meanwhile, halve carrot, turnip, leek and zucchini lengthwise. Slice into half-moons. Coarsely chop onion. Cut celery diagonally into $\frac{1}{2}$-inch (1 cm) thick pieces.

4. Add carrot, turnip, leek, onion, celery and salt to saucepan. Add enough water to cover vegetables by 2 inches (5 cm). Cook over medium heat for 20 minutes or until vegetables are tender. Stir in zucchini and green beans and cook for 10 minutes, adding a little more water if necessary to keep vegetables covered.

5. Remove basil leaves from stems. In a blender, combine basil leaves, garlic and oil. Add 1 or 2 ladlefuls of the soup. Blend until smooth. Stir back into remaining soup until well combined. Remove thyme.

6. Ladle into serving bowls. Serve immediately.

Miso Soup

By varying the seasonal vegetables you add, you can enjoy this miso soup throughout the year. In late summer, try carrots, daikon, chestnuts or winter squash. In the spring, try pungent tender greens and peas. Feel free to use leftover steamed or boiled vegetables to make the recipe more convenient. The fermented and flavorful miso calms the stomach and stimulates digestion.

MAKES 4 SERVINGS

Tips

If you like a more pronounced flavor, you can increase the miso to a maximum of ½ cup (125 mL).

If you're cooking vegetables specifically for this soup, steam each kind separately until very tender.

4 cups	Traditional or Vegetarian Dashi (see recipes, opposite)	1 L
6 tbsp	white miso	90 mL
2 tbsp	tamari or soy sauce (or 1 tsp/5 mL salt)	30 mL
2 cups	mixed cooked seasonal vegetables, warm or at room temperature	500 mL

1. In a medium saucepan, heat dashi until steaming. Whisk in miso and tamari and immediately remove from heat.

2. Stir in vegetables and serve immediately.

Health Tip

There are many types of miso, which may be made from a base of soybeans, rice, barley or other ingredients. Miso is inoculated with a fungal and bacterial culture called *koji* and fermented over a period of time, from a few months to years. It is a probiotic food, which adds beneficial bacteria to the gut, and has been a staple in Japanese cuisine for centuries. Be sure to add miso at the last minute and remove the pan from the heat right away; heating it to more than 100°F (38°C) destroys the beneficial bacteria.

Traditional Dashi

Dashi is a delicate broth used as a base for miso and other soups to give them a rich umami taste. The traditional version is flavored with katsuobushi (flakes of dried bonito) and kombu (dried kelp, a type of seaweed that is rich in glutamates and umami flavor). Look for both at Japanese grocery or health food stores.

MAKES 4 CUPS (1 L)

Tip

You can still use the kombu once it's been strained out of the dashi. Rinse it off and make Kombu Vinegar Pickle (page 428).

1	piece (3 inches/7.5 cm square) dried kombu	1
½ cup	katsuobushi	125 mL
1 tsp	salt	5 mL

1. In a large saucepan, bring 4 cups (1 L) water and kombu to a boil. Remove from heat and stir in katsuobushi.

2. Cover and let stand for 10 minutes. Strain through a fine-mesh sieve into a medium bowl, discarding kombu and katsuobushi. Stir in salt.

Vegetarian Dashi

If you don't eat fish, this vegetarian dashi is the answer. It gets its rich flavor from dried shiitake mushrooms and green onions, as well as the traditional kombu.

MAKES 4 CUPS (1 L)

Tip

See tip above.

6	dried shiitake mushrooms	6
2	green onions, sliced	2
1	piece (3 inches/7.5 cm square) dried kombu	1
1 tsp	salt	5 mL

1. Pour 5 cups (1.25 L) water into a medium bowl. Add shiitake mushrooms stem side down and let stand for 2 to 8 hours. If you are not ready to make the dashi, cover and refrigerate the mushrooms in their liquid for up to 2 days.

2. Using a slotted spoon, transfer mushrooms to a cutting board. Pour 4 cups (1 L) of the soaking liquid into a medium saucepan. Discard remaining liquid and sediment.

3. Remove mushroom stems and discard. Coarsely chop mushrooms and add to saucepan along with green onions and kombu. Bring to a boil. Remove from heat, cover and let stand for 10 minutes.

4. Strain through a fine-mesh sieve into a medium bowl, discarding vegetables and kombu (or see tip, above). Stir in salt.

Turkey Meatball and Watercress Soup

This is a variation on traditional Chinese lion's head soup, which is a rustic, hearty and delicious comfort food. Daikon radish gives a light sweetness to the tender turkey meatballs.

MAKES 4 SERVINGS

Tip

Turkey thigh meat is preferable in this recipe, as it is more flavorful than the breast.

Variation

If watercress is not available, substitute trimmed arugula.

1	piece (8 oz/250 g) daikon radish	1
4	green onions, minced	4
1	large egg, beaten	1
1 lb	ground turkey (preferably thighs)	500 g
1½ tsp	salt, divided	7 mL
2 oz	watercress, trimmed	60 g

1. Peel and coarsely grate daikon. One handful at a time, squeeze out liquid and place in a medium bowl. Add green onions, egg, turkey and ½ tsp (2 mL) of the salt. Mix until well combined. Shape into 16 meatballs and place on a large plate. Cover and refrigerate for 2 hours or for up to 24 hours.

2. In a medium saucepan, bring 4 cups (1 L) water to a boil. Add meatballs and remaining salt. Reduce heat to low and simmer, stirring gently once or twice, for 10 minutes.

3. Add watercress and cook for 2 to 3 minutes or until watercress is wilted and meatballs are no longer pink inside. Serve immediately.

Health Tip

Turkey is warming, sweet and slightly drying, and it supplements the *qi* and yang. If you often feel cold and lethargic, this soup can be beneficial. If you have a tendency toward feeling warm and dry, do not eat this soup; instead, try Tilapia and Arugula Soup (page 251).

Chunky Vegetable Bean Stew

Sweet root vegetables cooked with nutty-tasting adzuki beans makes this a very hearty stew. It's comforting to eat on a chilly day. This recipe makes more beans than you need; keep the leftovers in your fridge and stir them into other dishes for a protein boost.

MAKES 4 SERVINGS

Tips

For the root vegetables, try a mix of 2 or 3 of the following: carrot, parsnip, turnip, rutabaga, daikon radish or Asian sweet potatoes.

To make ginger juice, grate gingerroot and press it between your fingers or through a fine-mesh sieve.

Health Tips

Nourishing sweet root vegetables are beneficial to the stomach and spleen. The adzuki beans are sweet and sour in flavor; they improve digestion and help drain dampness and water from the body in cases of water retention. The sour, astringing flavor of the bean is also useful in some cases of diarrhea. This is an ideal dish for someone who wants a hearty vegetarian option or is looking to shed excess weight.

Adding kombu to the cooking beans helps increase their digestibility and reduces gas.

1 cup	dried adzuki beans	250 mL
1	piece (1 inch/2.5 cm square) dried kombu (optional)	1
2 tbsp	avocado oil	30 mL
6 cups	cubed peeled mixed root vegetables (see tips, at left)	1.5 L
½ cup	rice wine, such as sake	125 mL
2 tbsp	tamari or soy sauce	30 mL
1 tbsp	ginger juice (see tips, at left)	15 mL
1 tsp	salt	5 mL
2 tbsp	minced green onions	30 mL

1. In a large saucepan, combine 4 cups (1 L) water and adzuki beans and bring to a boil. Remove from heat, cover and let stand for 1 hour.

2. Drain and rinse beans well. Return to saucepan. Add 4 cups (1 L) fresh water and kombu (if using) and bring to a boil. Reduce heat to low, cover and simmer, stirring once or twice and adding more water if necessary, for 1½ to 2 hours or until beans are very tender. Remove from heat. Let cool in pan, uncovered, for 30 minutes. Drain well, discarding kombu.

3. About halfway through the bean cooking time, in a medium saucepan, heat oil over medium-high heat. Add root vegetables and cook, without stirring, for 2 minutes. Using tongs, turn vegetables and cook for 2 minutes or until browned on both sides.

4. Add 1 cup (250 mL) water, wine, tamari, ginger juice and salt. Bring to a simmer. Reduce heat to low, cover and simmer for 10 to 15 minutes or until vegetables are almost tender.

5. Uncover pan, increase heat to high and cook, shaking pan often, for 1 to 2 minutes or until almost no liquid remains.

6. To serve, gently stir in 1 cup (250 mL) of the beans and sprinkle with green onions. Cover and refrigerate remaining beans for up to 3 days.

Nourishing Vegetable Treasures

This is a variation on the traditional vegetarian dish called Buddha's Delight. It has lovely, subtle flavors and combines a number of contrasting textures. The variety of ingredients is important to this dish; however, if some of them are unavailable, feel free to leave them out and increase the amounts of others.

> **MAKES**
> **4 TO 6 SERVINGS**

Tips

If you can't find roasted peanuts, buy raw ones and toast them at home. In a small dry skillet, toast peanuts over low heat, stirring often, for 5 minutes or until golden and fragrant.

Tapioca flour is sometimes labeled tapioca starch. It's the same thing just under a different name.

It's best to buy the water-packed tofu sold in the refrigerated section of your supermarket. To store tofu, cover it with water in an airtight container and keep it refrigerated for up to 1 week, changing the water every day.

4 cups	warm water, divided	1 L
½ cup	dried shiitake mushrooms (about 4), stems removed	125 mL
½ cup	dried daylily bulbs	125 mL
½ cup	dried lotus seeds	125 mL
4 oz	lotus root, peeled	125 g
½ cup	tamari or soy sauce	125 mL
1 tsp	tapioca flour or arrowroot starch	5 mL
2 tbsp	avocado oil	30 mL
8 oz	snow peas, trimmed	250 g
½	small jicama (about 8 oz/250 g jicama), peeled and thinly sliced	½
4	baby bok choy, trimmed and halved lengthwise (or 2 cups/500 mL sliced regular bok choy, napa cabbage or green cabbage)	4
4 oz	drained canned whole bamboo shoots, cut into snow pea-size pieces	125 g
½ cup	rice wine, such as sake	125 mL
1	package (14 oz to 1 lb/420 to 500 g) extra-firm tofu, drained and cut into 1-inch (2.5 cm) cubes	1
½ cup	unsalted roasted peanuts	125 mL

1. In a medium bowl, combine 2 cups (500 mL) of the warm water and mushrooms. In another medium bowl, combine remaining warm water, daylily bulbs and lotus seeds. Let stand for 2 hours or cover and refrigerate for up to 24 hours. Drain well, discarding soaking liquid. Cut mushrooms into quarters and set aside.

2. In a medium saucepan, bring 2 cups (500 mL) water to a boil. Add daylily bulbs and lotus seeds. Reduce heat and simmer for 10 minutes. Drain.

Tip

If you are sensitive to sulfites, check the packaging on the mushrooms, lotus seeds and daylily bulbs. For sulfite-free ingredients, try Gold Mine Natural Food Co. at www.goldminenatural foods.com.

3. Cut lotus root into $1/8$-inch (3 mm) thick slices. Place in a small bowl and cover with water. Set aside.

4. In another small bowl, stir tamari with tapioca flour until dissolved. Set aside. Drain lotus root.

5. In a large skillet, heat oil over medium-high heat, swirling to coat bottom of pan. Add lotus root, snow peas, jicama and bok choy. Sauté for 3 to 4 minutes or until lotus root is translucent and bok choy is wilted.

6. Add daylily bulbs, lotus seeds, mushrooms, bamboo shoots and rice wine to pan. Sauté for 2 minutes.

7. Stir tamari mixture and add to pan. Cook, stirring often, until sauce is glossy. Remove from heat. Gently stir in tofu and sprinkle with peanuts. Serve immediately.

Health Tips

The mix of vegetables in this dish clears out heat and detoxifies the body. It is helpful for people who are transitioning away from more animal-based diets.

Bamboo shoots are cold in thermal nature and are especially beneficial for people who eat larger amounts of meat and other animal foods. Bamboo shoots moderate the warming effects of meat.

Lotus seeds, daylily bulbs and bamboo shoots all help calm the mind, so try this dish if you suffer from anxiety.

Mixed Mushroom Sauté

Mushrooms are rich in flavor and offer potent protection for the immune system. This quick sauté has more character and texture if you use at least two kinds of mushrooms. Nutmeg enhances their earthy and savory taste.

MAKES 4 SERVINGS

Tips

If you would like to use delicate mushrooms, such as morels or chanterelles, add them after the other mushrooms have cooked for 3 to 4 minutes.

You can use whatever kind of chives you have on hand. Both Chinese chives and regular garden chives commonly found in Western supermarkets are delicious.

2 lbs	mixed fresh mushrooms, such as oyster, shiitake, cremini or button (see box, below)	1 kg
2 tbsp	avocado oil	30 mL
1 tsp	salt	5 mL
¼ tsp	ground nutmeg	1 mL
2 tbsp	minced chives (see tips, at left)	30 mL

1. Trim off and discard mushroom stems. Cut caps into ¼-inch (0.5 cm) thick slices.

2. In a large skillet, heat oil over medium-high heat, swirling to coat bottom of pan. Add mushrooms, salt and nutmeg. Sauté for 8 to 10 minutes or until mushrooms are softened and no liquid remains.

3. Spoon onto serving plates and sprinkle with chives. Serve immediately.

Health Tip

The pungent chives and nutmeg add a warming aspect to this dish.

Different Mushrooms, Different Benefits

- Oyster mushrooms are sweet and slightly warming. They reinforce the spleen, can increase urination and calm muscle spasms. Studies have found that they lower blood sugar in people with diabetes, and reduce cholesterol and triglyceride levels when eaten over long periods of time.

- Shiitake mushrooms, also known as fragrant mushrooms, are sweet, neutral and most beneficial for reinforcing *qi*, which helps in cases of poor appetite or fatigue.

- Common button mushrooms and cremini mushrooms are sweet and slightly cooling. They replenish *qi*, moisten mucous membranes and dissolve phlegm.

Coconut Fish Curry

This colorful curry is very mild and creamy. Its simple flavors are highlighted by the pungent and warming curry spices. This dish is perfectly cozy and nourishing during seasonal transitions.

Tips

Pure coconut milk is used in this recipe, not coconut milk beverage. Look for a brand that is preservative-free — it will have better flavor.

An equal amount of another tender green, such as spinach, will work well if you can't find Swiss chard.

Health Tip

If you tend to feel cold, this curry will warm your body and move stagnant *qi* without being too drying. Coconut's warming and lubricating actions on the body counter the pungent and dispersing effect of the curry, which is often made from turmeric, fenugreek, cumin, coriander, cinnamon, cardamom, ginger and pepper — all pungent, aromatic and warming spices.

2 tbsp	avocado oil, divided	30 mL
½	large onion, thinly sliced	½
1 tsp	curry powder	5 mL
2 cups	cubed peeled sweet potatoes (½-inch/1 cm cubes)	500 mL
2 cups	coconut milk (see tips, at left)	500 mL
1 tsp	grated lime zest	5 mL
1 tbsp	freshly squeezed lime juice	15 mL
1 tsp	salt	5 mL
1 lb	Swiss chard	500 g
1 tsp	grated gingerroot	5 mL
1 lb	boneless skinless mild fish fillets (such as cod or sole)	500 g
1	lime, cut into wedges	1

1. In a medium saucepan, heat 1 tbsp (15 mL) of the oil over medium-low heat. Add onion and cook, stirring constantly, for 5 to 7 minutes or until golden brown. Stir in curry powder and cook for 30 seconds or until fragrant.

2. Stir in sweet potatoes, coconut milk, lime zest, lime juice and salt and bring to a simmer. Simmer for 10 minutes or just until potatoes are tender. Remove from heat and set aside.

3. Cut Swiss chard stems off leaves and chop coarsely. Set aside. Chop leaves coarsely and set aside separately.

4. In a medium skillet, heat remaining oil over medium-high heat. Add chard stems and ginger and cook, stirring, until translucent. Add chard leaves and cook, stirring, for 5 to 7 minutes or until wilted and tender. Remove from heat and keep warm.

5. Cut fish into 1-inch (2.5 cm) pieces. Return curry mixture to medium-high heat and bring to a boil, uncovered. Gently stir in fish and turn off heat. Let stand on burner for 5 minutes or until fish is opaque.

6. Spoon chard mixture into serving bowls and top with curry. Serve with lime wedges.

Grilled Squid

Squid is enjoyed in many different cuisines all over the world, especially in coastal communities around the Mediterranean, in Russia and the Philippines, and around the rest of Asia. When grilled well, it is simply perfect. If you don't like coconut, serve the squid over Simple Sautéed Greens (page 263).

MAKES 4 SERVINGS	

Tips

Buying already cleaned fresh squid is the easiest and quickest way to enjoy this dish. Of course, you can clean whole squid yourself if you like. Save the tentacles for another use.

If it's not grilling weather, you can broil the squid instead. Preheat broiler. Pat squid dry with paper towels and arrange on a foil-lined rimmed baking sheet. Broil, about 3 inches (7.5 cm) from heat, for 2 minutes per side or just until opaque.

- **Preheat barbecue to high**

1 lb	cleaned squid tubes (see tips, at left)	500 g
2 tsp	salt, divided	10 mL
2 lbs	summer squash, trimmed and coarsely grated	1 kg
2 cups	coconut milk (see tips, previous page)	500 mL
1/4 tsp	grated lime zest	1 mL
1/4 cup	coarsely chopped fresh cilantro or basil	60 mL

1. In a resealable plastic bag, combine squid tubes and 1 tsp (5 mL) of the salt. Seal and shake to combine. Refrigerate for 2 hours or up to 24 hours.

2. In a medium bowl, toss squash with remaining salt. Let stand for 30 minutes.

3. Drain squash. One handful at a time, squeeze out excess moisture. In a large skillet, combine squash, coconut milk and lime zest and bring to a boil. Reduce heat and simmer, uncovered, for 15 minutes or until squash is soft and liquid is slightly reduced.

4. Drain squid and pat dry with paper towels. Place on greased grill on preheated barbecue and grill for 2 minutes per side or just until opaque. (Overcooking makes squid tough and dry.)

5. Transfer to a cutting board and cut into 1/4-inch (0.5 cm) wide rings. Divide squash mixture among serving bowls. Top with squid and sprinkle with cilantro. Serve immediately.

Health Tip

Squid is neutral, sweet and salty. It is quite nourishing to the yin, *qi* and blood. It is useful for those who feel weak or suffer from low back pain due to rheumatism.

Shredded Pork and Vegetables with Tamarind Glaze

Tamarind gives recipes a complex, tangy brightness. Here, it balances the meat and the sweetness of the cabbage in an easy stir-fry.

MAKES 4 SERVINGS

Tip

Prep your ingredients before you start sautéing. It goes quickly once you begin.

Health Tips

Tamarind has a wonderful sweet-and-sour flavor and is cooling. It can be helpful with constipation. In China, tamarind cooked with crataegus (dried hawthorn fruit) and barley malt is recommended for indigestion.

According to Chinese medicine, pork, which is neutral in nature, will not contribute to dampness in the body — except if eaten in excess (it is not recommended for someone with circulatory or weight issues). It is one of the few meats indicated for dry conditions, such as constipation, dry cough or being underweight, as it nourishes the yin.

- **Blender or food processor**

¼ cup	unsweetened tamarind pulp	60 mL
1 cup	hot water	250 mL
1 lb	lean boneless pork, such as pork loin	500 g
½	Chinese cabbage (about 1 lb/ 500 g cabbage)	½
1 lb	small green beans	500 g
3 tbsp	avocado oil, divided	45 mL
¼ cup	palm sugar	60 mL
1 tsp	salt	5 mL

1. Break tamarind pulp into walnut-sized lumps and place in a small bowl. Stir in hot water and let stand for 30 minutes. In blender, purée tamarind mixture until smooth and thickened. Using a spatula, press through a fine-mesh sieve into a small bowl. Discard solids.

2. Cut pork into ¼-inch (0.5 cm) thick slices. Stack a few slices at a time and cut crosswise into ¼-inch (0.5 cm) wide strips. Core and cut cabbage into ¼-inch (0.5 cm) wide strips. Trim and halve green beans crosswise.

3. In a large skillet, heat 2 tbsp (30 mL) of the oil over medium-high heat, swirling to coat bottom of pan. Add green beans and cabbage and sauté just until tender. Transfer to a plate and set aside.

4. Add remaining oil to skillet and heat over medium-high heat. Add pork and sauté for 3 to 5 minutes or until no longer pink inside but not browned. Increase heat to high and stir in tamarind purée, palm sugar and salt. Cook, stirring, for 3 to 5 minutes or until sauce is translucent and glossy.

5. Return green beans and cabbage to pan and stir to coat. Serve immediately.

Tangy Carrot, Beet and Potato Salad

This earthy salad is a modern take on traditional European flavors. Lightly fermenting the vegetables makes them tastier and easier to digest.

Tip

The carrots and beets are put into separate jars to keep their colors vibrant.

Health Tips

Transitional times of the year, when the seasons are beginning to change, are periods when you should nourish the central resources of the body; namely, the stomach and spleen network, where all of your food is transformed into useable energy for your body. Carrots, beets and potatoes are *qi*-tonic foods that offer nourishing energy.

Adding sauerkraut lightly ferments the vegetables in this dish and increases their benefits to the gut.

Caraway is a warming, digestive and carminative cooking spice that enhances the natural sweetness of this dish.

- **Two 2-cup (500 mL) canning jars or airtight containers with lids**

1 cup	unpasteurized sauerkraut (store-bought or homemade) with juices	250 mL
1 cup	coarsely grated peeled carrots	250 mL
1 cup	coarsely grated peeled beets	250 mL
1 tsp	salt	5 mL
1 lb	yellow-fleshed or red potatoes (unpeeled)	500 g
2 tbsp	avocado oil	30 mL
1 tsp	caraway seeds	5 mL

1. Divide sauerkraut and its juice equally between jars. Add carrots to 1 of the jars and beets to the other. Divide salt between jars. Cover, shake and refrigerate for 1 to 2 days.

2. Place potatoes in a medium saucepan and cover with water. Bring to a boil. Reduce heat to low, cover and simmer for 20 minutes or just until tender. Drain potatoes. Return to pan and let cool.

3. Peel and cut potatoes into $1/2$-inch (1 cm) cubes. Transfer to a serving bowl and set aside.

4. In a small skillet, combine oil and caraway seeds. Cook over medium heat, stirring occasionally, for 2 to 3 minutes or until fragrant. Pour seeds and oil over potatoes and gently toss to coat.

5. Spoon potatoes onto serving plates. Top with carrot and beet mixtures and any juices in jars.

Wakame Salad

Wakame is a type of seaweed that you'll most likely see floating in miso soup. Its delicate texture and subtle sweet-and-salty flavor are also excellent in a salad.

> **MAKES 4 SERVINGS**

Tips

This salad will keep in the fridge for up to 3 days. Eat as a side salad or condiment with other meals.

Dried wakame and other seaweeds can be stored for a long time. Keep them in sealed glass containers in a cool, dark, dry location.

Don't toss the trimmed center veins of your wakame — they are great fertilizer for your garden!

½ oz	dried wakame	15 g
½ cup	sesame seeds	125 mL
3	red radishes, quartered and thinly sliced	3
1	piece (4 oz/125 g) jicama, peeled and julienned	1
1	sprig fresh basil, leaves removed	1
2 tbsp	freshly squeezed lemon juice	30 mL
1 tbsp	extra virgin olive oil (optional)	15 mL
	Salt	

1. Place wakame in a medium bowl and pour in enough water to cover. Let stand for 10 minutes or until softened.

2. Meanwhile, in a small dry skillet, toast sesame seeds over low heat, stirring constantly, for 3 to 5 minutes or until fragrant and golden. Immediately transfer to a small bowl and let cool.

3. Cut thick center vein out of each wakame leaf (see tips, at left). Cut leaves into about 1-inch (2.5 cm) pieces and place in a serving bowl. Add radishes and jicama and toss to combine.

4. Stir in basil leaves, lemon juice and olive oil (if using). Season to taste with salt. Sprinkle sesame seeds over top and toss well to combine. Serve immediately.

> ## Health Tip
>
> Wakame is a blood and yin tonic and is high in calcium (just behind hijiki). It is useful for treating edema, and clears excess heat, mucous and phlegm from the body. Even though wakame is salty in flavor, it actually helps to regulate sodium in the blood.

Mixed Crunchy Lettuce Salad with Tofu Miso Dressing

To give this salad the right balance of flavors — salty, sour and sweet — make sure to include the bitter inner leaves and stems of the lettuces. This is a lovely, fresh and wonderfully crisp side dish.

MAKES
MAKES 2 TO 4 SERVINGS

Tip

To toast sesame seeds, place them in a small dry skillet. Toast over low heat, stirring constantly, for 3 to 5 minutes or until fragrant. Immediately transfer to a small bowl and let cool.

½	package (14 oz to 1 lb/420 to 500 g package) soft or medium tofu, drained	½
2 tbsp	white miso	30 mL
1 tbsp	toasted sesame oil	15 mL
1 tbsp	freshly squeezed lemon juice	15 mL
1	small head red leaf lettuce, torn into bite-size pieces	1
1	small head romaine lettuce, torn into bite-size pieces	1
2 tbsp	sesame seeds (preferably black), toasted	30 mL

1. In a medium bowl, whisk together tofu, miso, sesame oil and lemon juice until smooth.

2. In a serving bowl, combine red leaf lettuce and romaine lettuce. Pour dressing over top and toss gently to coat. Sprinkle with sesame seeds. Serve immediately.

Health Tips

This fresh green salad is perfect for anyone who often feels hot and experiences feelings of frustration and agitation. The cooling and cleansing action of slightly bitter lettuce makes it a good diuretic. Its heat-clearing action can help with a fever and is beneficial to the liver. Combined with the cooling and lubricating action of tofu, this crunchy lettuce makes a terrific salad for people who have robust digestive systems.

If you often feel cold, have an underactive thyroid and sluggish digestion, avoid this dish.

Tamarind-Dressed Chickpea Salad

This nourishing salad offers a rich blend of textures, and is full of wholesome plant protein and beneficial fats. The chickpeas and vegetables are complemented by the tangy-sweet tamarind dressing, which gives the salad a bright taste. It makes an excellent one-dish meal.

MAKES 4 SERVINGS

Tips

To cook dried chickpeas, soak them overnight in enough water to cover. Drain well, then transfer to a saucepan and cover with fresh water. Bring to a boil. Reduce heat, cover and simmer for $1\frac{1}{2}$ to 3 hours or until tender. If you don't have time to cook dried chickpeas from scratch, substitute two $15\frac{1}{2}$-oz (429 g) cans, drained and rinsed.

To make this salad ahead, prep all the ingredients except the avocado and refrigerate them until you're ready to eat. Just before serving, peel, pit and cube the avocado, and stir it into the salad.

- **Blender or food processor**

$\frac{1}{4}$ cup	unsweetened tamarind pulp	60 mL
1 cup	hot water	250 mL
1	disc (1 oz/30 g) palm sugar	1
1 tsp	grated gingerroot	5 mL
$\frac{1}{2}$ tsp	salt	2 mL
2 cups	cubed peeled broccoli stems	500 mL
1 cup	dried chickpeas, cooked, rinsed and drained (see tips, at left)	250 mL
2	avocados, peeled, pitted and cut into $\frac{1}{2}$-inch (1 cm) cubes	2

1. Break tamarind pulp into walnut-sized lumps and place in a small bowl. Stir in hot water and let stand for 30 minutes. In blender, purée tamarind mixture until smooth and thickened. Using a spatula, press through a fine-mesh sieve into a small bowl. Discard solids.

2. In a medium saucepan, combine tamarind purée, sugar, ginger and salt and bring to a simmer over medium heat. Cook, stirring occasionally, for 5 minutes or until thick and glossy. Remove from heat and let cool.

3. Pour enough water into another medium saucepan to come $\frac{1}{4}$ inch (0.5 cm) up side. Bring to a boil. Add broccoli stems, cover and steam for 2 minutes or just until tender. Uncover and cook, shaking pan often, for 3 to 5 minutes or until almost no liquid remains.

4. Using a slotted spoon, transfer broccoli stems to a serving bowl. Add chickpeas and tamarind mixture. Toss gently to coat. Gently stir in avocado. Serve immediately.

Health Tip

Chickpeas nourish and support the spleen and are beneficial to people who are trying to regulate their blood sugar. Avocados are an excellent source of healthy vegetable fat, which means they are a great food for vegans and vegetarians. They are also beneficial for people trying to gain weight. Their lubricating action also balances the drying effect of the beans.

Cauliflower with Basil Sauce

The green hue of this sauce is vibrant; and since you eat with your eyes first, this colorful dish can spark the appetite. The steamed cauliflower florets have a substantial texture that's very satisfying. Be sure to serve and eat the dish right away to enjoy the beautiful green of the basil, which fades as the dish cools.

**MAKES
4 TO 6 SERVINGS**

Tip

To test the texture of the cauliflower, spear it with a fork. When cauliflower is barely tender, the fork will go in but still meet resistance.

4	green onions, thinly sliced	4
½ cup	minced fresh basil	125 mL
2 tbsp	black or white sesame seeds (or a mixture)	30 mL
2 tbsp	avocado oil	30 mL
1 tsp	salt	5 mL
1	large head cauliflower (about 2 lbs/1 kg)	1

1. In a small bowl, whisk together green onions, basil, sesame seeds, oil and salt. Set aside.

2. Cut cauliflower into about 1-inch (2.5 cm) florets. Pour enough water into a large skillet to come about ¼ inch (0.5 cm) up side. Bring to a boil. Add cauliflower. Reduce heat, cover and simmer for 2 minutes or until cauliflower is barely tender.

3. Uncover pan and cook, shaking pan often and watching closely to prevent burning, for 3 to 5 minutes or until no liquid remains.

4. Spoon cauliflower into a serving bowl. Pour sauce over top and toss gently to coat. Serve immediately.

Health Tip

Cauliflower is sweet, slightly bitter, and neutral to cooling in nature. It cools stomach heat, meaning if you have a voracious appetite, this is a perfect dish for you. The sauce, made with pungent and warming basil and green onions, balances the dish, which enhances digestion.

Sautéed Celery and Cabbage Ribbons

These two humble vegetables are delicious sautéed together with fragrant ginger. The best part: this dish is quick and easy to prepare, so it can be your healthy, go-to weeknight side.

MAKES 4 SERVINGS

Tips

Take your time cooking the cabbage. Lightly browning the edges builds more flavor.

4	stalks celery	4
1/2	head cabbage (1 lb/500 g cabbage)	1/2
2 tbsp	avocado oil	30 mL
1 tbsp	minced gingerroot	15 mL
2 tbsp	tamari or soy sauce	30 mL

1. Cut celery into 1/8-inch (3 mm) slices on the diagonal. Core and cut cabbage into 1/4-inch (0.5 cm) thick slices.

2. In a large skillet, heat oil over medium-high heat, swirling to coat bottom of pan. Add celery, cabbage and ginger. Sauté for 5 to 7 minutes or until celery and cabbage are lightly browned on the edges and celery is tender.

3. Spoon into a serving bowl. Drizzle with tamari and gently toss to coat. Serve immediately.

Health Tips

The Greeks identified celery as a valuable nerve and blood tonic, which was a good remedy for hangovers. The Chinese have long used celery to bring down high blood pressure and cool liver congestion. Celery is slightly cooling, slightly salty and bitter. It cools stomach heat, moves liver *qi* and reduces hypertension.

Cabbage is a sweet vegetable that is of great benefit to the stomach and spleen, a center of the body's *qi*. Its juice, when lightly heated with honey, relieves abdominal spasms and pain.

Tea-Pickled Eggs

Fragrant and appetizing tea eggs, also called marbleized eggs, are a traditional Chinese snack food. They have been adapted and are now beloved across Asia. Tea eggs are often sold as street food and at convenience stores in China, and the real things are even better than what you can buy in stores. Fortunately, they are easy to make at home and give your kitchen a wonderful aroma. These eggs are perfect for a picnic or other portable meal.

	MAKES 4 EGGS	

Tips

A smoky Chinese tea, such as pu-erh, lapsang souchong or a black breakfast tea (such as English or Irish breakfast) will give the brine a rich flavor.

A 1-quart (1 L) canning jar is the perfect container for marinating the eggs.

2	black tea bags (or 2 tsp/10 mL loose black tea)	2
1	whole star anise	1
½ cup	tamari or soy sauce	125 mL
4	large eggs	4

1. In a small saucepan, bring 2 cups (500 mL) water to a boil. Remove from heat and add tea bags and star anise. Let stand for 5 minutes. Discard tea bags.

2. Stir in tamari. Pour into a 3- or 4-cup (750 mL or 1 L) container that is no larger than 4 inches (10 cm) in diameter. (This ensures the eggs will be submerged in the brine.) Cover and refrigerate until ready to use.

3. Place eggs in a medium saucepan and pour in enough water to cover. Bring to a boil. Reduce heat and simmer for 8 minutes.

4. Immediately drain eggs and run cold water over them until cool. Gently tap eggs to crack shells all over (do not remove shells).

5. Add eggs to brine and refrigerate for 8 hours or up to 5 days. To serve, peel eggs.

> ### Health Tip
>
> Eggs are so nourishing to both yin and yang. The melding of sweet, salty and pungent flavors makes this a satisfying snack.

Almond and Goji Berry Snack Mix

The licorice-flavored anise seeds bring out the sweetness of the goji berries and the toasty taste of the nuts in this mix. It is a good pick-me-up snack packed with energy, but isn't full of sugar like commercial trail mixes. If you like it, double or triple this recipe to be sure to have it on hand. You and your children will love it.

> **MAKES**
> **1 CUP (250 ML)**

Tip

To toast sliced almonds, preheat oven to 300°F (150°C). Spread almonds on a rimmed baking sheet or in a metal cake pan and toast, stirring once or twice, for 6 to 8 minutes or until light golden brown. Let cool on pan.

½ cup	dried goji berries	125 mL
½ cup	sliced almonds, toasted	125 mL
¼ tsp	anise seeds	1 mL
⅛ tsp	ground cloves	0.5 mL
Pinch	salt	Pinch

1. In a medium bowl, toss together goji berries, almonds, anise seeds, cloves and salt.

2. Transfer to an airtight container and store at room temperature for up to 2 weeks.

> **Health Tip**
>
> This nourishing snack fortifies and moistens the body's tissues, soothing coughs while boosting vital energy. Goji berries are used in Chinese herbal medicine to boost vision and to promote regenerative energy in the body.

Nourish the Qi and Blood Tea

This simple, sweet and earthy tea builds qi and vitality. It's quite simple to make; sip it daily whenever you need an energy boost.

> **MAKES**
> **2 TO 4 SERVINGS**

Tip

The herbs in this tea will most likely need to be purchased from an herbal supplier or Asian grocery store, most of which have an herbal section. Store the herbs in glass jars, tightly sealed, in a cool, dark place for up to 1 year.

8	dried pitted red dates	8
1 oz	dried astragalus root	30 g

1. Cut red dates in half. In a large saucepan, combine 6 cups (1.5 L) water, dates and astragalus root. Bring to a boil. Reduce heat, cover and simmer for 20 minutes.

2. Strain into teacups. Serve immediately.

> **Health Tip**
>
> Red dates build the blood, and strengthen the *qi* of the stomach and spleen. Astragalus increases *qi* and has an affinity for the heart and lungs.

Tame-the-Tension Tea

This light, subtly sweet and calming tea recipe was passed on to Ellen by one of her Chinese medicine teachers, Dr. Mengke Kou. She and her fellow interns would often sip this tea to soothe their graduate-school stress. If you are feeling worked up, take a break and steep a cup for an effective tension buster.

MAKES 2 SERVINGS

Tip

Always store herbs in glass jars, tightly sealed, in a cool, dark place. They will keep for up to 1 year — no longer.

1 tbsp	dried chrysanthemum flowers	15 mL
1 tbsp	dried honeysuckle flower buds	15 mL
1 tbsp	dried goji berries	15 mL

1. In a small saucepan, bring 2 cups (500 mL) water to a boil.

2. Stir in chrysanthemum flowers, honeysuckle flower buds and goji berries. Reduce heat, cover and simmer for 5 to 10 minutes or until flavors are infused.

3. Strain into teacups. Serve immediately.

Health Tips

Chrysanthemum flowers and honeysuckle flower buds are both cooling in nature and slightly pungent in flavor. They disperse heat in the body and calm the liver.

Goji berries are sweet and nourishing and considered a general nutritive tonic with added benefits for vision and longevity. The goji berries add a grounding element to this tea. If you have a tendency toward stress, often feeling physically tense and overheated, this is an excellent tea you can drink on a regular basis with no adverse effects.

Red Date, Almond and Cinnamon Liquor

Herbal liquors and wines are traditional remedies around the world. A couple of sips of this velvety, sweet liquor is ideal after a meal and satisfies any desire you might have for a sweet dessert. The combination of ingredients is nourishing, adds warmth, boosts vitality and activates blood circulation.

MAKES
8 TO 10 SERVINGS

Tip

Don't let the ingredients steep in the liquor for more than 4 weeks. The liquor will become bitter and unpleasant.

- **1-quart (1 L) canning jar**

¼ cup	raw almonds (with skins)	60 mL
	Hot water	
1 cup	high-quality vodka	250 mL
1 tbsp	liquid honey	15 mL
20	dried pitted red dates	20
1	piece (2 inches/5 cm long) cinnamon stick	1

1. Place almonds in a medium bowl and pour in enough hot water to cover. Let stand for 1 hour. Drain and remove skins.

2. In canning jar, combine almonds, vodka, honey, red dates and cinnamon stick. Seal jar and shake to combine. Let stand in a cool, dark place, shaking every 2 to 3 days, for 2 weeks or for up to 4 weeks. To store for a longer period, strain the liquor into a small bottle. (Strained liquor will keep for years.)

3. To serve, pour into small glasses, such as a shot glasses or sake cups.

Health Tip

This liquor offers a number of different health benefits. Red dates, also known as jujubes, nourish the blood and *qi*. Almonds are lubricating and help the lungs. Cinnamon is pungent, sweet and warming; it also aids the kidneys. And alcohol, in the form of vodka, is pungent, increases circulation and is very warming.

Strawberries with Blackberry Coulis

This simple, healthful mixed-berry dessert is a delight. Sweet, pure blackberry and strawberry flavors make it perfect for special occasions when you want a light dessert.

MAKES 4 SERVINGS

Tip

If they are in season, you can substitute 1 pint (2 cups/500 mL) fresh blackberries. Thawed frozen blackberries make a thicker, silkier sauce than fresh blackberries.

• **Blender or food processor**

2 cups	thawed frozen blackberries (about 12 oz/375 g)	500 mL
1 tbsp	freshly squeezed lemon juice	15 mL
2 tbsp	liquid honey	30 mL
4 cups	fresh strawberries (1½ lbs/750 g), hulled and sliced	1 L

1. In blender, purée blackberries with lemon juice until as smooth as possible. Using a rubber spatula, press purée through a fine-mesh sieve into a medium bowl. Discard seeds.

2. Stir in honey. Cover and refrigerate until ready to use.

3. In a serving bowl, gently toss strawberries with blackberry coulis. Serve immediately.

Health Tips

This dessert can be a nice treat when you're suffering from a sore throat, hoarseness, a dry cough and/or a lack of energy. Blackberries are sweet-tart and warming like their relatives, raspberries, and can act as a liver and kidney tonic, nourishing vital energy. The Romans used blackberries as a treatment for gout.

Strawberries, on the other hand, are cooling, sweet-tart and often used to soothe a burning sore throat or ease a dry cough. They are beneficial for hoarseness as well as indigestion.

Asian Pears with Tangy Rose Hip Sauce

Sweet and sour is the theme for many fruits and desserts in late summer, a time of seasonal transition. Beautiful, deep red rose hips have a tangy flavor akin to that of cranberries. They make this sauce thick and velvety.

MAKES 4 SERVINGS

Tip

Rose hips are available where bulk spices and teas are sold, and online.

½ cup	unsweetened apple juice	125 mL
¼ cup	dried rose hips (1 oz/30 g)	60 mL
¼ cup	unsweetened cranberry juice	60 mL
1 tbsp	liquid honey	15 mL
¼ tsp	rose water	1 mL
2	large Asian pears (nashi)	2

1. In a small saucepan, combine apple juice, rose hips and cranberry juice and bring to a boil. Reduce heat to medium-low and simmer for 5 minutes or until rose hips are very soft. Using a rubber spatula, press mixture through a fine-mesh sieve into a medium bowl. Discard solids.

2. Stir in honey and rose water. Cover and refrigerate until ready to use or for up to 1 week.

3. Quarter and core pears. Cut into ¼-inch (0.5 cm) thick slices. In a serving bowl, gently toss pears with rose hip sauce. Serve immediately.

> ## Health Tip
>
> Pears are good for the lungs, as they help break up congestion and reduce coughing. Sweet-and-sour rose hips contain high levels of vitamin C, which stimulates the immune system and reduces water retention in the body.

Maple Tapioca Pudding with Toasted Nuts

This homey pudding — made with delicately chewy, soothing tapioca — is totally retro and delicious. The nuts are a nice, crunchy contrast to the maple-laced pudding. This dessert is delicious warm or cool.

MAKES 4 SERVINGS

Tips

You can substitute hemp milk for the rice milk.

To toast walnuts and pecans, preheat oven to 300°F (150°C). Spread nuts on a rimmed baking sheet and or in a metal cake pan and toast, stirring once or twice, for 8 to 10 minutes or until slightly darkened. Let cool on pan.

3 tbsp	small pearl tapioca	45 mL
Pinch	salt	Pinch
2½ cups	rice milk	625 mL
½ cup	pure maple syrup	125 mL
¼ tsp	ground nutmeg	1 mL
½ cup	coarsely chopped walnuts, toasted	125 mL
½ cup	coarsely chopped pecans, toasted	125 mL

1. In a medium saucepan, combine tapioca and salt. Slowly stir in rice milk and maple syrup. Place pan over medium heat and bring to a simmer, stirring constantly. Simmer for 15 minutes, stirring constantly, or until tapioca is translucent

2. Stir in nutmeg. Remove pan from heat and let cool for 15 minutes. (Or let cool completely. Cover and refrigerate for up to 3 days.)

3. In a small bowl, toss walnuts with pecans. Spoon pudding into serving bowls and sprinkle with nut mixture.

> ### Health Tip
>
> If you want an easy-to-digest dessert, tapioca is for you. Don't fret if you are feeling run-down or fatigued — grab a bowl of this pudding. It offers nourishment from the warming nuts, which are rich in lubricating oils.

Apple Honey Cake

The honey brings out the fragrance of the spices in this festive gluten-free cake.
The tang of the apples is a perfect match with sweet cinnamon, nutmeg and cloves.

MAKES 8 SERVINGS

Tips

The apple measurement is important; make sure you get a full 1 cup (250 mL) of lightly packed shredded peeled apple. You'll need about 2 apples (12 oz/375 g) to make this amount — buy an extra one just in case your apples are on the small side. You can always enjoy any leftovers as a snack!

This deeply flavorful cake is even better a day or two after baking, when the flavors have had a chance to develop.

Health Tip

Desserts are a special treat, and this gluten-free cake is a healthy one. A sweet treat calms and soothes the spirit — and a slice of this lovely cake does just that without making you feel heavy or bloated afterwards.

- **Preheat oven to 350°F (180°C), with rack positioned in lower third**
- **9-inch (23 cm) round cake pan**
- **Stand mixer fitted with paddle attachment**

½ cup + 2 tbsp	avocado oil	155 mL
1 cup	liquid honey	250 mL
2	large eggs	2
1 cup	brown rice flour	250 mL
1 cup	lightly packed shredded unpeeled apples (see tips, at left)	250 mL
½ cup	coarsely chopped walnuts	125 mL
½ cup	raisins	125 mL
1 tsp	baking powder	5 mL
1 tsp	ground cinnamon	5 mL
½ tsp	baking soda	2 mL
½ tsp	ground nutmeg	2 mL
¼ tsp	ground cloves	1 mL
¼ tsp	salt	1 mL

1. Lightly oil sides of cake pan and line bottom with parchment paper. Set aside.

2. In mixer bowl, combine oil, honey and eggs. Beat at medium speed for 4 minutes or until lightened in color.

3. Add flour, apples, walnuts, raisins, baking powder, cinnamon, baking soda, nutmeg, cloves and salt. Beat just until smooth. Scrape into prepared pan.

4. Bake in preheated oven for 30 minutes. Reduce heat to 325°F (160°C) and bake for 15 to 20 minutes more or until a toothpick inserted in the center comes out clean. Transfer pan to a wire rack and let cool.

5. To serve, cut into wedges. To store, cover and refrigerate for up to 5 days; let come to room temperature before serving.

Autumn Seasonal Menus

Menu 1
Salmon on Ginger-Braised Kale with Toasted Pine Nuts
Barberry and Winter Squash Pilaf

Menu 2
Chicken and Chestnut Fried Rice
Arame Sauté with Carrots and Broccoli

Menu 3
Braised Beef Brisket with Shiitakes
Roasted Beet Salad with Pickled Mustard Greens

Autumn Recipes

Sautéed Banana Crêpes

These grain-free vegan crêpes are nutritious and satisfyingly tangy because they are lightly fermented. The addition of sautéed bananas with vanilla makes them wonderfully sweet. Everyone will love them!

> **MAKES 12 CRÊPES, ENOUGH FOR 4 SERVINGS**

Tip

Lentils don't normally require soaking, but they do in this recipe to ensure they liquefy properly in the batter.

- **Blender or food processor**
- **2 large rimmed baking sheets, lined with parchment paper**

½ cup	dried red lentils or yellow split peas, rinsed	125 mL
1 cup	almond flour	250 mL
1 cup	warm water	250 mL
1 tbsp	plain non-dairy coconut yogurt or other yogurt	15 mL
¼ cup	avocado oil	60 mL
½ tsp	salt	2 mL
1 tsp	baking powder	5 mL

Sautéed Bananas

2	large firm ripe bananas	2
2 tbsp	ghee, walnut oil or avocado oil	30 mL
¼ tsp	vanilla extract	1 mL

1. In a medium bowl, combine 2 cups (500 mL) water and lentils; cover (see tip, at left). In another medium bowl, combine almond flour, warm water and yogurt; cover. Let both mixtures stand at room temperature for at least 4 hours or up to 24 hours.

2. Preheat oven to 400°F (200°C), with racks positioned in upper and lower thirds. Lightly oil parchment paper on baking sheets.

3. Drain and rinse lentils. Drain again. Transfer to blender and add almond flour mixture (undrained), oil and salt. Blend for 1 to 2 minutes or until very smooth. Add baking powder and blend just until combined.

Tip

The crêpes can be cooked ahead of time, layered between parchment paper and refrigerated for up to 3 days. (Cut up the parchment sheets on which the crêpes were baked to save paper.) To reheat, brush a medium skillet with a little oil and add crêpes; warm over medium-high heat.

4. Measure $1/4$ cup (60 mL) of the batter. Pour and spread into a 6-inch (15 cm) circle on 1 of the prepared baking sheets. Repeat to make a total of 6 circles on the two pans.

5. Bake on upper and lower racks in preheated oven, rotating and switching pans halfway through, for 6 to 8 minutes or until crêpes look dry, are slightly browned at the edges and are firm enough to peel gently off the parchment. Slide the parchment paper, with the crêpes in place, off the pans.

6. Line each baking sheet with another sheet of parchment paper and lightly oil the paper. Repeat steps 4 and 5 with the remaining batter. Slide the parchment paper, with the crêpes in place, off the pans.

7. *Sautéed Bananas:* Cut bananas into $1/4$-inch (0.5 cm) thick slices. In a large skillet, heat ghee over medium-high heat, swirling to coat bottom of pan. Add bananas and cook for 3 minutes or just until edges are browned. Turn and cook until bananas are lightly browned on bottoms. Remove from heat and drizzle with vanilla.

8. To serve, peel crêpes off paper. Fold each crêpe in half around some of the banana filling. Serve immediately.

Health Tip

Bananas are, of course, sweet but they are also cold. They will clear heat and moisten dry conditions. If you are suffering from constipation or a dry throat, they can be useful. However, if you suffer from a cold with lots of phlegm or any type of stomach ulcer or other digestive inflammation, you may choose to skip the bananas and substitute pears instead.

Scatter-the-Cold Congee

There are infinite variations on congee that can satisfy and support health and healing. The souplike consistency of this dish makes it easy to digest. Here, the addition of green onions and ginger enlivens the taste and is perfect when you are feeling achy due to an oncoming cold. Make this congee and then get under the covers; you might break a sweat.

1 cup	sweet (glutinous) brown rice (or brown Arborio rice)	250 mL
4	green onions, finely chopped	4
3 tbsp	minced gingerroot	45 mL

MAKES 4 SERVINGS

Tip

Enjoy this congee once a day, like soup with a meal. It makes a savory, satisfying breakfast.

Variations

Substitute an equal amount of millet, barley or sweet (glutinous) white rice for the brown rice.

Health Tip

When you're sick, you can use herbal tea or vegetable broth in place of some or all of the water to cook the rice. Cooking the congee with an herbal tea or broth infuses the dish with healing ingredients, making it truly tasty medicine.

1. In a large saucepan, bring 8 cups (2 L) water to a boil. Add rice and return to a boil. Reduce heat to low, cover and simmer, stirring occasionally, for 2 hours. The congee should have a souplike consistency; if there is not enough liquid left in the pan, add up to $1/2$ cup (125 mL) water.

2. Stir in green onions and ginger; simmer for 10 minutes, then stir well.

3. Serve immediately or transfer to an airtight container and refrigerate for up to 3 days. Warm in a small saucepan over low heat before serving.

Condiments for Congee

If you are well and simply want to make congee, in place of the green onions and ginger, you can stir one or more of the following condiments into your congee for a change of pace:

- Braised, sautéed, roasted, boiled or pickled vegetables
- Eggs cooked sunny side up, scrambled or hard-cooked
- Toasted nuts or seeds
- Chopped pungent herbs, such as parsley or basil

See Condiment Recipes (pages 422 to 465) for more delicious ideas.

Goji and Lily Bulb Beneficial Congee

This nourishing and soothing congee offers support to the immune and respiratory systems as we move indoors in autumn. The sweetness of the rice mixes with the sweet, slightly starchy and bitter lily bulb and goji berries for an harmonious combination.

MAKES 4 SERVINGS

Tip

Use sulfite-free lily bulbs; see Resources (page 466) for sources.

½ cup	sweet (glutinous) brown rice (or brown Arborio rice)	125 mL
½ cup	dried lily bulbs, rinsed	125 mL
½ cup	dried goji berries	125 mL
Pinch	salt	Pinch
½ cup	chopped toasted almonds	125 mL
4 tsp	liquid honey (optional)	20 mL

1. In a medium saucepan, combine 5 cups (1.25 L) water and rice and bring to a boil. Reduce heat to low, cover and simmer for 1 hour.

2. Stir in lily bulbs. Cover and simmer for 1 hour. Stir in goji berries and salt. The congee should have a souplike consistency; if there is not enough liquid left in the pan, add water as needed. Cover and let cool for 10 minutes.

3. Serve immediately or transfer to an airtight container and refrigerate for up to 3 days. Warm in a small saucepan over low heat before serving.

4. To serve, spoon congee into serving bowls. Sprinkle with almonds and drizzle with honey (if using).

Health Tips

The combination of lily bulb, honey and almonds, along with the soupy consistency of congee, makes this an excellent dish for anyone with a tendency toward a dry cough or other lung issues that arise in autumn.

Lily bulbs are beneficial to the lungs and heart and are often used to calm the mind.

Goji berries are one of Chinese medicine's longevity foods, supporting the *jing* (the essence and foundation of *qi*) and the immune system; they have been used for millennia to promote good vision.

Hato Mugi and Cinnamon Twig Congee

Here, hato mugi (Job's tears) enhances the earthy quality of the rice. The cinnamon twig adds a nice sweetness without the spiciness of ground cinnamon. Together, they create a lovely sweet congee that makes a warming immune-supportive breakfast.

MAKES 4 SERVINGS

Tip

To toast pecans, place them in a medium skillet. Toast over low heat, stirring or shaking pan frequently, for 5 to 7 minutes or until fragrant.

¼ cup	sweet (glutinous) brown rice (or brown Arborio rice)	60 mL
¼ cup	hato mugi (Job's tears)	60 mL
¼ cup	sliced cinnamon twig	60 mL
½ cup	chopped pitted dates	125 mL
Pinch	salt	Pinch
½ cup	chopped toasted pecans	125 mL

1. In a medium bowl, combine rice and hato mugi. Pour in enough water to cover. Set aside.

2. In a medium saucepan, bring 5 cups (1.25 L) water to a boil. Turn heat off but leave pan on burner. Add cinnamon twig, cover and let stand for 2 hours.

3. Strain cinnamon twig mixture through fine-mesh sieve into a medium bowl. Discard solids. Return tea to pan. Drain rice mixture, discarding soaking water, and add to tea. Bring to a simmer over medium-high heat. Reduce heat, cover and simmer for 2 hours.

4. Stir in dates and salt. The congee should have a souplike consistency; if there is not enough liquid left in the pan, add water as needed. Cover and let cool for 10 minutes.

5. Serve immediately or transfer to an airtight container and refrigerate for up to 3 days. Warm in a small saucepan over low heat before serving.

6. To serve, spoon congee into serving bowls. Sprinkle with pecans.

Health Tip

Decocting the cinnamon twig tea separately extracts the full benefits of this herb. Cinnamon twig is the foundation of the Chinese herbal tea *gui zhi tang*, which is used to combat the onset of a cold. Cinnamon twig is warming, sweet and pungent, and it benefits the extremities.

Essential Seed and Nut Porridge with Almonds

Autumn's nut and seed porridge combination supports and moistens the lungs with the addition of the venerable almond. Make this ahead of time for a quick and nutritious breakfast — it's even tastier with the addition of fruit or vegetables (see next page).

MAKES 4 SERVINGS

Tip

Check the package to make sure the plantain chips are cooked in a healthy oil and don't contain added sugar.

Health Tips

This combination of nuts and seeds ensures this porridge is packed with omega-3 fatty acids, which are essential for the immune and nervous systems. The nuts and seeds have an anti-inflammatory effect on the body.

Almonds and Brazil nuts are beneficial to the lungs, so this is a perfect dish to eat if you have a cough.

- **Blender**

2 cups	boiling water	500 mL

Porridge Mix

3 tbsp	flax seeds	45 mL
3 tbsp	shelled raw pumpkin seeds (pepitas)	45 mL
2 tbsp	chia seeds	30 mL
½ cup	sliced almonds	125 mL
½ cup	Brazil nuts	125 mL
1 cup	unsweetened roasted plantain chips	250 mL
½ tsp	salt	2 mL

1. *Porridge Mix:* In a large dry skillet, toast flax, pumpkin and chia seeds over medium-low heat, stirring often, for 5 minutes or until fragrant. Transfer to a heatproof plate and spread out; let cool completely.

2. Add almonds and Brazil nuts to pan. Toast over medium-low heat, stirring often, for 8 to 10 minutes or until fragrant. Transfer to a separate heatproof plate and spread out; let cool completely.

3. In blender, combine seed mixture and plantain chips and grind until the texture of brown sugar. Add nut mixture and salt and grind to the texture of brown sugar. (Porridge mix can be made up to this point and refrigerated in an airtight container for up to 2 weeks.)

4. In a medium bowl, stir porridge mix with boiling water. Cover and let stand for 5 minutes.

5. Spoon porridge into serving bowls. Serve immediately.

Essential Seed and Nut Porridge with Spiced Pears and Toasted Almonds

Pears are the go-to fruit for a wet cough with congestion. They are sweet and sour, soothing and slightly cooling — and they taste delightful. Adding ginger brings out the slightly spicy, floral flavor of the pears.

> **MAKES 4 SERVINGS**

Tip

To toast sliced almonds, place them in a medium dry skillet. Toast over low heat, stirring or shaking pan often, for 3 to 5 minutes or until fragrant.

1	batch Essential Seed and Nut Porridge with Almonds (previous page)	1
2	large firm ripe pears (preferably Bartlett or Williams)	2
1 tbsp	ghee	15 mL
1 tbsp	freshly squeezed lemon juice	15 mL
1 tbsp	liquid honey	15 mL
½ tsp	ground cinnamon	2 mL
¼ tsp	ground ginger	1 mL
½ cup	sliced almonds, toasted	125 mL

1. Make porridge according to instructions (previous page). Keep warm.

2. Meanwhile, peel, quarter and core pears. Cut into ¼-inch (0.5 cm) thick slices.

3. In a large skillet, heat ghee over medium-high heat. Add pears and cook, stirring, for 2 to 3 minutes or until almost tender. Stir in lemon juice, honey, cinnamon and ginger.

4. Spoon porridge into serving bowls. Top with pear mixture and almonds. Serve immediately.

> ### Health Tips
>
> If you are battling a dry cough and have heat symptoms, omit the ground ginger, as it is too warming and drying.
>
> Pears are the perfect fruit for a cough. They are cooling and help clear out phlegm. The addition of ginger and cinnamon helps balance the cooling nature of the fruit.
>
> Honey is a lubricating and especially helpful addition to this porridge if you have a dry cough.

Mushroom Immune Broth

Mushrooms are known for their immune-boosting potency and deep umami flavor. Enjoy this deeply satisfying broth on its own as a booster, or use it as the base for other dishes.

Variation

For a different taste and effect, substitute oyster mushrooms for the button mushrooms. They taste much like maitake mushrooms but they're much less expensive! Oyster mushrooms are sweet and slightly warm. Taken with hato mugi (you can add 1/3 oz/10 g to this soup), they drain away dampness and are said to help with painful joints.

Health Tip

Drink this broth weekly during times when you feel your immune system is under stress, such as during cold and flu or allergy season.

- **1-quart (1 L) canning jar**

1/2 cup	dried shiitake mushrooms (4 to 6)	125 mL
	Warm water	
1	leek	1
1	carrot	1
8 oz	button or cremini mushrooms, trimmed	250 g
1 tbsp	avocado oil	15 mL
1 tsp	grated gingerroot	5 mL
1 tsp	salt, or to taste	5 mL

1. Place shiitake mushrooms in jar. Pour in enough warm water to fill. Seal with lid and let stand, shaking once or twice, for at least 8 hours or up to 24 hours.

2. Using a slotted spoon, transfer shiitake mushrooms to a medium bowl (try to avoid swirling soaking liquid). Using kitchen scissors, trim off and discard stems and cut shiitake caps into 1/8-inch (3 mm) thick slices. Slowly pour soaking liquid from jar into a small bowl, discarding the last 1/2 cup (125 mL) or so of liquid with its sediment. Set aside.

3. Trim roots and dark green leaves off leek and discard. Cut leek into 2-inch (5 cm) long pieces, then thinly slice pieces lengthwise. Rinse very well in 2 changes of water to remove grit. Drain well. Peel carrot and cut into matchsticks. Cut button mushrooms into 1/8-inch (3 mm) thick slices.

4. In a medium saucepan, heat oil over medium-high heat. Add shiitake caps, leek, carrot, button mushrooms, ginger and salt; cook, stirring, until leeks are browned and limp, about 10 minutes.

5. Stir in reserved mushroom soaking liquid and bring to a simmer over medium heat, skimming off any foam. Reduce heat to low, cover and simmer for 30 minutes or until leek and carrot are very tender. Taste and season to taste with more salt, if desired.

6. Strain broth through a fine-mesh sieve into a large bowl. Discard solids. Use immediately or transfer to airtight containers, let cool and refrigerate for up to 5 days.

Creamed Cauliflower Soup with Aromatic Chive Condiment

There is nothing like a puréed soup for providing comfort and ease. Cauliflower has a subtle but distinct flavor and a rich texture, making this soup a satisfying light meal. The Aromatic Chive Condiment draws out the cauliflower's subtlety.

**MAKES
4 TO 6 SERVINGS**

Variation

For a richer texture, add a chopped parsnip or carrot to the pot along with the cauliflower.

- **Blender, food processor or immersion blender**

1 tbsp	avocado oil or olive oil	15 mL
1	medium to large onion, coarsely chopped	1
4 cups	water or reduced-sodium vegetable broth, divided	1 L
1	medium to large head cauliflower, cut into small pieces	1
	Salt and freshly ground black pepper	
¼ cup	Aromatic Chive Condiment (see recipe, opposite)	60 mL

1. In a large saucepan, heat oil over medium heat. Add onion and cook, stirring, for 5 to 7 minutes or until starting to soften. Add enough of the water to cover by 1 to 2 inches (2.5 to 5 cm) and bring to a boil. Reduce heat and simmer, stirring occasionally, for 10 minutes or until onion is soft.

2. Stir in cauliflower and remaining water and return to a simmer. Simmer for 10 to 15 minutes or until cauliflower is soft.

3. Working in batches if necessary, transfer soup to blender (or use immersion blender in the pan) and blend until very creamy. Return soup to pan (if necessary) and season to taste with salt and pepper.

4. Ladle soup into serving bowls. Serve immediately, sprinkled with Aromatic Chive Condiment.

> ## Health Tip
>
> Cauliflower is considered neutral to cooling, and clears stomach and lung heat. The nutmeg, chives and miso in the condiment support digestion and serve to warm the middle *jiao*, or digestive network. This soup is good for anyone who has a poor appetite or cough and needs a soothing soup that is easy to digest.

Aromatic Chive Condiment

Delicious with the soup on the opposite page, this digestion-supporting condiment is also a peppy complement to simply prepared mild vegetables.

MAKES ABOUT ¼ CUP (60 ML)

Tips

To toast sesame seeds, place them in a medium skillet. Toast over low heat, stirring or shaking pan often, for 3 to 5 minutes or until fragrant.

To dry chives, preheat oven to 300°F (150°C). Wash 1 bunch fresh chives and dry well, rolling in a paper towel and squeezing to absorb moisture. Mince chives and spread on a sheet of parchment paper. Place on a rimmed baking sheet and bake in preheated oven for 20 to 30 minutes or until leathery. Let cool on pan; chives should be crisp and lightly browned. Freeze any leftover dried chives in an airtight container for up to 2 months.

- Preheat oven to 200°F (100°C)
- Rimmed baking sheet, lined with parchment paper
- Large mortar and pestle, or food processor

2 tbsp	white miso (or ½ tsp/2 mL salt)	30 mL
2 tbsp	sesame seeds (preferably black), toasted	30 mL
1 tbsp	dried chives (see tips, at left)	15 mL
¼ tsp	ground nutmeg	1 mL
½ tsp	toasted sesame oil	2 mL

1. Spread miso in a very thin layer on prepared pan. Bake in preheated oven for 10 to 15 minutes or until leathery. Let cool completely on pan.

2. Peel dried miso from paper and place in mortar. Add sesame seeds, chives and nutmeg. Using pestle, grind until a coarse powder forms.

3. Transfer powder to a small bowl. Stir in oil until well combined. Serve immediately.

Health Tip

Chives are warming and pungent. They are beneficial if you often feel cold. This herb benefits the yang and the kidneys.

Boost-the-Qi Chicken Soup

This classic tonic chicken soup is chock-full of pleasant and neutral-tasting herbs. The marriage of chicken stock, herbs and vegetables will make this a favorite in your home.

> **MAKES
> 4 TO 6 SERVINGS**

Tips

The amount of garlic, ginger and salt can be adjusted to your taste; the amounts in the ingredient list will give the soup a mild flavor.

All of the herbal ingredients are edible except for the astragalus, which is too fibrous and should be removed before serving.

If you want to freeze the soup, first strain out all the solids, leaving a simple tonic chicken broth. Ladle individual portions into airtight containers and freeze for up to 3 months.

Buy your herbs from a Chinese herb supplier. See Resources, page 466.

2 lbs	bone-in chicken pieces, skinned	1 kg
6	thin slices gingerroot, lightly crushed	6
2	cloves garlic, lightly smashed	2
1 tsp	salt	5 mL
⅔ oz	dried goji berries	20 g
⅔ oz	dried longan fruit	20 g
½ oz	dried astragalus root	15 g
½ oz	dried codonopsis	15 g
½ oz	dried Chinese yam (dioscorea)	15 g
½ oz	dried lotus seeds	15 g
½ oz	dried Solomon's seal	15 g
½ oz	hato mugi (Job's tears)	15 g
½ oz	dried wood ear mushrooms (black fungus)	15 g
1 cup	dried shiitake mushrooms	250 mL
1	piece (1 inch/2.5 cm square) dried kombu	1
2 cups	mixed chopped seasonal vegetables (see box, opposite)	500 mL
1 tbsp	tamari or soy sauce	15 mL
1 tsp	sesame oil	5 mL
1 tsp	rice wine, such as sake (or mild vinegar)	5 mL

1. Place chicken in a large saucepan. Pour in enough water to cover by 2 to 3 inches (5 to 7.5 cm). Bring to a boil, skimming off any foam.

2. Add ginger, garlic, salt, goji berries, longan fruit, astragalus, codonopsis, Chinese yam, lotus seeds, Solomon's seal, hato mugi, wood ears, shiitakes and kombu; return to a gentle boil. Reduce heat to low, cover and simmer for 50 to 60 minutes or until chicken breasts are no longer pink inside and/or juices run clear when chicken legs or thighs are pierced.

Variations

For a vegetarian version, omit chicken. Use 1 package (1 to 1½ lbs/500 to 750 g) firm or extra-firm tofu, drained and cut into small cubes, for the chicken. Add tofu in Step 3 and simmer 5 to 10 minutes before serving.

For a pescetarian version, substitute 1 to 2 lbs (500 g to 1 kg) boneless skinless fish fillets, such as salmon, trout, arctic char or black cod, cut into 1- to 2-inch (2.5 to 5 cm) pieces, for the chicken. Simmer for 5 to 10 minutes.

You can also substitute an equal weight of fish heads and bones for the chicken. Simply simmer the fish heads and bones, in enough water to cover, for 2 to 3 hours over low heat. Strain broth through a fine-mesh sieve and return to the pan. Add the herbs and vegetables and cook as directed.

3. Stir in mixed vegetables, tamari, sesame oil and rice wine. Simmer for 15 to 20 minutes or until softened. Remove from heat and discard astragalus.

4. Ladle into serving bowls. Serve immediately.

Health Tip

There are three types of tonic herbs in this soup: *qi*, blood and yin. The astragalus, codonopsis (known as poor man's ginseng) and Chinese yam (dioscorea) support digestion, help transform food to *qi* and enhance vitality. Goji berries and dried longan fruit are blood tonics; they support sleep and are used to nourish the eyes and the essence. Lotus seeds nourish the heart and lungs. Hato mugi supports the spleen and drains away dampness, which accumulates in the body when the spleen's *qi* and yang are insufficient. This can cause digestive disturbances, difficulty losing weight and lethargy. The wood ear mushrooms and Solomon's seal nourish the yin and help moisten lung tissue.

Seasonal Vegetable Options

- For a warming effect, include sliced green onions, chopped onions and/or chopped seeded winter squash.

- For a more neutral effect, include 2 carrots, chopped; 1 stalk celery, chopped; 1 chayote, chopped; mixed leafy greens, such as Swiss chard, spinach, kale or napa cabbage; and/or trimmed snow peas.

Spinach and Egg Drop Soup

Soup is the wonder comfort food: modest, harmonious in flavor and a type of medicine unto itself. This silky soup is a simple pleasure; it's easy to prepare and an antidote to autumn dryness.

Health Tips

Spinach is cooling and lubricating, so it will help anyone who experiences an overwhelming feeling of dryness. Spinach also enriches the yin and blood, so it is a wonderful vegetable for vegetarians.

Eggs supplement *qi* and blood while nourishing the body's yin. If you are recovering from a cold, this soup will boost your *qi*.

1 tbsp	avocado oil	15 mL
2	green onions, cut into 1-inch (2.5 cm) pieces	2
½ cup	cherry tomatoes, cut in half	125 mL
½ cup	rice wine, such as sake	125 mL
8 oz	spinach, trimmed	250 g
3 tbsp	tamari or soy sauce	45 mL
2	large eggs, beaten	2

1. In a large saucepan, heat oil over medium heat. Add green onions and cook, stirring, for about 1 minute or until fragrant. Add cherry tomatoes and rice wine; cook for 3 minutes.

2. Stir in 4 cups (1 L) water and bring to a boil. Reduce heat, stir in spinach and tamari and simmer for 3 to 5 minutes or until spinach is wilted.

3. Turn off heat. Gently drizzle eggs around the edge of the pan into soup, stirring once or twice until egg is just cooked.

4. Ladle into serving bowls. Serve immediately.

Pork Lion's Head Soup with Bok Choy

In this simple, nourishing, almost-classic version of lion's head soup, the sweet potatoes add tenderness and flavor to the mild and slightly salty pork.

MAKES 4 SERVINGS

Tip

Asian sweet potatoes are milder in flavor and a little firmer when cooked than Western-style ones are.

1 lb	bok choy	500 g
4	green onions, minced	4
1 cup	coarsely grated peeled Asian or Western-style orange sweet potatoes	250 mL
1 lb	ground pork	500 g
1	large egg, beaten	1
1½ tsp	salt, divided	7 mL

1. Cut leaves off bok choy and then cut into shreds. Mince enough of the stems to make ½ cup (125 mL). Cut remaining stems crosswise into thin slices. Set aside.

2. In a medium bowl, combine minced bok choy stems, green onions, sweet potatoes, pork, egg and ½ tsp (2 mL) of the salt. Shape into 16 meatballs. Place in an airtight container and refrigerate for at least 2 hours or for up to 24 hours.

3. In a medium saucepan, bring 4 cups (1 L) water to a simmer over medium-high heat. Add meatballs and remaining salt. Reduce heat and simmer, stirring gently once or twice, for 10 minutes. Add reserved bok choy stems and leaves; cook until bok choy leaves are wilted and meatballs are no longer pink inside, about 5 minutes.

4. Ladle into serving bowls. Serve immediately.

Health Tips

This is an ideal soup for people who have a difficult time keeping their weight up. The pork nourishes the yin and blood. It is especially good for women who suffer from very light menstrual periods. The yin-nourishing aspect of pork is also good for people who suffer from dry skin or a dry throat. If you are obese or overweight, consuming large amounts of pork is contraindicated.

Bok choy moderates the effect of the pork by cooling and detoxifying the body.

Brothy Sweet Potato Noodles with Asian Vegetables

The beauty of this dish is its simplicity. The ingredients complement one another in a very harmonious way, allowing the down-to-earth flavors to shine and bestowing a feeling of calm.

MAKES 4 SERVINGS

Tip

If you are sensitive to sulfites, check the packaging on the lily bulbs. For sulfite-free ingredients, try Gold Mine Natural Food Co. at www.goldminenaturalfoods.com.

Variation

If baby bok choy is not available, substitute 4 cups (1 L) coarsely chopped tender greens, such as napa cabbage, tatsoi, choy sum, mustard greens or shepherd's purse. These greens have a slightly pungent flavor that complements the other ingredients.

¼ cup	dried lily bulbs	60 mL
8 oz	dried sweet potato noodles (see page 180)	250 g
1 tbsp	toasted sesame oil	15 mL
4 cups	Pork Broth with Ginger (page 418) or Mushroom Immune Broth (page 329)	1 L
4	baby bok choy, quartered	4
¼ cup	tamari or soy sauce	60 mL
¼ cup	black sesame seeds, toasted (see tip, page 445)	60 mL
4	green onions, minced	4

1. Place lily bulbs in a medium bowl and pour in enough water to cover. Let stand for 30 minutes. Drain and set aside.

2. In a large saucepan, bring 8 cups (2 L) water to a boil. Add noodles and cook, stirring once or twice, for 10 minutes or until completely limp. Drain and return to pan. Stir in sesame oil.

3. Meanwhile, in a medium saucepan, bring broth to a simmer over medium-high heat. Add lily bulbs and bok choy; simmer for 5 minutes or until bok choy is tender.

4. Divide noodles among serving bowls. Add 1 tbsp (15 mL) of the tamari to each. Divide bok choy, lily bulbs and broth evenly among bowls. Sprinkle with sesame seeds and green onions. Serve immediately.

> ### Health Tip
>
> Don't omit the lily bulbs; they have an earthy flavor and fragrance that helps calm the mind and nourish the lung yin.

Steamed Egg Custard with Mushrooms and Green Onions

This delectable savory steamed egg custard is a perfect small, light main dish. It's especially good if you are feeling tired and just need a simple meal. Serve it with sautéed or steamed greens.

Tips

Be careful not to steam the custard for too long, or it will dry out.

If your pot is too small to hold all of the ramekins at once, steam the custards in batches.

Rubber-tipped tongs are great for transferring the ramekins to the steamer pot. If you don't have them, you can wrap thick rubber bands around the tips of regular metal tongs.

Health Tip

Eggs are revitalizing, because they nourish both yin and yang. Mushrooms add sweetness, and green onion has a pungent, warming nature. Are you feeling weak after a cold, without much appetite? This dish will be easy to digest and will help you recover your energy.

- **Six ¹⁄₂- to ³⁄₄-cup (125 to 175 mL) ramekins or custard cups**
- **Large pot with steamer rack (about 1 inch/ 2.5 cm above bottom of pot)**

1 tbsp	avocado oil	15 mL
1 cup	sliced mushrooms, such as button, cremini or stemmed shiitake	250 mL
1¼ tsp	salt, divided	6 mL
1	green onion, thinly sliced	1
4	large eggs, beaten	4
3 cups	Traditional or Vegetarian Dashi (page 297), at room temperature	750 mL
1 tbsp	tamari or soy sauce	15 mL

1. In a small skillet, heat oil over medium heat. Add mushrooms and cook, stirring, for 8 to 10 minutes or until mushroom liquid is almost evaporated and mushrooms are fairly dry. Sprinkle with ¼ tsp (1 mL) of the salt and divide among ramekins. Top with green onion.

2. In a 4-cup (1 L) glass measuring cup, whisk together eggs, dashi, tamari and remaining salt. Strain and gently pour into ramekins.

3. Pour enough water into pot to come scant 1 inch (2.5 cm) up side. Place steamer rack in pan over water. Bring to a boil.

4. Arrange ramekins on rack, cover tightly and steam for 15 to 20 minutes or until custard is barely set in the center (it will be jiggly but not liquid).

5. Serve warm or at room temperature. Or cover and refrigerate for up to 3 days; let come to room temperature for an hour before serving.

Salmon on Ginger-Braised Kale with Toasted Pine Nuts

In this simply cooked dish, the richly flavored salmon sits atop freshly braised greens with a hint of ginger. Try it with fresh salmon from either the Pacific Northwest or the Atlantic.

MAKES 4 SERVINGS		

Tips

If flat-leaf kale is not available, use another sturdy green, such as collard greens.

To toast pine nuts, spread them in a shallow metal baking pan and bake in a preheated 350°F (180°C) oven, stirring once, for 5 to 7 minutes or until fragrant.

The salmon can be seasoned and refrigerated for up to 24 hours before cooking.

Health Tip

Salmon is slightly warming, unlike many other varieties of seafood. It has a sweet, slightly salty flavor and is rich in essential fatty acids necessary for nervous system and brain function. This dish will nourish *qi* and blood, and warm you up if you feel cold. The ginger mellows the fish flavor and supports the stomach.

- **Mortar and pestle, or spice grinder**

2 tsp	Sichuan peppercorns, shiny black seeds removed (see tip, page 219)	10 mL
1½ tsp	salt, divided	7 mL
2 tbsp	coconut sugar	30 mL
1 lb	boneless skinless salmon fillet, cut into 4 pieces	500 g
2 tbsp	avocado oil, divided	30 mL
1	large bunch flat-leaf kale (preferably lacinato or Tuscan), stemmed and coarsely shredded	1
1 tbsp	grated gingerroot	15 mL
¼ cup	pine nuts, toasted (see tips, at left)	60 mL

1. In mortar with pestle, grind Sichuan peppercorns with 1 tsp (5 mL) of the salt. Stir in coconut sugar. Press all over salmon to adhere. Set aside.

2. In a medium saucepan, heat 1 tbsp (15 mL) of the oil over medium-high heat. Add ½ cup (125 mL) water, kale and ginger. Cover and bring to a boil. Boil for 3 to 4 minutes. Stir, cover again and boil for 3 to 5 minutes or until kale is very tender. Stir in remaining salt.

3. Meanwhile, in a large skillet, heat remaining oil over medium-high heat. Add salmon and cook for 3 to 5 minutes or until deep brown on bottom. Turn and cook for 3 to 5 minutes or until fish is opaque.

4. Divide kale among serving plates and top with salmon. Sprinkle with pine nuts. Serve immediately.

Chicken and Chestnut Fried Rice

Chestnuts have long been a part of culinary traditions around the world. They have been used in Chinese cuisine since Neolithic times and are also a popular food in Europe. They have a sweet and nutty flavor that complements the sweetness of the chicken. This dish is nice any time of day, for breakfast, lunch or dinner!

**MAKES
4 TO 6 SERVINGS**

Tip

To cook chestnuts, using a sharp knife, cut an X in the back of each. In a medium saucepan, combine 4 cups (1 L) water and chestnuts and bring to a boil. Boil for 20 minutes or until tender. Drain and let cool enough to handle. Peel off outer peel and inner skin. Refrigerate for up to 2 days.

Health Tip

If you tend to feel cold or are feeling run-down, the hardy chestnut will warm and invigorate you — it is an excellent remedy for autumn and winter weather. Its sweetness is nourishing. It has a slight astringent action, so it can help stop diarrhea and has been used medicinally to improve circulation and stanch bleeding. Its warming nature encourages circulation of *qi* and blood. Be moderate in your chestnut intake; too many can cause stagnation, bloating and indigestion.

1 cup	red cargo rice or brown basmati rice	250 mL
¼ cup	avocado oil, divided	60 mL
8 oz	boneless skinless chicken thighs, cut into ¾-inch (2 cm) pieces	250 g
1 cup	finely shredded trimmed kale leaves	250 mL
2 tbsp	tamari or soy sauce	30 mL
8 oz	cooked peeled chestnuts (see tip, at left)	250 g
2 tbsp	thinly sliced green onion	30 mL

1. In a medium saucepan, combine $2\frac{1}{2}$ cups (625 mL) water and rice. Bring to a boil over high heat. Reduce heat to low, cover with a tight-fitting lid and simmer for 30 to 40 minutes or until almost tender. Turn off heat and let pan stand, covered, on burner for 15 minutes. Transfer rice to a flat container and let cool completely. Cover and refrigerate for at least 2 hours.

2. In a large skillet, heat 2 tbsp (30 mL) of the oil over medium-high heat. Add chicken and kale; cook, stirring, for 3 to 4 minutes or until juices run clear when chicken is pierced. Transfer chicken mixture to a bowl and stir in tamari.

3. In the same skillet, heat remaining oil over medium-high heat. Using a spatula, spread rice in skillet to cover bottom of pan. Cook, without stirring, for 1 minute or until bottom is lightly browned. Turn rice and cook for 1 minute or until lightly browned. (Avoid stirring the rice, as that will make it gummy.)

4. Return chicken mixture to pan and gently stir in chestnuts. Remove from heat and sprinkle with green onion.

5. Spoon into serving bowls. Serve immediately.

Braised Beef Brisket with Shiitakes

This hearty dish is a homey reminder of Ellen's grandma's brisket, which was served on cold nights. Using a classic mirepoix (a mixture of carrots, celery and onion) along with the mushrooms and chayote adds great depth of flavor.

**MAKES
6 TO 8 SERVINGS**

Tip

The meat will be easier to slice and will taste best if you make it at least a day ahead of time. Trim the fat off the cooked brisket and refrigerate meat separately from the vegetables and cooking liquid. When they are cold, skim the fat off the cooking liquid and slice meat. To reheat, place beef slices, vegetables and cooking liquid in a large skillet and warm over medium heat, shaking pan once or twice (but not stirring) until steaming.

- **1-quart (1 L) canning jar**
- **Large heavy ovenproof saucepan**

1 cup	dried shiitake mushrooms (8 to 12)	250 mL
	Warm water	
2 tbsp	avocado oil	30 mL
1	piece beef brisket (flat or point), 3 to 4 lbs/1.5 to 2 kg	1
2	carrots, minced	2
2	stalks celery, minced	2
1	large onion, minced	1
1 cup	rice wine, such as sake	250 mL
2 tbsp	unseasoned rice vinegar	30 mL
2	chayotes, peeled, seeded and cut into 1/4-inch (0.5 cm) thick slices	2
1/2 cup	tamari or soy sauce	125 mL
1/4 cup	minced fresh chives	60 mL

1. Place shiitake mushrooms in jar. Pour in enough warm water to fill. Seal with lid and let stand, shaking once or twice, for at least 8 hours or up to 24 hours.

2. Preheat oven to 300°F (150°C).

3. Using a slotted spoon, transfer shiitake mushrooms to a medium bowl (try to avoid swirling soaking liquid). Using kitchen scissors, trim off and discard stems and cut shiitake caps into quarters. Slowly pour soaking liquid from jar into a small bowl, discarding the last 1/2 cup (125 mL) or so of liquid with its sediment. Set aside.

4. Heat ovenproof saucepan over medium-high heat until a drop of water sizzles. Add oil and swirl to coat bottom of pan. Place brisket in pan and cook, turning once, for 2 minutes per side or until browned all over. Transfer to a plate.

5. Add carrots, celery and onion to pan. Cook, stirring often, for 5 minutes or until lightly browned.

6. Return brisket and any accumulated juices to pan. Add mushrooms, reserved soaking liquid, rice wine and vinegar; bring to a simmer. Cover with a tight-fitting lid or seal with foil. Transfer to preheated oven and bake for 2 hours.

7. Turn brisket in pan and add chayotes and tamari. Cover and bake, adding a little water if necessary to prevent scorching, for 1 to 2 more hours or until beef is very tender.

8. Transfer brisket to a cutting board. Skim fat off cooking liquid. Trimming off and discarding fat, cut brisket across the grain into slices.

9. Arrange in serving bowls. Top with cooking liquid and mushrooms. Sprinkle with chives. Serve immediately.

> ### Health Tips
>
> Beef is neutral to warming in its thermal nature. Cooked here with carrots and onions, it strengthens the spleen, *qi* and blood.
>
> Chayote is neutral in nature, mild in taste and soothing to the respiratory tract. In this recipe, the chayote moderates the warming effect of the beef.

Arame Sauté with Carrots and Broccoli

Introduce yourself to the wonders of seaweed with the mild flavor of arame, a type of kelp. This multi-textured, mineral-rich dish makes a marvelous side with dinner.

MAKES 4 SERVINGS

Tips

To julienne carrots and ginger, cut into ⅛-inch (3 mm) thick slices, and then cut slices into ⅛-inch (3 mm) wide strips.

To toast pine nuts, spread them in a shallow metal baking pan and bake in a preheated 350°F (180°C) oven, stirring once, for 5 to 7 minutes or until fragrant.

1 oz	dried arame	30 g
2 tbsp	avocado oil	30 mL
4	carrots, julienned (see tips, at left)	4
1 tbsp	julienned gingerroot	15 mL
½ tsp	salt	2 mL
½	bunch broccoli (about 12 oz/375 g), cut into thin florets	½
2	green onions, finely chopped	2
2 tbsp	pine nuts, toasted (see tips, at left)	30 mL

1. Rinse arame. Place in a small bowl and pour in enough water to cover. Let stand for 5 minutes. Drain and cut into thin strips if necessary (some dried arame comes already cut).

2. In a large skillet, heat oil over medium-high heat, swirling to coat bottom of pan. Add arame, carrots, ginger and salt; cook, stirring, for about 5 minutes or until carrots are just tender. Add broccoli and cook, stirring, for about 3 minutes or until bright green and just tender.

3. Spoon into serving dish. Top with green onions and pine nuts. Serve immediately.

Health Tip

Seaweed ought to be part of everyone's diet. This traditional food has been eaten by coastal peoples around the globe for millennia. Seaweeds are rich in a plethora of minerals. Thanks to their calcium and magnesium content, they are very beneficial for women who suffer from cramps if consumed just prior to the beginning of menstruation. In Chinese medicine, seaweeds are used to clear out excesses in the body and aid in detoxification. Their salty flavor acts on the body to moderate hardened areas and soften masses, such as noncancerous cysts. However, seaweeds should never be eaten in excess. Always check your seaweed sources to ensure they are high-quality. See Resources (page 466) for reliable sources.

Pan-Roasted Honey Carrots with Aromatic Spices

Nothing is more welcome in autumn than the arrival of sweet root vegetables that, when roasted, are bursting with flavor. This dish has a nice balance of sweetness from the carrots and honey, and a pungency and astringency from the seeds and shallots that is gently soothed by the yogurt.

MAKES 4 SERVINGS

Tip

For the mixed aromatic seeds, choose any two of the following: fennel seeds, coriander seeds, dill seeds or mustard seeds.

1 tbsp	avocado oil	15 mL
2 lbs	carrots (about 5 large), cut into 1-inch (2.5 cm) chunks	1 kg
2	shallots (or ½ red onion), thinly sliced lengthwise	2
2 tsp	mixed aromatic seeds (see tip, at left)	10 mL
1 tsp	minced turmeric root or gingerroot	5 mL
½ tsp	salt	2 mL
1 tbsp	liquid honey	15 mL
½ cup	plain sheep's or goat's milk yogurt	125 mL

1. In a medium skillet, heat oil over medium heat. Add carrots and cook, stirring, for 2 minutes. Add shallots, seeds, turmeric and salt; cook, stirring, for 5 to 7 minutes or until shallots are lightly browned.

2. Stir in ¼ cup (60 mL) water and honey; cover and cook for 5 minutes or just until carrots are tender. Uncover and cook, shaking pan often, until almost no liquid remains.

3. Spoon into a serving dish. Serve warm or at room temperature, drizzled with yogurt.

Health Tips

The seeds in this dish support digestive function, while the honey adds lubrication, supporting elimination.

Both sheep's milk and goat's milk yogurt are sweet and warming, and add beneficial bacteria to the gut, which boosts digestive and immune function. In Chinese medicine, they are noted to strengthen stomach function as well. Many people do not tolerate cow's milk, but if you do, you can use plain full-fat dairy yogurt instead.

Carrot Burdock Kinpira

This simple nourishing side dish is a great addition to an autumn menu. It is a common Japanese dish that Ellen learned years ago when studying macrobiotics. You may come to love its crunchy texture, and earthy, sweet flavor.

	MAKES 4 SERVINGS	

Tip

To retain their texture and flavor, don't overcook the carrots and burdock.

Variation

If you run hot, leave out the hot pepper flakes. You can substitute ginger juice; just grate 1 tbsp (15 mL) gingerroot and squeeze the juice into the dish. It will soothe the stomach and aid digestion.

2	large carrots	2
1	burdock root, 18 inches (45 cm) long (about 8 oz/250 g)	1
1 cup	Traditional or Vegetarian Dashi (page 297)	250 mL
¼ cup	rice wine, such as sake	60 mL
2 tbsp	tamari or soy sauce	30 mL
½ tsp	hot pepper flakes (optional)	2 mL
1 tbsp	avocado oil	15 mL

1. Peel carrots and burdock root, then cut into matchsticks. Set aside separately.

2. In a medium saucepan, combine burdock root, dashi, rice wine, tamari and hot pepper flakes (if using). Bring to a simmer over medium-high heat. Reduce heat to low, cover and simmer for 10 minutes.

3. Add carrots. Cover and simmer for 5 to 7 minutes or until burdock root and carrots are almost tender. Stir in oil. Increase heat to high and cook, uncovered and shaking pan often, for 1 to 2 minutes or until almost no liquid remains.

4. Spoon into a serving dish. Serve immediately.

Health Tip

Burdock root grows wild across North America and Europe. It has long been used therapeutically to support detoxification; adding ginger to a burdock dish will enhance the detoxifying powers of the root. Burdock can act as a gentle diuretic, reduce blood sugar and clear toxic heat (infection). It also has anti-inflammatory effects and is often included in skin salves. Burdock can be pickled or even steeped as a tea on its own.

Braised Fennel

Fennel is a sweet, slightly pungent vegetable with a refreshing hint of anise flavor. It is delicious on its own, added to soups or salads, or roasted with root vegetables. Braising fennel brings out its rich flavor. Once you discover this vegetable, we are sure you will love it.

MAKES 4 SERVINGS

Tip

This dish can be served at any temperature, so it makes a convenient side dish for company. It also makes a delicious lunch with toasted almonds or another source of protein.

1 tbsp	avocado oil	15 mL
1	large fennel bulb (12 oz/375 g), cored and cut lengthwise into ¼-inch (0.5 cm) thick slices	1
½ tsp	grated lemon zest	2 mL
1 tbsp	freshly squeezed lemon juice	15 mL
½ tsp	salt	2 mL
¼ tsp	dill seeds	1 mL

1. In a medium skillet, heat oil over medium-high heat. Add fennel and cook, stirring, for 2 to 3 minutes or until almost tender.

2. Stir in 2 cups (500 mL) water, lemon zest, lemon juice, salt and dill seeds. Cover and bring to a boil. Boil for 5 minutes. Uncover and cook, stirring often, for 4 to 6 minutes or until almost no liquid remains.

3. Spoon into a serving dish. Serve immediately or let cool to room temperature.

Health Tip

Dill seeds, much like fennel seeds, are used in Chinese medicine to ease abdominal pain, treat bloating, stimulate digestion and expel cold in the abdomen. Fennel bulb is warming; it is a yin and *qi* tonic. It is used to help stimulate lactation and menstruation. Fennel bulb is rich in the flavonoid quercetin, an antioxidant.

Black Soybeans and Kabocha with Walnuts

The contrast between the black soybeans and the orange squash is visually stunning, and it's reflected in the flavor contrast between the earthy beans and the sweet, creamy squash.

MAKES
MAKES **4 TO 6 SERVINGS**

Tip

Leftovers of this dish can be added to congee or served as a side dish with an egg for breakfast the next day.

Health Tip

Black soybeans are sweet, with a delicate flavor, thanks to the fat they contain. They nourish the kidney yin, move the blood, promote urination, improve lipid metabolism and build the blood and *qi*. Rich in isoflavones, black soybeans benefit women. Combining them with winter squash and walnuts makes for a perfectly balanced recipe that nourishes both yin and yang. The walnuts also contribute to the warming aspect of this dish.

- **1-quart (1 L) canning jar**

½ cup	dried black soybeans	125 mL
½	small kabocha or buttercup squash (1½ to 2 lbs/750 g to 1 kg)	½
1 cup	Traditional or Vegetarian Dashi (page 297)	250 mL
2 tbsp	tamari or soy sauce	30 mL
1 cup	walnut halves	250 mL
2 tbsp	avocado oil	30 mL

1. In jar, combine 2 cups (500 mL) water and soybeans. Cover and let stand for 8 to 12 hours. Drain well. Add 2 cups (500 mL) fresh water and drain well again.

2. In a large saucepan, combine 6 cups (1.5 L) water and soybeans. Bring to a boil. Reduce heat to low, cover and simmer, stirring once or twice and adding more water if necessary, for 2 hours or until very tender. Uncover and let cool for 30 minutes. Drain well.

3. Meanwhile, peel and seed squash and cut into 1-inch (2.5 cm) chunks. In a medium saucepan, combine squash, dashi and tamari; bring to a simmer over medium-high heat. Reduce heat to low, cover and simmer for 10 to 15 minutes or until squash is almost tender. Uncover, increase heat to high and cook, shaking pan often, for 1 or 2 minutes or until almost no liquid remains. Remove from heat.

4. In a large skillet over medium heat, combine walnuts and oil. Cook, stirring, for 3 to 4 minutes or until fragrant. Transfer nuts to a bowl.

5. Return skillet to medium heat. Add soybeans and squash and cook, stirring gently, for 2 to 4 minutes or until warmed through. Serve sprinkled with walnuts.

Roasted Winter Squash

Roasting winter squash brings out its full flavor, making it comforting, hearty and nourishing. This vegan dish is simply and wonderfully satisfying.

MAKES 4 SERVINGS

Tip

We have used kabocha or buttercup squash in this recipe, but feel free to substitute any of the winter squash varieties that are available in your region.

Variations

Sprinkle the squash with aromatic herbs and/or spices — such as rosemary, sage, thyme, nutmeg or cinnamon — when tossing it with the oil.

Serve the squash topped with toasted nuts for a mix of contrasting textures.

- **Preheat oven to 400°F (200°C)**
- **Rimmed baking sheet, lined with parchment paper**

1	small kabocha or buttercup squash (about 2 lbs/1 kg), see tip, at left	1
3 tbsp	avocado oil	45 mL
1 tbsp	toasted sesame oil	15 mL
½ cup	shelled raw pumpkin seeds (pepitas)	125 mL
1 tsp	coarse or sea salt	5 mL

1. Cut squash in half. Scoop out seeds and discard. Cut into 1-inch (2.5 cm) wide wedges.

2. In a large bowl, stir avocado oil with sesame oil. Add squash and toss gently to coat. Arrange squash wedges, on their sides, on prepared pan. Roast in preheated oven for 20 minutes.

3. Turn squash. Sprinkle pumpkin seeds over top. Bake for 15 minutes or until squash is very tender and browned.

4. Sprinkle squash wedges with salt. Spoon into a serving bowl. Serve warm or at room temperature.

Health Tip

Winter squash and pumpkin share many of the same therapeutic powers: they are both wholesome and sweet, and nourishing to the stomach and spleen, benefiting digestion. Winter squash is beneficial for anyone who has a sweet tooth — this hardy vegetable actually helps balance blood sugar levels.

Barberry and Winter Squash Pilaf

This is comfort food with a bright spot of flavor, thanks to the barberries and the fragrant rosemary. This is a variation on the beloved typical Iranian rice dish known as zereshk polow.

MAKES 4 SERVINGS

Tip

Barberries have a long culinary history in the Middle East, Europe and Russia. They often appear in jams (because of their high pectin levels), and meat and rice dishes.

- **Preheat oven to 350°F (180°C)**
- **Medium ovenproof saucepan with lid**

2 tbsp	ghee or avocado oil	30 mL
2 cups	diced seeded peeled winter squash, such as buttercup or butternut	500 mL
1 tsp	salt	5 mL
1 cup	long-grain brown rice or brown basmati rice	250 mL
½ tsp	finely crumbled dried rosemary	2 mL
½ cup	dried barberries	125 mL
½ cup	chopped toasted pistachios (see tips, page 284)	125 mL

1. In ovenproof saucepan, heat ghee over medium-high heat. Add squash and salt, and cook, stirring often, for 5 minutes. Add rice and rosemary; cook, stirring, for 2 minutes or until rice is coated and translucent. Add 2¼ cups (550 mL) water and bring to a simmer.

2. Cover and bake in preheated oven for 45 minutes. Remove from oven and stir in barberries. Cover and let stand for at least 15 minutes or for up to 1 hour.

3. Spoon into a serving dish. Sprinkle with pistachios. Serve immediately.

Health Tip

Barberries, also known by the Latin name *Berberis vulgaris*, are notable for their antibacterial and antimicrobial properties. These berries are used often in Western herbology to treat common colds and flu, as well as gastrointestinal disorders that feature inflammation and bacterial overgrowth. The tartness of the barberries stands out in this dish; it is nourishing and protective dish for autumn.

Roasted Beet Salad with Pickled Mustard Greens

The lightly fermented, pungent mustard greens contrast nicely with the sweet, earthy beets in this great digestive salad. Salted and pickled mustard greens are a typical, featured ingredient in many Chinese dishes that originated in Sichuan province.

MAKES 4 SERVINGS

Tip

To toast sunflower seeds, spread them in a shallow baking pan and bake in a preheated 350°F (180°C) oven, stirring once, for 5 to 7 minutes or until fragrant.

Health Tips

Sauerkraut and its juices kick off the fermentation of the pungent mustard greens, clearing heat and adding beneficial bacteria to your gut.

Beets are sweet and nourishing. They are recommended to help build the blood in cases of mild anemia. They benefit the liver, help move stagnant *qi* and support this organ's detoxification. Beets are also good for the blood and heart. In addition, they moisten and lubricate the large intestine, making them handy for treating constipation. Beets help promote menstruation, as well.

- **2-cup (500 mL) canning jar**
- **13- by 9-inch (33 by 23 cm) glass baking dish**

1 cup	packed finely shredded stemmed mustard greens	250 mL
½ tsp	kosher or non-iodized sea salt	2 mL
1 cup	unpasteurized sauerkraut (store-bought or homemade; see next page) with juice	250 mL
2 lbs	whole beets (unpeeled)	1 kg
½ cup	hulled sunflower seeds, toasted (see tip, at left)	125 mL

1. In jar, combine mustard greens and salt. Spoon sauerkraut and juice over top, without mixing. Press down firmly with the back of a spoon to compress greens. Cover and refrigerate for at least 4 hours or until greens are wilted, or for up to 24 hours.

2. Preheat oven to 350°F (180°C).

3. Place beets in baking dish and add ½ inch (1 cm) water. Cover with foil, crimping around the edges of the dish to seal. Bake for 1 hour or until beets are fork-tender. Uncover and let cool completely. Peel beets and cut into ¾-inch (2 cm) chunks.

4. Drain mustard greens and sauerkraut, discarding liquid. Transfer to a serving bowl. Add beets and toss gently to combine. Sprinkle with sunflower seeds. Serve immediately.

Sauerkraut

Sauerkraut, which is the German word meaning "sour cabbage," has its origins in China, and was brought to the Western world by migrating peoples. It is rich in digestive enzymes and flavor, so its crunchy, vibrant tang makes an enlivening addition to your meal.

**MAKES
2 CUPS (500 ML)**

Tip

Sauerkraut will be slightly tangy when it is first refrigerated and will become increasingly sour over the course of 2 weeks. Keep sauerkraut covered with liquid; if it develops any off flavors, a pink color or fuzziness, discard it.

- **2-cup (500 mL) canning jar**

2 cups	thinly sliced cabbage or mustard greens	500 mL
1 tsp	fennel or caraway seeds (optional)	5 mL
1 tsp	kosher or non-iodized sea salt	5 mL
1 tbsp	sauerkraut juice (from unpasteurized store-bought or homemade sauerkraut)	15 mL

1. In jar, combine cabbage, fennel seeds and salt. Pour sauerkraut juice over top. Cover and let stand at room temperature for 24 hours.

2. With the back of a spoon, press down cabbage so it is covered by liquid. Eat immediately or refrigerate for up to 2 weeks.

Health Tips

Cabbage is a sweet and pungent vegetable that is highly beneficial to your digestion and helps constipation. Through fermentation, it becomes a consummate probiotic-rich immune-boosting food. A little bit every day can support the digestive and immune systems.

Traditionally, pounded or grated cabbage leaves have been used as a poultice for swelling due to injury, skin eruptions and redness. Fresh cabbage juice is an old-fashioned remedy for stomach ulcers and abdominal pain, and was once used by the Romans as a hangover cure.

Wilted Cabbage and Red Lentil Salad with Pomegranate Dressing

In this excellent main course salad, the red lentils dissolve into a hearty sauce. The finished dish looks fancy and is still delicious at room temperature, so it's nice for a potluck.

Tip

This dish is good warm or at room temperature. Just keep the toppings separate from the cabbage mixture and add them just before serving.

Health Tips

Cabbage is neither cooling nor warming. In Chinese medicine, it is said to help relieve spasms and pain. Turmeric is anti-inflammatory. The addition of astringent pomegranate juice activates all the flavors and promotes hydration.

½ cup	dried red lentils, rinsed	125 mL
¼ cup	sliced or slivered almonds	60 mL
2 tbsp	avocado oil, divided	30 mL
1	onion, thinly sliced lengthwise	1
1½ tsp	salt, divided	7 mL
½	head green cabbage (about 3 lbs/ 1.5 kg cabbage), cored and cut into 1-inch (2.5 cm) chunks	½
1 tbsp	finely chopped turmeric root	15 mL
Pinch	ground cinnamon	Pinch
1 cup	unsweetened pomegranate juice	250 mL
1 tsp	coconut sugar	5 mL
¼ cup	plain sheep's milk yogurt, stirred until smooth (optional)	60 mL

1. In a large bowl, combine lentils and 4 cups (1 L) water; let stand for 2 to 8 hours. Drain well.

2. Place almonds in a large dry skillet over medium heat. Toast, stirring or shaking pan often, for 2 to 3 minutes or until lightly browned. Spread out on a plate and let cool.

3. Add 1 tbsp (15 mL) of the oil to the skillet, swirling to coat bottom of pan. Add onion and cook, stirring often, for 10 to 15 minutes or until browned. Stir in ½ tsp (2 mL) of the salt. Transfer to a bowl and set aside.

4. Add remaining oil to skillet, swirling to coat bottom of pan. Add cabbage, turmeric and cinnamon; cook, stirring, for 1 minute. Add lentils and 2 cups (500 mL) water; reduce heat, cover and simmer for 30 minutes or until lentils have completely broken down. Uncover, add remaining salt and cook, shaking pan often to prevent scorching, for 4 to 6 minutes or until almost no liquid remains.

5. Meanwhile, in a medium skillet, bring pomegranate juice and coconut sugar to a simmer over medium heat. Simmer, stirring occasionally, for 10 to 20 minutes or until syrupy and reduced by three-quarters.

6. Transfer cabbage mixture to a wide serving bowl. Top with onion and almonds. Drizzle with pomegranate syrup and yogurt (if using).

Grilled Romaine Lettuce with Anchovy Sauce

Most people are incredulous if you mention grilling romaine. Grill lettuce? Yes! It is delicious, especially with this lemony anchovy sauce. So much so that this side dish may become a regular on your table.

MAKES 4 SERVINGS

Variation

If you are a vegan or do not like anchovies, the dressing is still delicious without them.

- **Preheat broiler, with rack placed 4 inches (10 cm) below element**
- **Large rimmed baking sheet**

2	medium (or 1 large) heads romaine lettuce	2
2 tbsp	minced green onion	30 mL
½ tsp	grated lemon zest	2 mL
1 tbsp	freshly squeezed lemon juice	15 mL
¼ tsp	freshly ground black pepper	1 mL
1	can (2 oz/57 g) anchovies, drained	1
1 tbsp	avocado oil	15 mL
¼ cup	chopped toasted pistachios (see tips, page 284)	60 mL

1. Trim root ends off romaine but do not remove stems. Cut heads in half lengthwise. (If using a single large head, cut halves lengthwise into quarters.)

2. In a small bowl, combine green onion, lemon zest, lemon juice and pepper. Using a fork, mash in anchovies to make a chunky sauce.

3. Pour oil onto baking sheet. Dip cut sides of lettuces in oil and place, cut side up, on sheet. Broil under preheated broiler for about 2 minutes or until edges are browned and slightly wilted.

4. Transfer lettuce to a serving platter. Drizzle anchovy sauce over top and sprinkle with pistachios. Serve immediately.

Health Tip

The bitterness of romaine lettuce clears heat, which may appear as irritability, easy frustration or even high cholesterol or blood pressure. These are all signs of what we describe in Chinese medicine as liver *qi* stagnation. Romaine lettuce promotes urination, is beneficial for a fever and promotes mother's milk.

Edamame, Roasted Cherry Tomato and Blanched Escarole Salad

In the Chinese tradition, salads include wilted or lightly cooked vegetables served at room temperature. This salad includes all of the five flavors and several vibrant and palatable colors — it is a delight to put on your table. The varying textures make it a highly satisfying salad.

<table>
<tr><td colspan="3">MAKES 4 SERVINGS</td></tr>
</table>

Health Tip

The bitter flavor of the escarole is excellent for clearing heat. The sweet and sour tomatoes promote hydration of the body's tissues, nourishing the yin. The black and white sesame seeds nourish the kidney yin and yang.

- **Preheat oven to 400°F (200°C)**
- **Rimmed baking sheet**

1	head escarole	1
2 tbsp	avocado oil, divided	30 mL
12 oz	cherry tomatoes (about 2 cups/500 mL)	375 g
2 tbsp	sesame seeds (preferably a mix of black and white)	30 mL
2 tbsp	white miso	30 mL
1 tsp	grated lemon zest	5 mL
2 tbsp	freshly squeezed lemon juice	30 mL
1 tsp	coconut sugar	5 mL
2 cups	frozen shelled edamame	500 mL

1. Cut off and reserve escarole stems. Cut escarole leaves into 2-inch (5 cm) pieces. Cut stems into 1/4-inch (0.5 cm) thick slices. Set leaves and stems aside separately.

2. Place 1 tbsp (15 mL) of the oil on baking sheet, add cherry tomatoes and roll to coat. Roast in preheated oven for 10 minutes. Move tomatoes to edges of pan and spread sesame seeds in center. Roast for 5 minutes.

3. In a large heatproof bowl, whisk together remaining oil, miso, lemon zest, lemon juice and coconut sugar. Scrape tomatoes and sesame seeds into bowl and toss gently to coat with dressing. Set aside.

4. In a large saucepan, bring 8 cups (2 L) water to a boil. Add escarole leaves and edamame; cook for 1 minute. Drain well.

5. Arrange escarole leaves and edamame in a large, shallow serving bowl or on a platter. Top with tomato mixture and escarole stems.

Roasted Sweet Potato Salad

This salad features a nice contrast between the caramelized chewiness at the edges of the sweet potatoes and the smooth, creamy dressing.

MAKES 4 SERVINGS

Tip

To toast sesame seeds, place them in a small dry skillet. Toast over low heat, stirring or shaking pan constantly, for 3 minutes or until fragrant. Immediately transfer to a small bowl and let cool.

Variation

If you are allergic or sensitive to soy, skip this dish and try Roasted Chunky Root Vegetables with Tangy Tahini Dressing (page 395) instead.

- **Preheat oven to 400°F (200°C)**
- **Rimmed baking sheet, brushed with avocado oil**

½	package (14 oz to 1 lb/420 to 500 g package) soft or medium tofu, drained	½
2 tbsp	white miso	30 mL
1 tbsp	toasted sesame oil	15 mL
1 tbsp	freshly squeezed lemon juice	15 mL
2 lbs	sweet potatoes, peeled and cut into 1-inch (2.5 cm) chunks	1 kg
¼ cup	minced green onions	60 mL
2 tbsp	sesame seeds (preferably black), toasted	30 mL

1. In a small bowl, whisk together tofu, miso, sesame oil and lemon juice. Set aside.

2. Arrange sweet potatoes in a single layer on prepared baking sheet. Roast in preheated oven, turning once halfway through, for 30 minutes or until tender.

3. In a large bowl, gently toss potatoes with dressing to coat. Sprinkle with green onions and sesame seeds.

Health Tip

Sweet potatoes are beneficial to digestion, help stabilize blood sugar levels and ease constipation. They are often eaten to combat fatigue or constipation. The tofu and miso dressing balances the dish and incorporates protein into the salad. If you feel full easily, this dish is not recommended, as sweet potatoes can cause a feeling of fullness.

Roasted Peanuts with Tangerine Peel

Peanuts came to China via America as early as the 16th century. They are even more delicious when toasted and spiced, as they are here. This tasty recipe mixes sweet, salty and sour for a zesty flavor — the nuts make a great snack at a party.

> **MAKES ABOUT
> 1¾ CUPS (425 ML)**

Tips

Always choose organic peanuts and other nuts. Stay away from moldy peanuts, which are said to have a carcinogenic effect.

When you're grating citrus zest, don't press too hard. You just want the colored part, and not the bitter white pith beneath.

4 oz	unsalted raw peanuts	125 g
2 tbsp	coconut sugar	30 mL
2 tsp	grated gingerroot	10 mL
½ tsp	grated tangerine zest	2 mL
½ tsp	salt	2 mL

1. Place a sheet of parchment paper on a rimmed baking sheet or other heatproof surface.

2. In a medium skillet, toast peanuts over low heat, stirring often, for 5 to 7 minutes or until lightly browned and slightly oily.

3. Turn off heat and add coconut sugar, ginger, tangerine zest and salt, stirring until peanuts are coated. Spread out on parchment paper and let cool completely.

4. Store cooled peanuts in an airtight container at room temperature for up to 1 week.

> ### Health Tip
>
> Peanuts are lubricating. They nourish the blood, strengthen the lungs and stomach and increase overall *qi*. If you eat a handful of peanuts, it may help with constipation. Of course, roasting or toasting peanuts creates a more drying effect. The tangerine zest makes this snack a *qi* mover.

Fall Herbs and Cinnamon Tea

The combination of fragrant thyme and rosemary along with spicy cinnamon is surprisingly delicious. This warming, aromatic tea is a perfect digestive for cooler autumn days and nights.

Tip

While you can use dried herbs in this recipe, fresh herbs give it a vibrant and fresh aroma, which is always part of an infusion's magic.

3	sprigs fresh thyme (or 2 tsp/10 mL dried thyme)	3
2	pieces (2 inches/5 cm long each) cinnamon sticks	2
1	sprig rosemary (or 2 tsp/10 mL dried rosemary leaves)	1
	Liquid honey (optional)	

1. In a large saucepan, bring 4 cups (1 L) water to a boil. Remove from heat.

2. Stir in thyme, cinnamon sticks and rosemary. Cover and let stand for 10 minutes.

3. Strain into teacups. Stir in honey (if using) to taste.

> **Health Tip**
>
> Digestive teas are common in most cultures. The harmonious combination of warming cinnamon bark, rosemary and thyme is delightful. Thyme relieves indigestion and benefits the lungs and mind. Rosemary is a sweet and warming pungent herb that nourishes the heart.

Clear-the-Lungs Tea

This sweet and aromatic hot beverage is great when you are finished with a cold but want to clear excess mucus and soothe a slight cough.

Tip

If you don't have loose tea, cut open a tea bag and measure out the correct amount.

1½ tbsp	chopped raw almonds, rinsed	22 mL
1 tsp	anise seeds	5 mL
½ tsp	loose green tea	2 mL
	Liquid honey (optional)	

1. In a large saucepan, combine 4 cups (1 L) water, almonds and anise seeds and bring to a boil. Reduce heat and simmer for 10 minutes.

2. Strain liquid into a small bowl. Return to pan. Add green tea, cover and let stand for 3 minutes.

3. Strain into teacups. Stir in honey (if using) to taste.

Autumnal Sweet-and-Sour Tea

This herbal tea unites East and West with sweet da zao (red dates) and sour rose hips, with just a hint of ginger to keep you warm. Ellen often enjoyed picking rose hips near where she lived in the Veneto area of Italy.

MAKES 2 SERVINGS

Tip

Red dates, known as *da zao* or *hong zao* in Mandarin, are available in Asian herbal or grocery stores, or online.

10	dried red dates	10
2	slices (quarter-size) gingerroot	2
1 tsp	crushed dried rose hips	5 mL
	Liquid honey (optional)	

1. In a large saucepan, combine 3 cups (750 mL) water, dates, ginger and rose hips. Bring to a boil. Reduce heat and simmer for 5 minutes.

2. Remove from heat. Cover and let stand for 5 minutes.

3. Strain into teacups. Stir in honey (if using) to taste.

Health Tip

Da zao are precious red dates known for their sweet flavor and nourishing qualities. They are added to many herbal formulas to harmonize the herbal prescription. On their own, they serve to strengthen the *qi* and build energy. Rose hips are known in the West for their high vitamin C content. Ginger is warming to the stomach and aids digestion.

Cranberry-Apple Rooibos Tea with Star Anise

This is quite different from the usual spiced teas, but is absolutely lovely. The rooibos adds a toasty note, and the star anise a licorice flavor. The sweet-and-sour apple and cranberry juices make it a great thirst-quenching drink. You can enjoy this tea warm or at room temperature.

**MAKES
4 TO 6 SERVINGS**

Tip

Star anise has an earthier flavor than anise seed; these two spices are generally not interchangeable in recipes.

1 cup	unsweetened cranberry juice	250 mL
3 cups	unsweetened apple juice	750 mL
4	rooibos tea bags (or 4 tsp/20 mL loose rooibos tea)	4
1 or 2	whole star anise	1 or 2

1. In a large saucepan, combine cranberry juice and apple juice. Bring to a boil.
2. Turn off heat and stir in rooibos tea and star anise. Cover and let stand on burner for 10 minutes.
3. Strain into teacups.

Health Tip

Rooibos, also known as red bush tea, is made from the leaves of the *Aspalathus linearis* tree, which grows in South Africa. The tree's leaves are fermented to make the tea. This national drink of South Africa is caffeine-free, sweet and fragrant, and is high in antioxidants and vitamin C.

Cardamom and Ginger Digestive Liquor

Liquors and medicinal wines were one of the first medicines, and were often made by fermenting or decocting a wide variety of herbs and foods to treat a wide variety of ailments. They were most often administered in the colder months. This spicy, fragrant wine is an excellent digestive, meant to be drunk in very small amounts after a meal. It is marvelous on a cool evening.

> **MAKES
> 2 CUPS (500 ML)**

Tips

Drink this liquor in small quantities, using shot glasses or sake cups. Serve after dinner to aid digestion.

Make sure to strain the liquor when it achieves the flavor you desire. The spices will make the vodka increasingly bitter over time.

- **2-cup (500 mL) canning jar**
- **2-cup (500 mL) glass bottle**

2 cups	vodka	500 mL
20	green cardamom pods	20
10	slices (quarter-size) gingerroot, gently crushed	10
2 tbsp	liquid honey	30 mL

1. In jar, combine vodka, cardamom, ginger and honey. Seal with lid and shake well to combine. Let stand in a cool, dark place, shaking every few days, for 2 weeks.

2. Taste the mixture. (It should be fragrant, warming and spicy.) If you want a fuller flavor, let it stand for a few more days.

3. Strain through a fine-mesh sieve into bottle. Store in a cool, dark place for up to 6 months.

> ### Health Tip
>
> Cardamom and ginger are two warming digestives. Both ginger and cardamom warm the stomach and improve circulation.

Autumn Fruit Salad with Rose Syrup

This fragrant and fresh fruit dessert, alive with color, highlights each distinct flavor. The sweetness of the grape juice and apple is well balanced by the astringency of the pomegranate and the floral rose water.

1 cup	unsweetened pomegranate juice (freshly squeezed or store-bought)	250 mL
1 cup	unsweetened white grape juice	250 mL
1/4 tsp	rose water, or to taste	1 mL
2	nonastringent persimmons (such as Fuyu), peeled and cut into thin slices	2
1	large apple, cored and cut into thin slices	1
1 cup	pomegranate seeds (arils)	250 mL
	Food-grade fresh or dried rose petals (optional), see tips, at left	
1/2 cup	chopped toasted pistachios (see tips, page 284)	125 mL

MAKES 4 SERVINGS

Tips

If persimmons are not available, use another sweet fruit, such as late-season peaches or bananas.

Culinary rose water is available at Indian and Middle Eastern grocery stores. It is potent, so use only small amounts.

The syrup can be doubled. Extra syrup may be stored for up to 1 week in the refrigerator.

Use rose petals from roses that have not been sprayed with pesticides or herbicides.

1. In a nonreactive medium skillet, combine pomegranate juice and grape juice. Bring to a simmer over medium-high heat. Reduce heat and simmer for 10 to 20 minutes or until reduced by three-quarters. Remove from heat and let cool completely. Stir in rose water to taste.

2. In a medium bowl, combine persimmon and apple slices. Drizzle with rose water mixture. Gently stir in pomegranate seeds. Sprinkle with rose petals (if using) and pistachios. Serve immediately.

Health Tip

Rose is beneficial for the nervous system and can help move liver *qi*. In ancient Chinese alchemy, the bright red juice of pomegranates was regarded as analogous to human blood, and pomegranates were considered a fruit of immortality. They are sweet and sour in flavor and can soothe a dry throat. Persimmons are cooling and sweet. They clear lung heat and phlegm, and can soothe mucous membranes in the digestive tract and lungs. If you feel dry and parched, persimmons can help to quench thirst.

Velvety Pears with Anise Seeds, Lemon and Honey

The pears and their juice may be enjoyed together, or you can eat the pears as a dessert and warm the juice to sip as a soothing tea.

	MAKES 4 TO 6 SERVINGS	

Tips

Use a saucepan that is wider than it is tall.

If you like, you can add these pears to plain rice congee for breakfast.

1 cup	unsweetened white grape juice	250 mL
1 tsp	grated lemon zest	5 mL
2 tbsp	freshly squeezed lemon juice	30 mL
1 tbsp	liquid honey, or to taste	15 mL
1 tsp	anise seeds	5 mL
4	large firm-ripe pears, such as Bartlett (Williams) or Bosc, peeled, cored and quartered	4

1. In a medium shallow saucepan (see tips, at left), combine grape juice, lemon zest, lemon juice, honey and anise seeds, adding up to 1 tbsp (15 mL) more honey, if desired. Add pears and bring to a boil. Reduce heat to medium, cover and boil gently for 10 minutes.

2. Uncover; if any pears are above the liquid, push them under the other pears. Simmer, uncovered, for 5 minutes or until pears are completely translucent.

3. Spoon into serving bowls. Serve warm or let cool to room temperature. Refrigerate for up to 1 week.

> ## Health Tip
>
> Pears are the fruit to eat when you're suffering from a cough with phlegm. They are not a substitute for treatment, but their cooling nature will soothe and help clear any excess mucus. If you want to increase the potency of this action, grate 1/2 tsp (2 mL) gingerroot and squeeze the juice into the pear cooking liquid and drink it as a warm tea.

Quinces in Schisandra Syrup

This delightfully intriguing dish can be eaten on its own as a simple compote. You can also enjoy the syrup stirred into water or tea.

MAKES
MAKES **6 TO 8 SERVINGS**

Tip

Don't try nibbling the berries as a snack; they have a hard seed in the center.

- **Preheat oven to 350°F (180°C)**
- **13- by 9-inch (33 by 23 cm) glass baking dish**

1 cup	unsweetened white grape juice	250 mL
2 tbsp	dried schisandra berries	30 mL
2 tbsp	liquid honey	30 mL
2 lbs	quinces, quartered and cored	1 kg

1. In a small saucepan, combine grape juice and schisandra berries. Bring to a boil over medium-high heat. Remove from heat, cover and let stand for 10 minutes.

2. Strain grape juice mixture through a fine-mesh sieve into baking dish, pressing hard with the back of a spoon to extract most of the pulp from the berries. Scrape the outside of the sieve with a spatula and add pulp to the dish (discard seeds from berries). Stir in honey.

3. Place quince quarters, cut side down, in syrup and cover dish tightly with foil.

4. Bake in preheated oven for 45 minutes or until tender. Uncover and bake for 15 minutes. Let cool in dish.

Health Tips

The common quince used in Western cuisine is different from the Chinese quince (*mu gua*). The common quince is sweet, sour, slightly bitter and astringent. (These are the quinces used in this recipe because they are available in Western grocery stores and farmers' markets.) Cooked into a compote, these fruits are especially effective at stopping diarrhea.

Schisandra is often called the "five-flavored seed," because it embodies all five flavors: sweet, sour, salty, pungent and bitter. It is a powerful adaptogenic tonic herb that can support the *qi*, build the blood and calm the shen. It has been used for millennia to build immunity, mental calm and focus.

Steamed Pumpkin Pudding

Pumpkin is one of the quintessential autumn foods. Just the thought of it makes North Americans think of autumn and yummy treats. Steaming is a quick, easy way to cook these individual puddings, which have a very traditional creamy spiciness.

MAKES 6 SERVINGS

Tips

To make purée, peel and seed pumpkin. Cut into 2-inch (5 cm) pieces. In a medium saucepan, combine pumpkin and ¼ cup (60 mL) water. Bring to a simmer over medium heat. Simmer, watching carefully and adding more water if mixture is drying out, for 1 hour or until very soft. Transfer pumpkin, in batches if necessary, to a blender or food processor and purée. You can also substitute canned 100% pumpkin purée (not pie filling).

If your pot is too small to hold all of the ramekins at once, steam the puddings in batches.

- **Six ½- or ¾-cup (125 or 175 mL) ramekins or custard cups**
- **Large pot with steamer rack (about 1 inch/2.5 cm above bottom of pot)**

2	large eggs	2
2 cups	pumpkin or squash purée (see tips, at left)	500 mL
1 cup	goat's milk	250 mL
½ cup	coconut sugar	125 mL
½ tsp	ground cinnamon	2 mL
¼ tsp	ground nutmeg	1 mL
¼ tsp	ground ginger	1 mL
⅛ tsp	ground cloves	0.5 mL

1. In a medium bowl and using a fork, beat eggs well. Whisk in pumpkin, milk, coconut sugar, cinnamon, nutmeg, ginger and cloves. Divide mixture evenly among ramekins.

2. Pour enough water into pot to come scant 1 inch (2.5 cm) up side. Place steamer rack in pan over water. Bring to a boil.

3. Arrange ramekins on rack, cover tightly and steam for 15 to 20 minutes or until puddings are barely set in the center (they will be jiggly but not liquid).

4. Serve warm or at room temperature. Or cover and refrigerate for up to 3 days; let come to room temperature for an hour before serving.

Health Tips

Pumpkin is sweet and warming, reinforcing the digestive system and helping to regulate blood sugar. It is a perfect choice for those who love sweetness but want to stay away from sweets. Goat's milk adds a heart yang *qi* tonic to the mix. With the addition of warming aromatic spices, this is a beneficial dessert for those who are recovering from a long-term illness and are feeling tired, or feeling deficient in any way.

Coconut sugar is made from the sap obtained from the coconut tree's flower buds. It has a lower glycemic index than white or brown sugar, but it is still sugar, so enjoy it in moderation.

Crunchy Seed Cookies

Everyone needs a cookie every now and then. These yummy seed-packed cookies are mildly sweet and very crunchy.

MAKES 32 COOKIES

Health Tip

Nuts and seeds are incredibly beneficial foods. These grain-free cookies are an essence-building delight, nourishing the liver and kidneys. Sesame seeds are known as "longevity seeds" in China, are good for the skin and hair, and nourish the yin. Hemp seeds are beneficial for elimination.

- **Preheat oven to 300°F (150°C), with racks positioned in upper and lower thirds**
- **2 baking sheets, lined with parchment paper**

1 cup	almond flour	250 mL
1 cup	firmly packed coconut sugar	250 mL
½ cup	hulled hemp seeds	125 mL
½ cup	tahini	125 mL
2 tbsp	white sesame seeds	30 mL
2 tbsp	black sesame seeds	30 mL
2 tbsp	poppy seeds	30 mL
½ tsp	vanilla extract	2 mL
¼ tsp	salt	1 mL

1. In a medium bowl, combine almond flour, coconut sugar, hemp seeds, tahini, ½ cup (125 mL) water, white and black sesame seeds, poppy seeds, vanilla and salt. Stir until well combined.

2. Using a small ice cream scoop or 2 spoons, scoop 2-tbsp (30 mL) chunks of dough onto prepared baking sheets. Cover with a second sheet of parchment paper; press down on each cookie and flatten to ¼-inch (0.5 cm) thickness. Remove second sheet of paper.

3. Bake on upper and lower racks in preheated oven, switching and rotating pans halfway through, for 15 to 17 minutes or until cookies are firm and edges are golden. Let cool on pans on wire racks. Store in an airtight container for up to 1 week.

Cranberry and Apricot Crumble

This sweet and tangy fall dessert captures the flavors of the season and is grain-free.

Tips

To make buckwheat meal, process buckwheat groats in a blender until they are the texture of cornmeal.

If you like a sweeter crumble, you can increase the amount of coconut sugar to ½ cup (125 mL).

To make ahead: Follow instructions through Step 6 and then let crumble cool completely. Place paper towel over top and cover with plastic wrap. Refrigerate for up to 5 days. Crumble can be reheated over low heat, without stirring, for 5 minutes.

Health Tip

The combination of apricots, pear and cranberries supplements and moistens the lungs and throat while supporting a healthy appetite. The addition of almonds and almond flour makes this a beneficial dessert for people who want something sweet but may have a slight cough or cold.

- **8-cup (2 L) deep baking dish**
- **Rimmed baking sheet, lined with parchment paper**

2 cups	dried apricots, halved	500 mL
2 cups	unsweetened apple juice	500 mL
½ cup	unsweetened dried cranberries	125 mL
1	large pear (preferably Bartlett or Williams), peeled and cubed	1
3 tbsp	buckwheat meal (see tips, at left)	45 mL
2 tbsp	freshly squeezed lemon juice	30 mL
¼ cup	liquid honey	60 mL

Crumble

½ cup	sliced almonds	125 mL
½ cup	buckwheat meal	125 mL
6 tbsp	almond flour	90 mL
6 tbsp	firmly packed coconut sugar	90 mL
2 tbsp	ghee	30 mL
¼ tsp	ground cinnamon	1 mL
⅛ tsp	salt	0.5 mL

1. In a large bowl, combine apricots, apple juice and cranberries. Cover and let stand for at least 4 hours or until fruit is rehydrated and plump, or for up to 12 hours.

2. Preheat oven to 400°F (200°C), with racks positioned in upper and lower thirds.

3. Transfer apricot mixture to baking dish. Stir in pear, buckwheat meal and lemon juice. Drizzle with honey.

4. Bake on lower rack in preheated oven for about 45 minutes, stirring once or twice, until juices are bubbling in the center.

5. *Crumble:* Meanwhile, in a large bowl, combine almonds, buckwheat meal, almond flour, coconut sugar, ghee, cinnamon and salt. Using a fork, stir until well combined. Spoon onto prepared baking sheet in a layer about ½ inch (1 cm) thick. Add to upper rack in preheated oven and bake for 6 to 8 minutes or until edges are browned.

6. When fruit is cooked, using a spatula, spoon crumble over fruit. Serve warm or at room temperature.

Winter Seasonal Menus

Menu 1
Bitter Melon with Shrimp
Creamy Cabbage Salad
Brown Rice

Menu 2
Roasted Chunky Root Vegetables with Tangy Tahini Dressing
Hijiki and Carrot Sauté with Ginger
Braised Mixed Greens with Lemon Rind Pickle and Eggs

Menu 3
Braised Duck with Lotus Seeds
Curly Endive and Apple Chopped Salad with Candied Walnuts

Winter Recipes

Breakfasts

Soups

Meats, Fish and Other Mains

Mostly Vegetables

Snack

Teas and Tonic Beverages

Desserts

Many Treasures Congee

This is a variation on a classic Chinese dish that translates as "longevity eight treasures congee." It includes simple, sweet winter tonic foods to build qi and blood first thing in the morning. This congee was traditionally eaten on the eighth day of winter in the lunar calendar, and offers a satisfying variety of textures and simple, well-balanced flavors.

| | MAKES 4 SERVINGS | |

Tip

To toast walnuts, place them in a medium dry skillet. Toast over low heat, stirring often, for 8 to 10 minutes or until fragrant.

2 tbsp	dried adzuki beans	30 mL
½ cup	sweet (glutinous) brown rice (or brown Arborio rice)	125 mL
2 tbsp	blanched almonds	30 mL
½ tsp	salt	2 mL
1 tbsp	chopped dried pitted red dates	15 mL
1 tbsp	chopped dried longan fruit	15 mL
1 tbsp	dried goji berries	15 mL
¼ cup	walnuts, toasted and chopped	60 mL

1. In a medium saucepan, combine 2 cups (500 mL) water and adzuki beans. Bring to a boil. Remove from heat, cover and let stand for 1 hour. Drain and rinse beans well.

2. In a large saucepan, combine beans, 5 cups (1.25 L) water, rice, almonds and salt. Bring to a boil. Reduce heat to low, cover and simmer, stirring occasionally, for 2 hours. The congee should have a souplike consistency; if there is not enough liquid left in the pan, add up to ½ cup (125 mL) more water as needed.

3. Stir in red dates, longan fruit and goji berries. Remove from heat, cover and let cool for 10 minutes. Serve immediately or transfer to an airtight container and refrigerate for up to 3 days. Warm in a small saucepan over low heat before serving.

4. Spoon into serving bowls and sprinkle with walnuts.

> ## Health Tip
>
> Tonic foods are considered treasures in Chinese medicine and are credited with protecting a person's health throughout the seasons. In this dish, blood- and *qi*-building tonics come in the form of goji berries (good for the liver and kidneys), longan fruit (good for the heart), red dates (good for the spleen), almonds (good for the lungs) and adzuki beans (good for the kidneys).

Savory Winter Congee

Each morning, our bodies awake with a few different needs: first we move and then we need to be nourished. Here, a simple, savory congee offers excellent nutritional support in winter — a perfect time to nourish the kidney qi and yin. The pork topping is optional.

Tip

If you're not using the optional pork topping, garnish the congee with $1/4$ cup (60 mL) toasted sesame seeds (white or black) before serving. Toast them in a medium skillet over low heat, stirring constantly, for about 3 minutes or until fragrant. White sesame seeds nourish the kidneys, are rich in omega-3 fatty acids and help prevent constipation.

Health Tips

Pork is a sweet, salty meat that nourishes the kidney yin. Often used in Chinese medicine, pork can be added in small amounts to recipes as a supplement to strengthen the low back and relieve dryness. It's very useful for women going through menopause.

The addition of shiitake mushrooms makes this congee an excellent immune-system tonic.

- **1-quart (1 L) canning jar**

4	dried shiitake mushrooms	4
	Warm water	
1	large leek	1
$1/2$ cup	sweet (glutinous) brown rice	125 mL
1 cup	diced peeled sweet potatoes	250 mL

Pork Topping (optional)

8 oz	pork shoulder or pork loin, trimmed	250 g
4 oz	tender greens, such as spinach or mustard, stemmed	125 g
1 tbsp	avocado oil	15 mL
1 tsp	salt	5 mL
1 tbsp	julienned gingerroot (optional)	15 mL

1. Place shiitake mushrooms in jar and pour in enough warm water to fill. Seal lid and let stand, shaking jar once or twice, for 2 to 8 hours.

2. Drain mushrooms. Trim off and discard stems. Coarsely chop mushrooms. Trim roots and all but 1 inch (2.5 cm) of the dark green leaves off leek and discard. Cut leek in half lengthwise, then cut crosswise into $1/2$-inch (1 cm) wide pieces. Rinse very well in 2 changes of water to remove grit.

3. In a medium saucepan, combine mushrooms, leek, 5 cups (1.25 L) water and rice. Bring to a boil. Reduce heat to low and simmer for $1^1/2$ hours. The congee should have a souplike consistency; if there is not enough liquid left in the pan, add up to $1/2$ cup (125 mL) more water as needed. Stir in sweet potatoes and simmer for 30 minutes.

4. *Pork Topping (if using):* Meanwhile, cut pork into $1/4$-inch (0.5 cm) thick slices. Stack a few slices at a time and cut into $1/4$-inch (0.5 cm) wide strips. Cut greens into thin shreds.

5. In a large skillet, heat oil over high heat, swirling to coat bottom of pan. Add pork, greens and salt and cook, stirring often, for 3 to 4 minutes or until pork is no longer pink inside and greens are wilted.

6. Spoon congee into bowls and garnish with pork mixture and ginger (if using). Serve immediately.

Essential Seed and Nut Porridge with Ghee and Honey

Of all the seasonal essential nut and seed porridges in this book, this is our favorite. We call it "The Queen." Walnuts are a winter nut; they are warming, with a hearty, bitter taste that is smoothed out by the ghee and honey.

MAKES 4 SERVINGS

Tips

If you like your porridge thinner, add up to 1 cup (250 mL) more water to the seed mixture.

Plantain chips are available in the bulk section of grocery stores, in packages in the dried fruit section or online.

Health Tips

Ghee, or clarified butter, has been used in Ayurvedic medicine for thousands of years to replenish vital energy, and treat allergy, skin and respiratory disorders. It is casein- and lactose-free, so it is easier for people with dairy sensitivities to digest. Ghee is rich in medium-chain fatty acids, moistens and balances hormonal function. According to Chinese medicine, ghee benefits and nourishes the *jing* and the kidneys.

- **Blender**

4 tsp	liquid honey or pure maple syrup	20 mL
4 tsp	ghee	20 mL
Porridge		
¼ cup	hulled hemp seeds	60 mL
2 tbsp	chia seeds	30 mL
2 tbsp	flax seeds	30 mL
½ cup	walnuts (2 oz/60 g)	125 mL
½ cup	unsalted raw cashews (2 oz/ 60 g)	125 mL
1 cup	unsweetened roasted plantain chips (3 oz/90 g)	250 mL
½ tsp	salt	2 mL
2 cups	boiling water	500 mL

1. *Porridge:* In a large dry skillet, toast hemp, chia and flax seeds over medium-low heat, stirring often, for about 5 minutes or until fragrant. Transfer to a small heatproof bowl and let cool completely.

2. Meanwhile, add walnuts and cashews to skillet and toast over medium-low heat, stirring often, for about 10 minutes or until golden and fragrant. Transfer to a large heatproof bowl and let cool completely.

3. In blender, combine seed mixture and plantain chips and grind until the texture of brown sugar. Return to small bowl.

4. Add nut mixture and salt to blender and grind to the texture of brown sugar or a little coarser. Return to large bowl and stir in seed mixture. Stir in boiling water, cover and let stand for 5 minutes.

5. Spoon porridge into serving bowls. Divide honey and ghee among bowls. Serve immediately.

Health Tips

Walnuts are the queens of nuts during the winter. They are warming and beneficial for the kidneys. They are considered a brain and longevity-promoting food.

Shrimp and Leek Steamed Egg Custard

This custard is gentle and delicately flavored with tamari. The warming shrimp and leek make it a favorite dish for chilly mornings.

> **MAKES 6 SERVINGS**

Tips

If your pot is too small to hold all of the ramekins at once, steam the custards in batches.

Rubber-tipped tongs are great for transferring the ramekins to the steamer pot. If you don't have them, you can wrap thick rubber bands around the tips of regular metal tongs.

Health Tips

Eggs are the perfect yin-yang food. When steamed, they are easy to digest and beneficial if you are recovering from an illness and feeling weak.

Leeks are a milder allium, and not as stimulating and warming as onions or their other stronger cousins. Their pungent, slightly sour flavor and astringent action help counter diarrhea.

Shrimp is warming and salty, with an affinity for the kidneys. It is considered a yang food, so this recipe specifically benefits the renal system.

- **Six $^1\!/_2$- or $^3\!/_4$-cup (125 to 175 mL) ramekins or custard cups**
- **Large pot with steamer rack (about 1 inch/2.5 cm above bottom of pot)**

1	leek	1
4	large eggs	4
3 cups	Traditional Dashi (page 297), at room temperature	750 mL
1 tbsp	tamari or soy sauce	15 mL
$^1\!/_2$ tsp	salt	2 mL
12	jumbo shrimp (25 count), peeled, deveined and cooked	12

1. Trim roots and all but 1 inch (2.5 cm) of the dark green leaves off leek and discard. Cut leek in half lengthwise, then cut crosswise into $^1\!/_2$-inch (1 cm) wide pieces. Rinse very well in 2 changes of water to remove grit.

2. In a medium saucepan, combine leek with $^1\!/_2$ cup (125 mL) water and bring to a simmer over medium-high heat. Reduce heat to low, cover and cook for about 5 minutes or until tender. Uncover and cook, stirring often, until no liquid remains. Let cool.

3. In a 4-cup (1 L) glass measuring cup, whisk together eggs, dashi, tamari and salt. Divide leek and shrimp equally among ramekins. Strain and gently pour egg mixture into ramekins.

4. Pour enough water into pot to come scant 1 inch (2.5 cm) up side. Place steamer rack in pan over water. Bring to a boil.

5. Arrange ramekins on rack, cover tightly and steam for 15 to 20 minutes or until custard is barely set in the center (it will be jiggly but not liquid).

6. Serve warm or at room temperature. Or cover and refrigerate for up to 3 days; let come to room temperature for an hour before serving.

Mushroom and Adzuki Bean Breakfast Fried Rice

Rich, woodsy mushrooms and earthy adzuki beans make this dish a hearty choice for breakfast, lunch or dinner. You can vary the types of mushrooms you use — this recipe is a great opportunity to explore new varieties you've never tried.

> **MAKES
> 4 TO 6 SERVINGS**

Tip

For a protein boost, beat 2 large eggs well. At the end of Step 5, move rice to 1 side of pan. Pour in eggs and cook, without stirring, for 30 seconds. Using spatula, flip eggs and cook for 30 seconds until set. Chop coarsely with spatula and mix into rice. Continue with recipe.

1 cup	dried adzuki beans	250 mL
1 cup	brown jasmine rice or brown basmati rice	250 mL
¼ cup	avocado oil, divided	60 mL
6 cups	minced mixed mushrooms, such as cremini, button, oyster, or fresh or soaked dried shiitake	1.5 L
1 oz	thinly sliced tender greens, such as spinach or baby kale	30 g
2 tbsp	tamari or soy sauce	30 mL
2 tbsp	thinly sliced green onions	30 mL

1. In a large saucepan, combine 4 cups (1 L) water and adzuki beans and bring to a boil. Remove from heat, cover and let stand for 1 hour. Drain and rinse beans well.

2. Return beans to saucepan. Add 4 cups (1 L) fresh water and bring to a boil. Reduce heat to low, cover and simmer, stirring once or twice and adding more water if necessary, for 1½ to 2 hours or until beans are very tender. Remove from heat. Let cool in pan, uncovered, for 30 minutes. Drain well.

3. In a medium saucepan, combine 2½ cups (625 mL) water and rice. Bring to a boil. Reduce heat to low, cover and simmer for 30 to 45 minutes or until almost tender. Turn off heat and let pan stand, covered, on burner for 15 minutes. Let cool. Refrigerate for 2 hours.

This fortifying sautéed dish contains a number of ingredients that strengthen different parts of the body: the immune system (mushrooms); stomach and spleen, which are responsible for building overall vitality (rice and mushrooms); kidney *qi* (adzuki beans); and liver (greens, which clear heat and detoxify, thereby supporting the liver's *qi*-regulating and detoxifying functions).

4. In a large skillet, heat 2 tbsp (30 mL) of oil over medium-high heat. Add mushrooms and sauté until browned and almost no liquid remains, about 8 minutes. Stir in greens and sauté for 2 to 3 minutes or until wilted and no liquid remains. Transfer mushroom mixture to a medium bowl and stir in tamari. Set aside.

5. In the same skillet, heat remaining oil over medium-high heat. Using a spatula, spread rice in skillet to cover bottom of pan. Cook, without stirring, for 1 minute or until bottom is lightly browned. Turn rice and cook for 1 minute or until lightly browned. (Avoid stirring the rice, as that will make it gummy.)

6. Gently stir in beans and mushroom mixture. Remove from heat and sprinkle with green onions.

7. Spoon into serving bowls. Serve immediately.

Turkey Lion's Head Soup

Lion's head soup is a traditional dish in the cuisine of eastern China. The name comes from the meatballs, which were said to resemble a lion's head, and the added vegetables, which look like its mane. It is an easy, tasty soup to make and enjoy. Sweet potato lightens up the texture of these turkey-based meatballs, and flavorful minced green onions give them a little color. Mustard greens add a nice fresh touch to the soup.

MAKES 4 SERVINGS

Tips

Mirepoix is the French name for a blend of celery, onion and carrot that serves as a base for many soups. When a recipe says to cut vegetables "into a mirepoix," it means they should be diced finely, into about ¼- to ½-inch (0.5 to 1 cm) pieces.

Not feeling like soup? In a large skillet, heat 1 tbsp (15 mL) avocado oil over low heat. Add meatballs and cook, turning often to prevent sticking, for about 15 minutes or until no longer pink inside. Serve with a green vegetable on the side.

1	small sweet potato (about 8 oz/250 g)	1
1	large egg, beaten	1
1 lb	ground turkey (preferably thigh)	500 g
1½ tsp	salt, divided	7 mL
4	green onions, minced	4
1	stalk celery, finely diced (see tips, at left)	1
1	small bunch (12 oz/375 g) mustard greens, thinly shredded crosswise	1

1. Peel sweet potato and shred coarsely. Squeeze out liquid and place in a medium bowl.

2. Add egg, turkey, ½ tsp (2 mL) of the salt and green onions. Shape into 16 meatballs and place on a large plate or baking sheet. Cover and refrigerate for 2 hours or until well chilled, or for up to 24 hours.

3. In a medium saucepan, bring 4 cups (1 L) water and celery to a boil. Reduce heat to low and add meatballs and remaining salt. Simmer, stirring gently once or twice, for 10 minutes.

4. Gently stir in mustard greens and cook for 2 to 3 minutes or until greens are wilted and meatballs are no longer pink inside.

5. Ladle into serving bowls. Serve immediately.

> ## Health Tip
>
> This soup supports recovery from illness.
>
> Turkey is warming, sweet and drying. However, the mixture of neutral and sweet vegetables in the meatballs counters this drying effect. The flavorful mustard greens are pungent and warming — good for clearing phlegm from the lungs.

Duck Broth with Tatsoi

This soup is so rich and tasty! The simple flavor of the rich duck broth mixed with the slight bitterness of the greens creates a beautifully balanced dish. Try sprinkling Black and White Sesame Furikake (page 445) or Dried Lime Furikake (page 446) on top for two delicious variations.

MAKES 4 SERVINGS

Tip

Tatsoi is a delicious Asian green vegetable in the cabbage family. If it is unavailable, you can substitute bok choy or another similar green. If you are shopping in an Asian grocery store, it's always fun to try a new leafy green vegetable.

2	duck leg quarters (about 1½ lbs/750 g)	2
8 oz	tatsoi (see tip, at left), trimmed and cut crosswise into 1-inch (2.5 cm) pieces	250 g
2 tsp	salt	10 mL

1. In a large saucepan, combine duck and 4 cups (1 L) water. Bring to a boil, skimming any foam off surface. Reduce heat to low, cover and simmer for 2 hours or until duck is very tender.

2. Using a slotted spoon, transfer duck to a cutting board. Cut meat into bite-size pieces, discarding bones. Return to soup along with tatsoi and salt. Simmer, uncovered, for 10 minutes or until greens are wilted and tender.

3. Ladle into serving bowls. Serve immediately.

Health Tip

Duck meat tastes sweet and salty. It is neutral and enriches the body's yin while reinforcing the spleen. Duck promotes urination, so this soup is excellent for people who suffer from mild edema.

If you have a fever due to yin deficiency, a cough or a dry throat, duck cooked with asparagus root (called *tian hua fen* in Mandarin) will clear out heat, nurture the yin and moisten the mucous membranes. Avoid if you suffer from diarrhea.

Another recipe you might like to try is Duck Soup with Cordyceps (page 415). It is a delicious, healthy blood tonic.

Warming Winter Squash Soup

Sweet, earthy, deep and pungent flavors are what make this winter soup so enormously satisfying. The crunchy seed garnish is a lovely contrast to the tender vegetables and broth.

MAKES 4 SERVINGS

Tips

The baking pan dimensions aren't critical for toasting the seeds, so use whatever size you have in your cupboard.

If you like, you can use shelled raw pumpkin seeds (pepitas) instead of the seeds from the buttercup squash. Reduce roasting time to 10 minutes.

If napa cabbage is unavailable, use the regular green cabbage commonly found in North American grocery stores.

- **Preheat oven to 350°F (180°C)**
- **8-inch (20 cm) square metal baking pan (see tips, at left)**

¼ cup	buttercup squash seeds (see tips, at left)	60 mL
1	leek	1
2 tbsp	avocado oil	30 mL
4 cups	cubed peeled seeded buttercup squash	1 L
2 cups	coarsely chopped napa cabbage	500 mL
2 tsp	grated gingerroot	10 mL
2 tsp	salt	10 mL

1. Place seeds in baking pan. Roast in preheated oven for 15 minutes or until golden and fragrant. Let cool. Using clean pliers, remove shells from seeds and discard. (Or, using a rolling pin, gently tap seeds along edges to split open; discard shells.) Set seeds aside.

2. Trim roots and all but 3 inches (7.5 cm) of the dark green leaves off leek and discard. Cut leek in half lengthwise, then cut crosswise into ½-inch (1 cm) wide pieces. Rinse very well in 2 changes of water to remove grit.

3. In a medium saucepan, heat oil over medium-high heat. Add leek and sauté for about 5 minutes or until translucent and edges are lightly browned.

4. Add 4 cups (1 L) water, squash, cabbage, ginger and salt and bring to a simmer over medium-high heat. Reduce heat, cover and simmer for about 25 minutes or until squash is tender.

5. Ladle into serving bowls and sprinkle with seeds. Serve immediately.

Health Tips

Winter squash is a sweet, warming vegetable that nourishes and supports the digestive system. Warming, pungent leek and mild napa cabbage are also superior at promoting good digestion, while ginger is an outstanding herb for the stomach. This soup is a good remedy for people suffering from a cold, chills or a cough with clear phlegm. It also works well to combat indigestion.

Brothy Salmon and Ginger Soup

This comforting fish soup is subtly seasoned with fresh ginger. If you like your soup with more zip, increase the ginger juice to ¼ cup (60 mL).

MAKES 4 SERVINGS

Tip

To make ginger juice, grate fresh ginger and press it between your fingers or through a fine-mesh sieve into a bowl. Discard solids.

4 cups	Traditional Dashi (page 297)	1 L
2 tbsp	ginger juice (see tip, at left)	30 mL
2 tbsp	rice wine, such as sake	30 mL
2 oz	baby spinach	60 g
1 lb	boneless skinless salmon fillets, cut into 1-inch (2.5 cm) pieces	500 g

1. In a medium saucepan, bring dashi, ginger juice and rice wine to a simmer over medium-high heat.

2. Stir in spinach and cook for 2 to 3 minutes or just until wilted.

3. Remove from heat. Add salmon, cover and let stand for 5 minutes or until fish is just opaque.

4. Spoon into serving bowls. Serve immediately.

Health Tip

Salmon is rich in omega-3 fatty acids, which are anti-inflammatory and nourish the nervous system and brain. The warming and nourishing properties of this soup will benefit sluggish digestion, strengthen the *qi*, and enhance blood circulation. It is beneficial for people with diabetes, high cholesterol and high blood pressure, and for those who often feel cold and tired.

Tofu Vegetable Curry

This curry is delightfully sweet and mild, thanks to the winter squash and coconut milk. Serve it with your favorite chutney on the side — we recommend Endive, Raisin and Pine Nut Chutney (page 458).

MAKES 4 SERVINGS

Tip

The winter squashes we suggest have firm, dense flesh that holds up when cooked. Don't use acorn or delicata squash — they will turn to mush.

2 tbsp	avocado oil	30 mL
1 tbsp	curry powder	15 mL
1	clove garlic, minced	1
2 cups	cubed peeled seeded winter squash, such as buttercup, kabocha or turban	500 mL
4 oz	mixed baby greens, such as baby spinach, kale, bok choy, Swiss chard, beet greens or turnip greens	125 g
2 cups	coconut milk (see tips, page 303)	500 mL
2 tsp	salt	10 mL
1	package (14 oz to 1 lb/420 to 500 g) firm tofu, drained and cubed	1
¼ cup	coarsely chopped fresh cilantro or basil	60 mL

1. In a medium saucepan, heat oil over medium-low heat. Add curry powder and garlic and cook, stirring constantly, for 1 to 2 minutes or until garlic is fragrant and golden.

2. Stir in squash and cook, stirring often, for 5 minutes. Stir in greens and cook, stirring often, for 1 to 2 minutes or until greens are wilted and no liquid remains.

3. Stir in coconut milk and salt and bring to a simmer. Simmer, uncovered, for 12 to 15 minutes or until squash is tender. Gently stir in tofu cubes and remove pan from heat.

4. Spoon into serving bowls and sprinkle with cilantro. Serve immediately.

Health Tips

Tofu, a sweet and cooling food, is also considered a *qi* tonic. It is good, in small amounts, as a source of protein for vegetarians.

The warming winter squash, aromatic spices and garlic in this dish balance the cooling aspect of the tofu, making it an appropriate winter meal.

Trout Steamed with Green Peas and Lemony Herbed Rice

Steaming foods enhances their juiciness and flavor. It is a terrific way to cook fish, because it comes out moist and delectable. This light, fresh and warming dish is so welcome in the dark winter months.

MAKES 4 SERVINGS

Tip

The acid from the lemon juice will turn the herbs olive green, but they will still taste fresh.

1 cup	brown jasmine rice	250 mL
1/2 cup	packed chopped fresh parsley and/or trimmed arugula	125 mL
1 tbsp	minced fresh chives	15 mL
1/2 tsp	grated lemon zest	2 mL
1 tbsp	freshly squeezed lemon juice	15 mL
2 tsp	salt, divided	10 mL
1 tbsp	ghee	15 mL
2 cups	fresh shelled or thawed frozen green peas	500 mL
4	boneless skinless trout fillets (about 1 1/2 lbs/750 g)	4
4	lemon wedges	4

1. In a medium saucepan, combine $2\frac{1}{2}$ cups (625 mL) water and rice. Bring to a boil. Reduce heat to low, cover and simmer for 30 to 45 minutes or until almost tender. Turn off heat and let stand on burner for 15 minutes. Add parsley, chives, lemon zest, lemon juice and 1 tsp (5 mL) of the salt. Using a fork, gently fluff rice mixture.

2. Meanwhile, in a medium saucepan, heat ghee over medium heat. Add peas and lay trout over top. Cover and steam, shaking pan 2 or 3 times, for 3 to 4 minutes or until fish is just opaque. Uncover pan and remove from heat.

3. Divide rice among serving plates. Top with peas and trout. Sprinkle trout with remaining salt. Serve immediately with lemon wedges.

Health Tip

Trout is warming and sweet. It nourishes and supports *qi* and yang. This dish is beneficial for people who have poor appetite, feel weak and/or often have cold hands and feet. The peas are sweet and nourishing; the pungent herbs, and bitter and sour lemon, contribute to the light flavor and easy palatability of this delicious fish.

Braised Duck with Lotus Seeds

This simply seasoned duck with nutty lotus seeds banishes the chill on a cold day. Adding a chutney-style condiment or pickle that suits your preference is a nice complement to the rich meat — turn to pages 422 to 465 to find your favorite.

MAKES 4 SERVINGS

Tip

Many lotus seeds contain added sulfites; read ingredient labels carefully and avoid them. The best sources for sulfite-free lotus seeds are Chinese herb suppliers (see Resources, page 466).

½ cup	dried lotus seeds	125 mL
1 tbsp	avocado oil	15 mL
4	duck leg quarters (about 2 lbs/1 kg)	4
2 cups	duck broth or chicken broth	500 mL
½ cup	rice wine, such as sake	125 mL
¼ cup	tamari or soy sauce	60 mL
1 tbsp	slivered gingerroot	15 mL
2 tbsp	chopped fresh cilantro or green onions	30 mL

1. In a medium bowl, combine 2 cups (500 mL) water and lotus seeds. Cover and set aside.

2. In a large saucepan, heat oil over medium-high heat, swirling to coat bottom of pan. Add duck pieces and cook, turning once, until browned on both sides Reduce heat to medium-low, cover and cook, turning once or twice, for 30 minutes.

3. Transfer duck to a plate and drain fat from pan (do not wipe out). Return duck to pan along with broth, wine, tamari and ginger. Bring to a boil. Reduce heat to low, cover and simmer for 30 minutes.

4. Drain lotus seeds and add to duck mixture. Simmer, uncovered, for 30 minutes or until duck is very tender and sauce is lightly syrupy.

5. Spoon duck and sauce onto serving plates. Sprinkle with cilantro. Serve immediately.

Health Tip

Duck cooked with lotus seeds can help with difficult urination and mild edema. You can also add hato mugi (at the same time as the lotus seeds) to make this dish more effective at clearing dampness and water retention.

Spaghetti Squash with Aromatic Ground Beef

The vegetables take center stage in this hearty main dish. Spaghetti squash is a winter squash with a hard, pale yellow skin. When cooked, the flesh can be easily separated into thin, noodle-like strands. You only need half of the spaghetti squash for this recipe, so save the leftovers and serve them topped with your favorite pasta sauce another day.

MAKES 4 SERVINGS

Tip

If spaghetti squash is not available, roast a different kind of winter squash as described. Cut it into wedges and serve topped with the beef mixture.

Health Tips

Beef is very nourishing and warming. It enriches the *qi* and blood, so this dish is excellent for people who feel fatigued, weak and cold. The spaghetti squash is also sweet and nourishing to the stomach and spleen.

If you tend to run warm or hot, eat more vegetables and only condiment-sized portions of meat. Meat is warming and can aggravate warm or hot conditions.

- **Preheat oven to 350°F (180°C)**
- **13- by 9-inch (33 by 23 cm) glass baking dish**

1	spaghetti squash (4 lbs/2 kg)	1
1 lb	ground beef	500 g
½	large onion, minced	½
8 oz	snow peas, trimmed and halved crosswise	250 g
½ cup	thinly sliced tender greens, such as arugula or mustard	125 mL
2 tbsp	tomato paste	30 mL
2 tbsp	tamari or soy sauce	30 mL
1 tbsp	grated gingerroot	15 mL

1. Cut squash in half lengthwise and scrape out seeds. Place squash halves, cut sides down, in baking dish and add about ½ inch (1 cm) water. Bake in preheated oven for 1 hour or until squash collapses slightly and is tender.

2. Meanwhile, in a large skillet, cook beef and onion over medium-high heat, breaking up with a spoon, until beef is no longer pink and onions are soft.

3. Drain off any fat in pan. Stir in snow peas, greens, tomato paste, tamari and ginger. Reduce heat to medium and cook, stirring often, for about 5 minutes or until snow peas are tender-crisp.

4. Using a fork, scrape out insides of 1 of the squash halves, discarding skin. (Save the other squash half for another use). Spoon squash strands onto serving plates and top with beef mixture. Serve immediately.

Nourishing Lamb Stew with Butternut Squash and Dang Gui

This nourishing and comforting lamb stew is perfect if you often tend to feel cold. The addition of warming and aromatic spices further enhances its healing qualities. The recipe was inspired by and adapted from a recipe by Nina Simonds in her book A Spoonful of Ginger. We've added herbs that are typical in Chinese medicinal soups; they are especially beneficial for women and people with circulation issues. Serve as-is or over steamed brown rice.

MAKES 6 SERVINGS

Tips

We like to use grass-fed lamb in this recipe. If you want a meatier dish, you can increase the amount to 3 lbs (1.5 kg).

Heating the spices in oil builds a deep flavor base for the stew. We remove the Sichuan peppercorns after this step so that you don't end up biting into a nugget of numbing, spicy pepper in the finished dish.

Dang gui and Sichuan peppercorns are available online, and in Asian grocery stores, Chinese medicinal herb stores and specialty spice shops. Dang gui is usually sold dried and sliced.

2 lbs	trimmed cubed lamb shoulder or lamb stewing cubes (1½-inch/ 4 cm cubes)	1 kg
1 oz	dried dang gui (see tips, at left)	30 g
1	butternut squash (about 2 lbs/1 kg), peeled, seeded and cut into 1½-inch (4 cm) cubes	1
1	bunch Swiss chard (12 oz/375 g), stemmed and cut into 2-inch (5 cm) wide ribbons	1

Sauce Mixture

¼ cup	tamari or soy sauce	60 mL
¼ cup	rice wine, such as sake	60 mL
1 tbsp	coconut sugar or Demerara sugar	15 mL

Spice Mixture

1 tbsp	coconut oil or avocado oil	15 mL
1 tsp	Sichuan peppercorns, shiny black seeds removed	5 mL
9	slices (quarter-size) gingerroot, lightly crushed	9
8	green onions, trimmed and cut into 1-inch (2.5 cm) pieces, lightly crushed	8
3	cloves garlic, smashed and thinly sliced	3
2	pieces (2 inches/5 cm long each) cinnamon sticks	2
2	whole star anise	2

1. *Sauce Mixture:* In a medium bowl, stir together 5 cups (1.25 L) water, tamari, wine and coconut sugar. Set aside.

2. *Spice Mixture:* In a Dutch oven, heat oil over medium heat. Add Sichuan peppercorns and cook, stirring, for 15 to 30 seconds or until grayish. Using a slotted soon, remove Sichuan peppercorns and discard. Add ginger, green onions, garlic, cinnamon sticks and star anise to pan and cook, stirring, for about 15 seconds or until fragrant.

Variation

Ellen discovered this vegan variation while teaching (vegetarian) students to cook with medicinal herbs. It is nourishing, aromatic and rich tasting. Substitute two 15½-oz (439 g) cans chickpeas, drained and rinsed, for the lamb. Or cook them from scratch: soak 1½ cups (375 mL) dried chickpeas in 5 cups (1.25 mL) water overnight or for up to 8 hours. Drain and rinse well. In a large saucepan, combine chickpeas, 4 cups (1 L) fresh water and 1 piece (1 inch/2.5 cm square) dried kombu. Bring to a boil. Reduce heat to low and simmer for 1½ hours or until tender. Reserving cooking liquid, drain chickpeas well. Use reserved cooking liquid in place of some of the water in Step 1. To cook the stew, complete Steps 1 and 2. Stir in chickpeas. Reduce cooking time in Step 4 to 15 minutes. Add squash in Step 5 and reduce cooking time to 20 to 30 minutes. Continue with recipe.

3. Add lamb to spice mixture. Cook, turning often, for about 5 to 7 minutes or until browned on all sides.

4. Pour in sauce mixture and bring to a boil. Reduce heat and stir in dang gui. Partially cover and simmer, stirring every 30 minutes and skimming off any foam or fat that rises to the surface, for 2 hours or until lamb is fork-tender.

5. Stir in squash. Partially cover and cook, stirring occasionally and skimming off any foam or fat that rises to the surface, for 30 to 60 minutes or until squash is tender. Discard cinnamon sticks, ginger and star anise.

6. Stir in Swiss chard. Partially cover and cook for 5 minutes or until wilted and tender.

7. Spoon into serving bowls. Serve immediately.

Health Tips

Lamb is a warming, blood-building meat, and long cooking enhances these effects. In Chinese medicine, blood is considered a woman's essence, so this is a great dish for promoting female health. It is also excellent for anyone who habitually feels cold in the winter. However, if your body tends to run hot, it may be best to skip this stew.

The herb dang gui is used in Chinese herbal medicine to nourish, warm and enhance circulation, and is often administered to treat menstrual disorders. The herb is added to stews, soups, teas or tonic wines to support the yin and blood.

The ginger and dang gui in this stew echo the ingredients in a traditional Chinese medicinal lamb soup called *qian jin yao fang*, which was given to postpartum women experiencing cold in the abdomen.

The longer you cook this stew, the stronger its therapeutic value. The meat will also break down and be easier to digest and absorb.

Sake-Braised Shiitake Mushrooms with Vegetables and Kombu

This is a variation on nishime, a traditional Japanese simmered dish. It is usually sweet, served as a complement to bitter or astringent foods. The earthy and savory flavors of the shiitake and kombu harmonize with the root vegetables to make this a delicious one-pot meal.

MAKES 4 SERVINGS

Tip

You can substitute other root vegetables, such as rutabagas or turnips, for the carrots, parsnips or daikon.

Health Tip

This dish is especially harmonizing for the body; it supports and builds *qi* and the immune system.

- **1-quart (1 L) canning jar**

1 cup	dried shiitake mushrooms (8 to 12)	250 mL
	Warm water	
2	pieces (each 4 inches/10 cm square) dried kombu	2
2	large carrots	2
2	large parsnips	2
½	large daikon radish (1½-lb/750 g radish)	½
½ cup	rice wine, such as sake	125 mL
2 tbsp	tamari or soy sauce	30 mL
1 tsp	toasted sesame oil	5 mL
2 tbsp	white sesame seeds, toasted (see tip, page 387)	30 mL

1. Place shiitake mushrooms in jar and pour in enough warm water to fill. Seal lid and let stand, shaking jar once or twice, for 6 to 8 hours.

2. Reserving 2 cups (500 mL) of the soaking liquid, drain mushrooms. Trim off and discard stems. Cut caps into quarters and place in a medium bowl. Set aside.

3. In a medium saucepan, combine 4 cups (1 L) water and kombu. Bring to a boil. Turn off heat and let stand on burner for 10 minutes. Drain and cut kombu into 1-inch (2.5 cm) squares.

4. Peel and cut carrots, parsnips and daikon into 1-inch (2.5 cm) chunks. In a medium saucepan, combine mushrooms, reserved soaking liquid, kombu, carrots, parsnips, daikon, wine and tamari. Bring to a simmer over medium-high heat. Reduce heat to low and cook, stirring often, for 5 to 7 minutes or until carrots are almost tender.

5. Increase heat to high and cook, shaking pan often, for 1 to 2 minutes or until almost no liquid remains.

6. Spoon into serving bowls. Drizzle with sesame oil and sprinkle with sesame seeds. Serve immediately.

Bitter Melon with Shrimp

Bitter melon is an extraordinary food that is — as the name implies — very bitter. As Ellen's first herbalist said, "The stronger the bitter flavor, the better." Blanching the slices diminishes that a bit to make this dish more delicious, especially when accompanied by shrimp and pungent herbs. Serve this intensely flavored combination with a bland side, such as rice or water-sautéed vegetables, to balance it.

MAKES 4 SIDE-DISH SERVINGS

Tip

There are two varieties of bitter melon. One is shiny and light green, with smooth, elongated bumps. The other is darker green with sharp, pointy bumps. We prefer the latter for its firmer texture.

Caution

Pregnant women and nursing mothers should avoid bitter melon, as it's contraindicated for them. If you are trying to conceive, be moderate in your bitter melon intake. Eating too much can cause digestive issues, such as bloating, diarrhea or abdominal cramping. In pregnancy, the medicinal element, *Momordica charantia*, can cause toxicity in some people. It also can disturb the fetus and cause premature labor.

---

8 oz	bitter melons (2 or 3 small)	250 g
1 tsp	salt	5 mL
2 tbsp	avocado oil	30 mL
2 tsp	minced gingerroot	10 mL
2 tbsp	minced fresh basil	30 mL
1	clove garlic, minced	1
2 tbsp	tamari or soy sauce	30 mL
8 oz	cooked peeled deveined shrimp, chopped	250 g

1. Cut bitter melons in half lengthwise and scrape out seeds and white pulp. Cut crosswise into $1/8$-inch (3 mm) thick slices. In a medium bowl, toss bitter melon slices with salt and let stand for 30 minutes.

2. In a medium saucepan, bring 4 cups (1 L) water to a boil. Drain bitter melon and add to pan. Return to a boil. Remove from heat and drain well.

3. In a large skillet, heat oil over medium-high heat. Add bitter melon, ginger, basil and garlic and cook, stirring often, for 5 to 7 minutes or just until bitter melon is tender.

4. Stir in tamari and cook for 3 to 5 minutes or until almost no liquid remains. Remove from heat and stir in shrimp.

5. Spoon into serving dishes. Serve immediately.

Health Tips

The famous Chinese medicine book *Shen Nong Ben Cao Jing* (*The Divine Farmers' Materia Medica*) states that "bitter gourd is bitter in taste, cold in nature and has the ability to clear the body of summer heat." Its main therapeutic use is in the treatment of diabetes. In Asia it is also eaten as a treatment for malaria. It clears liver heat, purifies the blood and is a digestive stimulant.

Bitter melon is a powerfully bitter food that is wonderful to eat — once you have acquired a taste for it. Stick with it if you don't like it at first. It may take a few tries, but you will welcome it!

Kimchi and Lotus Root Salad

Adding some healthy probiotic foods to your diet is easy when you have this recipe. The mild sweetness and crunchiness of the lotus root is complemented by the tart funkiness of the fermented kimchi. It's delicious as a condiment with cooked sweet vegetables, such as winter squash.

> **MAKES GENEROUS 1 CUP (250 ML), ABOUT 2 SERVINGS**

Tips

When we say to let a food stand at room temperature, that is about 68°F (20°C). It's fine if it is cooler in your kitchen, but if it is warmer, only let the mixture stand for 2 hours, then refrigerate.

Although kimchi can be very spicy, only a small amount is used in this recipe, so it is relatively mild.

- **2-cup (500 mL) canning jar**

8 oz	lotus root	250 g
2 tbsp	finely chopped unpasteurized kimchi (radish or cabbage type)	30 mL
¼ tsp	kosher or non-iodized sea salt	1 mL

1. Pour enough water into a medium saucepan to come 2 inches (5 cm) up side. Bring to a simmer.

2. Trim ends off lotus roots and peel. Immediately immerse in simmering water and cook for 25 to 30 minutes or until tender. Drain and let cool to room temperature.

3. Cut lotus root into ⅛-inch (3 mm) thick slices. In jar, combine lotus root, kimchi and salt. Seal lid and gently shake jar to make sure lotus root is evenly coated with juice and salt. Cover jar mouth with a paper towel and let stand at room temperature for 24 hours (see tips, at left).

4. Remove paper towel and seal jar with lid. Shake vigorously to mix. Refrigerate for at least 2 hours before serving or for up to 1 week.

> ### Health Tip
>
> Fermented foods like kimchi add beneficial bacteria to your gut, boosting immunity and improving digestion. Add small amounts of them to your diet daily.
>
> Lotus root benefits digestion and is cooling.

Creamy Cabbage Salad

Cabbage is so delightful, sweet and mild when it's cooked. The tart creaminess of the dressing complements its light sweetness in this highly nutritious salad.

MAKES 4 SERVINGS

Tip

To toast sesame seeds, place them in a medium dry skillet over low heat. Toast, stirring or shaking pan constantly, for about 3 minutes or until fragrant.

- **Blender or food processor**

½	package (14 oz to 1 lb/420 to 500 g package) soft or medium tofu, drained	½
2 tbsp	mashed pitted umeboshi (see health tips, below)	30 mL
2 tbsp	white miso	30 mL
2 tbsp	avocado oil	30 mL
1 tsp	coconut sugar	5 mL
½ tsp	salt	2 mL
1	small head green cabbage	1
2 tbsp	sesame seeds (preferably black), toasted (see tip, at left)	30 mL

1. In blender, combine tofu, umeboshi, miso, oil, coconut sugar and salt. Purée until smooth. Set aside.

2. Core cabbage and cut into 1-inch (2.5 cm) chunks. Meanwhile, in a medium saucepan, bring 4 cups (1 L) water to a boil. Add cabbage and cook for 3 to 4 minutes or just until tender. Drain well.

3. In a serving bowl, gently toss cabbage with dressing until coated. Sprinkle with sesame seeds. Serve immediately.

Health Tips

Cabbage is sweet, neutral and most beneficial for the stomach and spleen. It's especially good for soothing spasms and mild discomfort in the upper abdomen.

Tofu is cooling and lubricating, and adds excellent nourishment to this dish.

Umeboshi plums contain a large amount of citric acid, which aids digestion in the stomach by increasing the volume of hydrochloric acid it needs to work. Umeboshi help relieve indigestion and mild morning sickness; simply steep an umeboshi plum in boiling water and drink. These plums are extremely salty, so be prepared.

Curly Endive and Apple Chopped Salad with Candied Walnuts

Even in the dead of winter, we often crave crisp, fresh salads. This one focuses on curly endive, a bitter type of lettuce. Quickly blanched, it offers a tender contrast to the crunchy apples and walnuts.

MAKES 4 SERVINGS

Tip

Blanching not only softens the endive a bit but also makes it easier to digest.

- **1-quart (1 L) canning jar**

2 tbsp	unfiltered cider vinegar	30 mL
2 tbsp	avocado oil	30 mL
2 tbsp	roasted walnut oil or toasted sesame oil	30 mL
¼ tsp	salt	1 mL
¼ tsp	cayenne pepper	1 mL
2	large tart apples, such as Granny Smith or Pink Lady	2
1	head curly endive	1
1 cup	Candied Walnuts (see recipe, opposite)	250 mL

1. In jar, combine vinegar, avocado oil, walnut oil, salt and cayenne. Seal with lid and shake until well combined.

2. Quarter, core and cut apples into ½-inch (1 cm) cubes. Add to dressing and turn jar gently to mix.

3. Trim endive and cut crosswise into 1-inch (2.5 cm) wide slices. In a medium saucepan, bring 4 cups (1 L) water to a boil. Add endive, stir once and immediately drain. Let cool.

4. In a serving bowl, toss together endive, apple mixture and walnuts until coated. Serve immediately.

Health Tips

Apples are sweet and sour at the same time. Partnered with lightly bitter walnuts, pungent spices and salt, they help make this salad a very balanced dish. Be sure to eat it if you suffer from headaches, hypertension or high cholesterol.

Eating bitter foods in the winter helps the body store energy and provides a vent through which excess heat can clear out. Building internal warmth in the cold months is important to counter external cold, but balance is most important. Bitter foods help balance excessive heat from building up in the body, which can be too drying and thereby injure the yin.

Candied Walnuts

This recipe makes double the amount of walnuts you will need for the salad on this page. Enjoy the leftovers as snacks.

MAKES 2 CUPS (500 ML)			
1 tbsp	avocado oil		15 mL
2 cups	walnut halves		500 mL
2 tbsp	coconut sugar		30 mL
2 tbsp	liquid honey		30 mL
¼ tsp	salt		1 mL
¼ tsp	ground cinnamon		1 mL
¼ tsp	ground ginger		1 mL

1. Place a large piece of parchment paper or buttered foil on a heatproof surface.

2. In a large heavy skillet, heat oil over medium heat. Add walnuts and cook, stirring often with a heatproof spatula, for 2 minutes. Stir in coconut sugar, honey and salt and cook, stirring, for 2 minutes or until fragrant.

3. Remove pan from heat. Stir in cinnamon and ginger. Immediately spread nut mixture in a single layer on parchment paper. (Be careful, as the nuts and sugar mixture are very hot.) Let cool to room temperature.

4. Serve immediately or store in an airtight container for up to 1 week.

Braised Mixed Greens with Lemon Rind Pickle and Eggs

You can never eat too many leafy greens. And it's hard to get bored by them, because there are so many varieties to choose from. Here, simple wilted greens are perked up by a zippy citrus rind pickle and enhanced with fried eggs.

<table>
<tr><td>2 tbsp</td><td>avocado oil, divided</td><td>30 mL</td></tr>
<tr><td>8 oz</td><td>leafy greens (see tip, at left), stemmed and chopped</td><td>250 g</td></tr>
<tr><td>4</td><td>large eggs</td><td>4</td></tr>
<tr><td></td><td>Lemon Rind Pickle (see recipe, opposite)</td><td></td></tr>
</table>

MAKES 4 SERVINGS

1. In a large skillet, heat 1 tbsp (15 mL) of the oil over medium-high heat, swirling pan to coat bottom. Add greens and cook, stirring often, for 3 to 5 minutes or until wilted and tender. Remove from heat and divide among serving bowls. Keep warm.

2. Return pan to medium heat and heat remaining oil over medium-high heat. Break eggs into pan and cook to desired doneness.

3. Place 1 egg in each bowl and top with some of the pickle. Serve immediately.

Tip

Some of the more unusual varieties of leafy greens — such as amaranth, water spinach, pea shoots and Chinese broccoli (*gai lan*) — will work well in this recipe. The cooking time will vary depending on the variety, so watch carefully to avoid overcooking them.

Health Tip

Leafy greens are cooling, renewing and detoxifying. Their flavors range from slightly sweet to pungent to sour to bitter, so look for and try new varieties whenever possible. If you suffer from headaches or high blood pressure, include greens in your daily diet.

Lemon Rind Pickle

Try this tangy condiment to balance other dishes or to pep up plain foods.

- 1-cup (250 mL) canning jar

2 or 3	large lemons	2 or 3
¼ cup	chopped pitted dates	60 mL
1 tsp	salt	5 mL

1. Halve 2 of the lemons and squeeze juice into a bowl. Set aside. Using a metal spoon, scrape out membranes from lemon halves and discard, leaving white pith intact. Coarsely chop rinds and measure. If 2 lemons do not yield enough rind to make ½ cup (125 mL), use third lemon.

2. In a medium saucepan, combine 4 cups (1 L) water and lemon rind. Bring to a boil. Remove from heat, cover and let stand for 10 minutes. Drain and repeat twice, using fresh water each time.

3. In jar, combine blanched rind, 2 tbsp (30 mL) of the reserved lemon juice, the dates and salt. Seal with lid and shake well to combine. Serve immediately or refrigerate for up to 1 week.

Health Tip

Lemon rind is bitter and sour, so it cools and detoxifies the body. It is also rich in vitamin C, flavonoids and antioxidants. This lightly brined pickle contains beneficial bacteria and helps digestion.

Hijiki and Carrot Sauté with Ginger

Hijiki is packed with minerals and fiber. This dark, firm, yet subtly flavored seaweed has long been a staple in Japanese cuisine. It grows off the coasts of Japan, Korea and China but was only introduced into other countries in the last 50 years. Ellen learned how to make this easy, tasty and nutritious recipe when she was studying macrobiotics. It is a hearty, healthy small side dish.

> **MAKES 4 SERVINGS**

Tips

Some seaweed can contain unhealthy levels of contaminants. Hijiki has been found to sometimes contain a higher-than-normal level of inorganic arsenic. Be sure to check that your preferred brand has been tested for heavy metals and is safe to consume. See Resources, page 466.

Always rinse dried seaweed well before adding it to recipes.

½ cup	dried hijiki	125 mL
1 tsp	avocado oil	5 mL
2 tsp	chopped gingerroot	10 mL
2	small to medium carrots, julienned	2
1 tbsp	rice wine, such as sake	15 mL
1 tbsp	tamari or soy sauce	15 mL
1	green onion, finely chopped	1

1. Place hijiki in a medium bowl and cover with water. Let stand for 15 to 20 minutes or until rehydrated. Drain well, discarding soaking liquid.

2. In a medium skillet, heat oil over medium heat. Add ginger and cook, stirring, for about 30 seconds or until fragrant. Add carrots and cook, stirring often, for about 2 minutes or until softened.

3. Stir in hijiki and rice wine. Reduce heat, cover and simmer for 5 minutes. Stir in tamari and cook for 5 minutes or until flavors meld.

4. Spoon into serving dishes and sprinkle with green onion. Serve immediately.

> ### Health Tip
>
> Hijiki seaweed is salty, cooling and rich in minerals, including iodine (which is essential for hormonal health, particularly in the thyroid), iron, magnesium and calcium. It is touted for its health benefits because it lowers cholesterol as part of a balanced diet and detoxifies the body; it also nourishes hair, skin and nails. However, more is not better — seaweed is best consumed regularly in small, condiment-size amounts.

Sautéed Curly Endive and Chestnuts with Mushrooms

Bitter, sweet and comforting are the themes of this surprising winter dish. The earthiness of the chestnuts and mushrooms tempers the bitterness of the greens.

MAKES 4 SERVINGS

Tip

To prepare 3 oz (90 g) cooked peeled chestnuts, start with 6 oz (175 g) fresh chestnuts. Using a sharp knife, cut an X in the back of each. In a medium saucepan, combine 4 cups (1 L) water and chestnuts and bring to a boil. Boil for 20 minutes or until tender. Drain and let cool enough to handle. Peel off outer peel and inner skin. Refrigerate for up to 1 week.

1	head curly endive or escarole	1
2 tbsp	avocado oil	30 mL
8 oz	cremini or button mushrooms, stemmed and halved	250 g
1 tsp	grated gingerroot	5 mL
3 oz	cooked peeled chestnuts (see tip, at left)	90 g
1 tsp	salt	5 mL

1. Trim curly endive and cut crosswise into 1-inch (2.5 cm) pieces.

2. In a large skillet, heat 1 tbsp (15 mL) of the oil over medium-high heat. Add mushrooms and cook, stirring often, for 5 to 7 minutes or until almost no liquid remains. Transfer mushrooms to a plate and set aside.

3. Heat remaining oil in pan. Add endive and ginger. Cook, stirring often, for 3 to 5 minutes or until greens are wilted. Stir in mushrooms, chestnuts and salt. Remove from heat.

4. Spoon into serving bowls. Serve immediately.

Health Tips

Bitter greens should definitely be on your table during the winter. Curly endive is cooling in nature, with a specific affinity for the liver. It also builds the blood and enhances circulation. It contains high levels of inulin, a type of dietary fiber, which helps regulate blood sugar levels in people who have diabetes. In this dish, it's combined with the yang-building *qi* of chestnuts and the immune-boosting powers of mushrooms, and helps warm you up without requiring a ton of cooking.

Chestnuts are sweet and astringent, so they help remedy loose stools caused by cold weather or consumption of too many cold foods. They also soothe coughs and have been used to stanch nosebleeds. They are made into flour in many areas of the world due to their high carbohydrate and low oil content.

Roasted Chunky Root Vegetables with Tangy Tahini Dressing

Roasted vegetables are completely satisfying on days when you want something substantial but simple to prepare. The earthy sweetness of root vegetables is enhanced by the caramelization that occurs when they're roasted at a high temperature. The tangy dressing offers a nice contrast.

MAKES 4 SERVINGS		

- **Preheat oven to 400°F (200°C), with racks positioned in upper and lower thirds**
- **2 large rimmed baking sheets**

1	large turnip, cubed	1
1	large carrot, cubed	1
2 tbsp	avocado oil, divided	30 mL
1	Asian sweet potato, peeled and cubed	1
1	sweet potato (orange Western type), peeled and cubed	1
	Tangy Tahini Dressing (see recipe, opposite)	
2 tbsp	minced fresh parsley	30 mL

1. On 1 of the baking sheets, toss together turnip, carrot and 1 tbsp (15 mL) of the oil.

2. On remaining baking sheet, toss together Asian sweet potato, orange sweet potato and remaining oil. Roast in preheated oven, stirring 2 or 3 times, for about 20 minutes or until vegetables are tender. (Turnip and carrot may take slightly longer to cook than sweet potatoes.)

3. In a serving bowl, combine turnip, carrot, Asian sweet potato and orange sweet potato. Gently toss with dressing until coated. Sprinkle with parsley.

4. Spoon into serving bowls. Serve immediately.

Health Tip

Nourishing sweet vegetables boost *qi*, warm the stomach, and dispel congestion and dampness. The tahini dressing nourishes the blood and benefits the eyes. It is considered a yin tonic, which boosts breast-milk flow in nursing mothers and promotes regular bowel movements (as it is moistening and lubricating to the intestines). It also remedies weakness and is beneficial for people with anemia.

Tangy Tahini Dressing

This nutty, tangy and spicy dressing is also delightful on cooked winter vegetables, braised or steamed greens, or your favorite thin noodles with cooked greens on the side.

**MAKES ABOUT
3/4 CUP (175 ML)**

Tip

To make ginger juice, grate ginger and press it through a fine-mesh sieve into a bowl. Discard solids.

1/4 cup	tahini	60 mL
3 tbsp	unseasoned rice vinegar	45 mL
1 tbsp	toasted sesame oil	15 mL
2 tsp	coconut sugar	10 mL
1 tsp	ginger juice (see tip, at left)	5 mL
1/2 tsp	salt	2 mL

1. In a small bowl, whisk together 1/4 cup (60 mL) water, tahini, rice vinegar, sesame oil, coconut sugar, ginger juice and salt until smooth.

Aromatic Nut Mix

Unlike typical sweet-and-spicy nut mixes, this snack blend finds its balance between bitter and savory elements. As such, it is a lovely winter snack and accompaniment to beverages.

> **MAKES ABOUT**
> **3 CUPS (750 ML)**

Tip

When using rose petals in cooking, always make sure to choose unsprayed ones. This will keep unwanted pesticides and contaminants out of your food.

- **Mortar and pestle, or spice grinder**

2 tsp	caraway seeds	10 mL
2 tsp	food-grade dried red rose petals (see tip, at left)	10 mL
1 tsp	salt	5 mL
1 cup	unsalted raw peanuts	250 mL
1 cup	unsalted raw cashews	250 mL
1 cup	unsalted raw pistachios	250 mL
1 tbsp	ghee	15 mL
2 tsp	smoked paprika	10 mL

1. Place a large piece of parchment paper or lightly oiled foil on a heatproof surface.

2. In mortar with pestle, grind together caraway seeds, rose petals and salt until powdery. Set aside.

3. In a large dry skillet, toast peanuts, cashews and pistachios over medium-low heat, stirring often, for 5 to 10 minutes or until golden and fragrant.

4. Stir in ghee and caraway seed mixture. Cook, stirring constantly, for 30 seconds. Stir in paprika and remove from heat. Scrape nut mixture onto parchment paper and let cool completely.

5. Serve immediately or store in an airtight container at room temperature for up to 5 days.

> ### Health Tip
>
> In Chinese medicine, roses are used to move and regulate *qi*, as well as to move stagnant energy. Rose petals are often added to teas, syrups, spice mixtures, tinctures and wines. The mixture of fragrant roses, pungent and aromatic caraway and smoky paprika in this snack mix enhances the digestibility of the nuts. In Persian and other Middle Eastern cuisines, rose petals are often added to spice mixtures to give them a beautiful, floral fragrance and taste. Rose water — another delicious way to enjoy this flower — can be added to beverages, teas and desserts (try our Autumn Fruit Salad with Rose Syrup, page 360).

Ginger and Mint Tea

The robust, cooling aroma of mint balances the pungent, warming ginger in this tea. This combination makes it a beneficial digestive.

Tips

Peppermint is slightly less sharply flavored than spearmint, which you could use to make a variation.

Using ⅛ to ¼ tsp (0.5 to 1 mL) dried sliced ginger in place of fresh will yield a spicier, more warming tea.

It can be tough to find fresh peppermint in the dead of winter. Buy dried peppermint leaves in bulk and store them in a glass jar in a dark cool place so you have this herb on hand whenever you need it.

2	slices (quarter-size) gingerroot	2
2 tbsp	dried peppermint (or 12 fresh peppermint leaves)	30 mL
	Lemon wedges (optional)	
	Liquid honey (optional)	

1. Using the edge of a spoon or the back of a knife, crush ginger. In a small saucepan, combine 2 cups (500 mL) water and ginger. Bring to a boil.

2. Reduce heat and stir in mint.

3. Let stand for 5 to 10 minutes or until fragrant and light brown. (Do not steep for more than 10 minutes or the tea will taste slightly bitter.)

4. Strain into teacups. Add a squeeze of lemon and/or honey to taste (if using). Drink hot or let cool slightly.

Health Tips

Ginger and mint are beneficial digestives. They're also good at stopping an impending cold or sore throat in its tracks. If you are suffering from a sore throat, add honey to make the tea more soothing.

Peppermint is pungent and cooling. Because of its *qi*-moving properties, it is also good for calming stress, reducing muscle tension and soothing stomach pain or cramping.

Ginger is one of the queens of the herbal kitchen. It adds lively flavor to many foods and teas, and has potent medicinal properties. It improves digestion, and relieves nausea, headaches and colds. We like to always keep fresh ginger on hand — you never know when you might need it.

Ginger and Orange Rind Tea with Honey

This is a warming, digestive tea that smells heavenly, thanks to the aromatic fresh ginger and orange rind. It is simple to make and a wonderful drink to sip prior to or after a meal.

3	slices (quarter-size) gingerroot	3
1	piece (2 inches/5 cm long) orange or tangerine rind	1
	Liquid honey (optional)	

MAKES 2 SERVINGS

Tip

Orange peel contains fragrant and health-enhancing essential oil. Use a sharp vegetable peeler or paring knife to slice it, making sure not to include any of the bitter white pith.

1. In a small saucepan, bring 2 cups (500 mL) water to a boil. Stir in ginger and orange rind. Reduce heat and simmer for 5 minutes or until fragrant.

2. Strain into teacups. Add honey to taste (if using). Drink hot or let cool slightly.

Health Tips

Ginger is a champion when it comes to warming the body and easing stomach distress. It is the go-to remedy for nausea and indigestion, and orange or tangerine peel augments its digestion-supporting powers. Drink the tea as you wish, sweetened with honey or without. It's wonderful for young and old alike.

Dried orange peel and tangerine peel are often used in Chinese medicinal teas, but fresh is a delicious alternative. The peel is beneficial for people who suffer from mild bloating or belching after eating. It also can be helpful in clearing out phlegm if you have a cough.

Kumquat Electuary Tea

This slow-cooked electuary (see tips, below) of kumquat, honey and ginger is an adaptation of a tried-and-true home remedy for a cough. It is delicious on its own, but is most effective when added to hot water and drunk as a tea to clear up a wet cough.

1 lb	kumquats, cut crosswise into ¼-inch (0.5 cm) thick slices	500 g
½ cup	liquid honey	125 mL
1 tbsp	ginger juice (see tips, at left)	15 mL

1. In a small saucepan, combine kumquats, honey and 1 tbsp (15 mL) water. Cover and cook over low heat, stirring often to prevent sticking, for 30 minutes or until kumquats break down to a jam-like consistency.

2. Stir in ginger juice until well combined. Let cool. Transfer to a sealed glass jar and refrigerate for up to 2 weeks.

3. For each cup of tea, stir 1 tbsp (15 mL) of the kumquat mixture into 1 cup (250 mL) boiling water. Pour into a teacup and serve immediately. You can add a bit more of the kumquat mixture if you like a stronger taste.

Tips

Electuaries are made two ways. The first is to simply mix powdered herbs with liquid honey. The second is to cook nourishing or therapeutic foods with water and honey until they are condensed to a thick paste, which can be eaten on its own or mixed with hot water to make tea.

To make ginger juice, grate ginger and press it through a fine-mesh sieve into a small bowl. Discard solids.

Health Tips

Kumquats are pungent, sweet and sour. They are most effective for clearing out phlegm and soothing coughs. They are also useful in stimulating a poor appetite and encouraging healthy digestion.

If you have a cough with phlegm, drink this tea one to three times a day to help clear it up.

Goji Berry and Schisandra Tea

This is a delightful sweet-and-sour tea you can sip anytime. Goji berries and schisandra berries are two treasured herbs that have been used for thousands of years in Chinese herbal therapy as tonics to revitalize and nourish the body.

MAKES 2 SERVINGS		

Tip

The goji berries will naturally sweeten the tea, but you can always add a little more honey if you like your tea sweeter.

6 tbsp	dried goji berries	90 mL
¼ cup	dried schisandra berries	60 mL
	Lemon wedges (optional)	
	Liquid honey (optional)	

1. In a medium saucepan, bring 4 cups (1 L) water to a boil. Stir in goji berries and schisandra berries. Reduce heat and simmer for 10 minutes or until fragrant. Remove from heat, cover and let stand for 5 minutes.

2. Strain into teacups. Add a squeeze of lemon and/or honey to taste (if using). Drink hot or let cool slightly.

Health Tips

This tea invigorates vitality while calming the nervous system. The goji berries and schisandra berries are nourishing, cleanse the blood, promote a calm mind and are said to beautify the skin.

Goji berries are becoming more widely used in the West. They are delicious and can be eaten as-is, in small handfuls. They are considered a type of "super and longevity" food or herb because they benefit the liver, the eyes and the skin and build vitality.

Schisandra, which is also called five-flavor fruit, is said to include all the five flavors in one berry — sweet, sour, pungent, salty and bitter. It is easily assimilated by the body and enhances all functions.

Tonic herbs are good — but too much of them is not. Even though you can sip this tea regularly, enjoy it in smaller portions. Everything in moderation!

Walnut Chai

This creamy and satisfyingly rich chai is caffeine-free. Usually black tea gives masala (or spiced) chai a gentle bitterness. Here, that comes from the combination of warming spices and sweet walnuts, which have a mildly bitter aftertaste.

> ## MAKES 4 SERVINGS

Tip

True cinnamon gives chai a sweeter, less bitter taste, but you can substitute cassia cinnamon if you prefer. Most of the cinnamon sold in supermarkets is cassia cinnamon. See page 166 for more information.

- **Blender or food processor**

1 cup	walnut pieces or halves	250 mL
1	piece (2 inches/5 cm long) cinnamon stick	1
1 tsp	whole cloves	5 mL
6	green cardamom pods, crushed	6
2	slices (quarter-size) gingerroot	2
	Liquid honey	

1. In a medium dry skillet over low heat, toast walnuts, stirring often, for 10 minutes or until golden and fragrant.

2. Transfer to a medium saucepan and add 4 cups (1 L) water. Bring to a boil. Turn off heat and let stand on burner for 10 minutes.

3. Meanwhile, return skillet to low heat. Add cinnamon stick, cloves and cardamom pods and toast, shaking pan often, for about 5 minutes or until fragrant.

4. Drain walnuts. Rinse and drain well again. In blender, combine walnuts and 2 cups (500 mL) water. Blend until smooth. Pour into saucepan and add cinnamon mixture and ginger. Bring to a boil. Remove from heat and let stand for 10 minutes.

5. Strain into teacups. Add honey to taste. Drink hot or let cool slightly. Refrigerate for up to 3 days; warm in a small saucepan.

> ## Health Tip
>
> Walnuts are sweet and warming. They are moistening and beneficial for a dry cough or dry-type constipation. They are considered a tonic for the kidneys and low back, as well. Walnuts are not recommended for people who have symptoms caused by excessive heat in the body, including canker sores, facial flushing or the tendency to feel overheated.

Mulberry Spiced Wine

Many cultures have a tradition of enjoying spiced wine in the darker months of the year. Here, dried mulberries give the wine medicinal powers, so this drink not only tastes good — it also does good things for your body.

MAKES 2 SERVINGS

Tips

For an even more warming treat, try the wine gently heated.

A lighter, fruitier red wine is best for this recipe. It does not need to be expensive to be delicious.

Variation

You can also make this recipe with brandy in place of the wine. If you do, it will make 5 servings.

- **1-quart (1 L) canning jar**

1¼ cups	red wine (see tips, at left)	300 mL
½ cup	dried mulberries	125 mL
10	whole cloves	10
4	green cardamom pods, crushed	4
2	slices (⅛-inch/3 mm thick) gingerroot	2
1	piece (2 inches/5 cm long) cinnamon stick, broken into pieces	1
1	strip (4 inches/10 cm long) tangerine rind	1

1. In jar, combine wine, mulberries, cloves, cardamom pods, ginger, cinnamon stick and tangerine rind. Seal with lid and shake well to combine. Let stand at room temperature, shaking 1 or 2 times a day, for 2 days or refrigerate for up to 1 week.

2. To serve, strain through a fine-mesh sieve into glasses.

Health Tip

Mulberries, often mixed with other herbs, are traditionally used as a restorative tonic in Chinese herbal medicine and in other Asian medical practices. The fresh berries and juice quench thirst, and nourish the liver, kidneys, yin and blood. When mixed with wine and aromatic spices to make a warming and calming drink, mulberries can be a blood restorative.

Red Bean Soup with Tangerine Rind and Lotus Seeds

This recipe is based on the popular Chinese red bean soup that is served as a snack or dessert — most often around the lunar New Year celebration. These red beans are not kidney beans but rather smaller, sweeter red adzuki beans.

> **MAKES
> 4 TO 6 SERVINGS**

Tips

If you like a sweeter soup, you can increase the coconut sugar to ¾ cup (175 mL).

Lotus seeds are slightly sour and have a nut-like consistency. Look for them in Asian grocery stores or Chinese herbal pharmacies. You can soak them for 1 to 2 hours to soften them before adding them to the recipe, if you prefer.

1 cup	dried adzuki beans	250 mL
1	piece (1 inch/2.5 cm square) dried kombu	1
1	strip dried tangerine rind (or fresh orange or tangerine rind)	1
1 tbsp	dried lotus seeds	15 mL
½ cup	coconut sugar	125 mL

1. Place adzuki beans in a medium bowl and cover with water. Let stand overnight. Drain well.

2. Rinse beans and cover with fresh water. Let stand for 4 to 8 hours. Drain and rinse beans well.

3. In a medium saucepan, bring 4 cups (1 L) water to a boil. Add adzuki beans, kombu and tangerine rind. Reduce heat, cover and simmer, stirring occasionally, for 1 hour.

4. Stir in lotus seeds and simmer for 1 hour or until beans are tender and just starting to break apart. Stir in coconut sugar until dissolved.

5. Spoon into serving bowls. Serve immediately.

> ## Health Tips
>
> Adzuki beans are a yang, or warming, food. Dried tangerine peel aids digestion and adds a flavor kick to the beans.
>
> This dish is typically served as a dessert but you could also add it to your morning congee or one of our essential nut and seed porridges.
>
> Beans can be beneficial for people with varying blood sugar levels. The body digests beans slowly, which helps keep blood sugar steady.

Tea-Soaked Fruit with Chunky Walnut Florentines

This super fruit-packed dessert, served with warming walnut cookies, is as lovely for teatime as it is as a finish after a simple meal. The astringency of the tea and the tanginess of the lemon balance the sweet dried fruit.

MAKES 6 SERVINGS

Health Tip

Most desserts are eaten just for the simple pleasure they give. But if any dessert could actually be a yang and *qi* builder, it might be this one. The sweet flavors in these cookies calm and harmonize the body and mind. The warming, essence-building properties of goji berries, walnuts and ghee combined with the *qi*-building powers of dates and blood-building mulberries, cherries and apricots make this a nutritional power-house of a dessert.

- **1-quart (1 L) canning jar**

2 cups	unsweetened white grape juice	500 mL
4	black tea bags	4
½ cup	halved dried apricots	125 mL
½ cup	dried pitted cherries	125 mL
½ cup	dried goji berries	125 mL
½ cup	halved pitted dates	125 mL
½ cup	dried mulberries or raisins	125 mL
2 tbsp	freshly squeezed lemon juice	30 mL
	Chunky Walnut Florentine Cookies (see recipe, opposite)	

1. In a medium saucepan, bring grape juice to a boil. Remove from heat and add tea bags. Cover and let stand for 5 minutes. Discard tea bags.

2. Pour tea into jar. Add apricots, cherries, goji berries, dates, mulberries and lemon juice. Seal with lid and shake to combine. Refrigerate, shaking jar occasionally, for 1 to 5 days.

3. Serve fruit and syrup with cookies.

Chunky Walnut Florentine Cookies

The bitter and crisp walnuts in these cookies are balanced by the sweetness of the honey and coconut sugar.

MAKES THIRTY-SIX 2½-INCH (6 CM) COOKIES

- Preheat oven to 300°F (150°C), with rack positioned in upper third
- 2 rimmed baking sheets, lined with parchment paper

½ cup	liquid honey	125 mL
¼ cup	ghee	60 mL
2 tbsp	coconut sugar	30 mL
½ tsp	salt	2 mL
1 cup	almond flour	250 mL
½ tsp	vanilla extract	2 mL
3 cups	coarsely chopped walnuts	750 mL

1. In a medium saucepan, heat honey, ghee, coconut sugar and salt over low heat, stirring constantly, until completely smooth. Stir in almond flour and vanilla until combined.

2. Remove from heat. Stir in walnuts. Let cool for 30 minutes.

3. Spoon half of the dough by rounded 1 tbsp (15 mL) onto 1 of the prepared baking sheets, spacing cookies 2 inches (5 cm) apart. Bake on upper rack in preheated oven for 15 minutes or until edges of cookies are browned.

4. Transfer pan to a wire rack. Let cool completely on pan. Repeat with remaining dough.

Cocoa Crumble on Sliced Oranges

The bittersweet richness of this delicious cocoa crumble is amazing over fresh sweet-tart oranges. It makes a celebratory but luxuriously light dessert — and an elegant ending to a special holiday meal. The crumble will remind you of a crushed dark chocolate wafer cookie, just a bit healthier.

MAKES 4 SERVINGS

Tip

You can peel the oranges with your hands or use a sharp chef's knife. Try to remove as much of the white pith as you can.

Health Tips

Oranges, with their sweet, sour and cooling nature, moisten the body and quench thirst. Oranges are beneficial to people who tend to feel hot and have poor appetite. Combining them with cocoa powder, which is bitter, warming and stimulating, creates a delicious dessert that will lift your spirits on a cold, dark winter evening.

Researchers at the National Institute of Integrative Medicine in Melbourne, Australia, conducted a meta-analysis of 20 studies and found that the flavanols in cocoa had a slight, but statistically relevant, ability to reduce blood pressure. So cocoa might be your ally in the fight against hypertension!

- **Preheat oven to 300°F (150°C)**
- **Rimmed baking sheet, lined with parchment paper**

2	large oranges	2
1 tbsp	liquid honey	15 mL
1/2 cup	coconut sugar	125 mL
6 tbsp	unsweetened cocoa powder	90 mL
1/4 cup	almond flour	60 mL
1/4 cup	ghee	60 mL
1 tsp	vanilla extract	5 mL
1/2 tsp	ground cinnamon	2 mL
Pinch	salt	Pinch

1. Peel oranges and cut crosswise into 1/4-inch (0.5 cm) thick slices. Cut slices into quarters. In a medium bowl, gently toss oranges with honey. Cover and refrigerate for 2 to 24 hours.

2. In another medium bowl, stir together coconut sugar, cocoa powder, almond flour, ghee, vanilla, cinnamon and salt until well combined. Using a spatula, spread cocoa mixture in 1/4-inch (0.5 cm) thick layer on prepared pan.

3. Bake in preheated oven for 12 to 15 minutes or until very fragrant and edges look dry. Transfer pan to a wire rack and let cool completely.

4. Divide oranges among serving bowls. Using a spatula, scoop up cocoa mixture and scatter over oranges. Serve immediately.

Cardamom Shortbread

In India, cardamom has long been known as the "queen of spices," thanks to its deeply aromatic appeal. The cardamom flavor in these cookies will intensify for the first few days after baking, so they are even more delicious if you make them ahead. They are an especially tasty gift.

**MAKES
16 LARGE WEDGES**

Tips

The cardamom we use in this recipe is made from the little black seeds inside green cardamom pods. You can buy this spice already ground or crack the pods open and grind the seeds at home. Look for green cardamom pods in grocery stores and spice shops. Chinese medicine often calls for black cardamom, from the *Amomum* genus; in baking, however, we use green (or true) cardamom from the *Elettaria* genus.

If you don't have the right-size springform pans, you can substitute 8-inch (20 cm) round metal cake pans or 7-inch (18 cm) square metal baking pans.

- **Preheat oven to 300°F (150°C)**
- **Two 8-inch (20 cm) springform pans, bottoms lined with parchment paper**

1 cup	brown rice flour	250 mL
1 cup	almond meal	250 mL
1 cup	coconut sugar	250 mL
1 cup	ghee	250 mL
1 tsp	ground cardamom	5 mL
1/4 tsp	salt	1 mL
1	large egg	1
1/2 cup	pine nuts or chopped pistachios	125 mL

1. In a medium bowl, combine flour, almond meal, coconut sugar, ghee, cardamom, salt and egg. Stir until well combined.

2. Divide dough in half. Press 1 half into each of the prepared pans, using the back of a large spoon to create an even layer. Scatter pine nuts over top and press gently to adhere. Bake in preheated oven for 25 to 27 minutes or until fragrant and edges are browned.

3. Remove from oven. Using a thin, sharp knife, immediately cut each circle into 8 wedges. Let cool completely.

4. To remove, release side of pan and lift cookies off paper. Store in an airtight container for up to 2 weeks.

Health Tip

Cardamom is a highly aromatic herb, with an uplifting menthol-like fragrance. It warms the abdomen and helps soothe digestive disorders. It is also used to treat tooth and gum problems and to calm sore throats. In the dark days of winter, cardamom is a warming balm that counters the cold.

Fragrant Poached Quince with Fresh Ginger Cookies

The unusual, ancient quince deserves a comeback in the kitchen. Its pink hue and bright fragrance is so nice, especially when the fruit is poached and served with these spicy cookies.

MAKES 4 SERVINGS	½ cup	unsweetened apple juice	125 mL
	¼ cup	liquid honey	60 mL
	1 lb	quinces (about 2 medium)	500 g
		Fresh Ginger Cookies (see recipe, opposite)	

1. In a medium nonreactive saucepan, stir apple juice with honey. Quarter and core quince and cut into ¼-inch (0.5 cm) thick slices, adding to saucepan as you go so quince does not turn brown.

2. Bring to a boil. Reduce heat, cover and simmer, stirring often, for 20 minutes or until very tender. Serve immediately or refrigerate in an airtight container for up to 1 week. Warm before serving with cookies.

Health Tip

The quince is known for its sweetness and astringent action on the body, making it a perfect treat for someone suffering from a mild digestive disturbance, diarrhea or a lingering cough. The aromatic and pungent spices in the poaching liquid and cookies ensure that this dish will warm you as it supports digestion.

Do not eat too much of this dessert, as it can be drying and exacerbate constipation.

From a Western medical perspective, the large amount of pectin in this fruit makes it an excellent choice for adding fiber to the diet and lowering cholesterol.

Fresh Ginger Cookies

Eat these zippy ginger cookies soon after they are baked to enjoy maximum crispiness. They soften quickly when stored.

MAKES ABOUT THIRTY-TWO 2½-INCH (6 CM) COOKIES

Tip

Make sure to choose unsulphured molasses, which is made from ripe sugarcane. Sulphured molasses has a bitter aftertaste

- Preheat oven to 350°F (180°C), with racks positioned in upper and lower thirds
- 2 rimmed baking sheets, lined with parchment paper

1¼ cups	oat flour	300 mL
½ cup	coconut sugar	125 mL
¼ cup	ghee	60 mL
¼ cup	unsulphured dark (cooking) molasses (see tip, at left)	60 mL
2 tbsp	grated gingerroot	30 mL
1 tsp	baking soda	5 mL
1 tsp	ground cinnamon	5 mL
¼ tsp	ground cloves	1 mL
Pinch	salt	Pinch
1	large egg	1

1. In a large bowl, combine flour, coconut sugar, ghee, molasses, ginger, baking soda, cinnamon, cloves, salt and egg. Stir until well combined to make a soft dough. (The dough can be made up to this point, then wrapped in plastic wrap and refrigerated up to 3 days or frozen for up to 1 month. If frozen, thaw in the refrigerator before continuing.)

2. Scrape dough onto a cutting board. Form into a 1-inch (2.5 cm) thick rectangle. Cut lengthwise into quarters. Cut crosswise into eighths to make 32 equal pieces.

3. Roll each piece into a ball and arrange on prepared pans. Cover balls with parchment paper and press to flatten to scant ½-inch (1 cm) thickness. Remove top sheet of parchment.

4. Bake on upper and lower racks in preheated oven for 5 minutes. Rotate and switch pans and bake for 5 to 7 minutes more or until edges are lightly browned and tops look dry.

5. Transfer pans to wire racks and let cool completely.

Blood Tonic Recipes

Blood Tonic Basics

Blood tonic dishes are beneficial for woman after childbirth or for anyone recovering from surgery. A woman needs nutritional and physical support after childbirth so that her body can recover and she can spend time bonding with her newborn infant. Some cultures have traditionally encouraged a sort of quarantine of between 30 and 40 days post-birth so that a woman can rest and recover. Often, during that period of time, women ate special foods and herbs meant to address the unique needs of their postpartum state.

In China and other parts of Asia, some women adhere to the tradition of "sitting out the month." Called *zuo yuezi* in Chinese, this tradition began during the Song Dynasty (960–1279). During the first month postpartum, a woman stays inside the house and refrains from overexertion. In ancient times, to rebuild her essence — which is the blood and yang *qi* — she would avoid bathing, hair washing and drinking cold water, which inhibit that process. This latter prohibition was probably a leftover from the times when there was no indoor heating and plumbing.

In Chinese medicine, blood is considered a woman's essence. From a Chinese medicine perspective, the physical trauma of childbirth is the most taxing event in a woman's life, due to the simultaneous depletion of *qi* and blood. Indeed, women may experience many different negative outcomes after childbirth, which Chinese medicine sees as related to the depletion of *qi* and blood. Some examples of related conditions are postpartum fatigue, depression, hormone-induced thyroid problems, pain, hair loss, breast problems and difficulty lactating. The good news is that rest and nourishment, along with therapeutic foods, herbs and other health treatments, can restore a woman's health and vitality.

During *zuo yuezi*, a woman rebuilds a foundation for good health by eating foods that enrich and move the blood, and nourish the *qi* and yang. We recommend eating easy-to-digest dishes in the first weeks after childbirth to help the body heal and rebuild. In this chapter, we have included nourishing recipes that boost circulation, and rebuild a new mother's *qi* and blood. Because of these beneficial effects, these dishes are also recommended for people who are recovering from surgery.

To foster healing during this period, you should skip any dishes that are overly sweet or salty. Avoid spicy, cold, greasy and creamy foods; alcohol; and excessive sugar, which all disperse or stagnate *qi*.

Adzuki Bean Congee

This mild-tasting congee is easy to make and digest. It has a very light taste, so feel free to augment it with any of your favorite vegetables, condiments or animal proteins.

MAKES
6 TO 8 SERVINGS

Tip

The kombu, or kelp (a kind of seaweed), helps break down the oligosaccharides in the beans so that they are more digestible. You can remove it after 1 hour of simmering, or leave it in if you like the texture.

Variation

During the fall and winter, cook ½ cup (125 mL) peeled seeded diced winter squash in the congee to give it a sweeter flavor. Winter squashes, such as butternut, kabocha or acorn, are nourishing and good for the digestive system.

⅓ cup	dried adzuki beans	75 mL
1 cup	sweet (glutinous) brown rice (or brown Arborio rice)	250 mL
1	piece (1 inch/2.5 cm square) dried kombu	1
	Salt	
1 tbsp	grated gingerroot (optional)	15 mL

1. Place beans in a medium bowl and pour in enough water to cover. Cover and let stand overnight. Drain and rinse well.

2. In a large saucepan, combine 12 cups (3 L) water, beans, rice and kombu and bring to a boil. Season to taste with salt. Reduce heat to low, cover and simmer, stirring occasionally, for 2 hours. The congee should have a souplike consistency; if there is not enough liquid left in the pan, add water as needed. Serve immediately or transfer to airtight containers and freeze for up to 6 weeks. Thaw and warm in a small saucepan over low heat before serving.

3. Stir ginger (if using) into warm congee just before serving; or squeeze just the juice from the ginger into the congee if you prefer.

Health Tips

Adzuki beans help decrease any fluid retention in the body and support lactation.

Sweet brown rice and ginger are both warming, which supports the rebuilding of yang *qi*, an important action for people who often feel cold or have hypothyroidism.

Chicken Broth Congee

This ultra-simple congee rebuilds the qi and warms the body. It is a perfectly mild, soothing first meal to eat after childbirth. Serve with a condiment that is balancing, nourishing or warming, such as Gomashio (page 447), Black and White Sesame Furikake (page 445), Walnut and Black Sesame Sprinkle (page 451) or Nettle and Chive Seaweed Sprinkle (page 441).

MAKES 4 SERVINGS	6 cups	Chicken Broth (see recipe in Variation, page 418)	1.5 L
	½ cup	sweet (glutinous) brown rice or short-grain brown rice	125 mL

1. In a medium saucepan, combine broth and rice and bring to a boil. Reduce heat to low, cover and simmer, stirring occasionally, for 2 hours. The congee should have a souplike consistency; if there is not enough liquid left in the pan, add up to ½ cup (125 mL) water. Let cool for 10 minutes.

2. Serve immediately or transfer to an airtight container and refrigerate for up to 3 days. Warm in a small saucepan over low heat before serving.

Health Tip

Chicken meat is sweet, warming and nourishing. The *qi*- and blood-nourishing properties of the chicken broth are great for building up strength postpartum. This congee is especially beneficial for women who feel weak and are prone to abdominal cramps during their periods.

Duck Soup with Cordyceps

This soup has a delicate, slightly sweet flavor. Cordyceps mushrooms are widely hailed as a powerful qi and longevity tonic. They have a pleasant chewiness that contrasts nicely with the other textures in the dish.

<table>
<tr><td>½ cup</td><td>dried cordyceps mushrooms (½ oz/15 g)</td><td>125 mL</td></tr>
<tr><td>½ cup</td><td>dried lotus seeds</td><td>125 mL</td></tr>
<tr><td>1</td><td>whole duck (neck and giblets removed)</td><td>1</td></tr>
<tr><td>1 cup</td><td>dried pitted red dates</td><td>250 mL</td></tr>
<tr><td>5</td><td>slices (quarter-size) gingerroot</td><td>5</td></tr>
<tr><td>¼ cup</td><td>dried goji berries</td><td>60 mL</td></tr>
<tr><td>1 tbsp</td><td>salt, or to taste</td><td>15 mL</td></tr>
<tr><td>½ cup</td><td>minced green onions</td><td>125 mL</td></tr>
</table>

MAKES 6 TO 8 SERVINGS

Tip

Farmed cordyceps are easier to find and less expensive than wild ones. They are available online or through Asian herb suppliers (see Resources, page 466, for sources).

1. In a medium bowl, combine cordyceps and lotus seeds. Pour in enough water to cover. Cover and let stand while duck is cooking.

2. Cut duck into about 6 pieces. In a large saucepan, combine duck pieces, 12 cups (3 L) water, red dates and ginger and bring to a simmer over medium heat. Skim off any foam. Reduce heat to low and simmer, stirring occasionally, for 1½ hours.

3. Drain cordyceps and lotus seeds, discarding soaking liquid. Add to soup along with goji berries and 1 tbsp (15 mL) salt. Simmer for 30 minutes or until duck is very tender. Taste soup and season to taste with more salt, if desired.

4. Ladle soup into serving bowls and sprinkle with green onions. Serve immediately.

Health Tip

This tonic soup helps restore the essence, nourishes the kidneys and invigorates the lungs, enhancing *qi* and blood. It is also recommended for men who experience erectile dysfunction.

Cordyceps mushrooms, like ginseng, are one of the most treasured *qi* tonics. When added to this duck soup, they are most beneficial for postpartum women. Cordyceps also strengthen the immune system, soothe a dry cough and build the blood by building bone marrow (essence).

Silkie Chicken Soup with Lotus Seeds and Red Dates

This nourishing, deeply flavorful soup is perfect postpartum or post-surgery fare. The black-skinned silkie chicken has been part of medicinal lore in China for more than 1,000 years. It has a subtly deeper flavor than regular chicken and a firmer, chewier texture.

MAKES 4 TO 6 SERVINGS		

Tip

You'll often find black-skinned silkie chickens in Asian grocery stores. If they aren't available, substitute 2 lbs (1 kg) organic chicken legs or leg quarters.

½ cup	dried lotus seeds	125 mL
1	whole silkie chicken (neck and giblets removed)	1
½ cup	dried pitted red dates	125 mL
3	slices (quarter-size) gingerroot	3
¼ cup	dried goji berries	60 mL
2 tsp	salt, or to taste	10 mL
¼ cup	minced green onions	60 mL

1. Place lotus seeds in a medium bowl and pour in enough water to cover. Cover and let stand while chicken is cooking.

2. In a large saucepan, combine chicken, 8 cups (2 L) water, red dates and ginger and bring to a simmer over medium heat. Skim off any foam. Reduce heat to low and simmer, stirring occasionally, for 1 hour.

3. Drain lotus seeds, discarding soaking liquid. Add to soup along with goji berries and 2 tsp (10 mL) salt. Simmer for 30 minutes or until chicken is very tender. Taste soup and season to taste with more salt, if desired.

4. Gently break chicken into large pieces. Ladle soup and chicken into serving bowls and sprinkle with green onions. Serve immediately.

Health Tip

Lotus seeds, red dates and goji berries increase the *qi*- and blood-building qualities of this nourishing soup.

Silkie chicken (also called black-boned chicken) is indeed black and a member of the Bantam variety, even though there are non-Bantam silkies. It is traditionally used to supplement the liver and kidney. It is also useful for treating cases of blood deficiency and is often prescribed for women's gynecological issues, such as menstrual irregularities and anemia. It is sweet in flavor, neutral in nature and beneficial for the *qi*. It is also a powerful blood builder.

Qi Tonic Vegetable Broth

This vegan variation on qi-building chicken broth is a welcome addition for vegans and vegetarians. It is has a sweet and full flavor.

**MAKES
4 TO 6 SERVINGS**

Tips

All of the herbs are edible, so feel free to not strain them out of the broth and to eat this dish as a soup.

You can add tofu or fish to the broth, or use the broth as a base for congee, other soups or beans.

Health Tip

This vegetable broth is an immunity- and *qi*-building tonic. It is lovely for breakfast or to sip prior to a meal. It is good if you are feeling run-down and fatigued.

2 cups	dried shiitake mushrooms, stems removed	500 mL
	Hot water	
1	piece (3 inches/7.5 cm square) dried kombu	1
8	slices (quarter-size) gingerroot, lightly crushed	8
4	green onions, cut into 2-inch (5 cm) long pieces	4
3	stalks celery, coarsely chopped	3
1	large onion, coarsely chopped	1
1	large carrot, coarsely chopped	1
½	bulb fennel, cored and coarsely chopped	½
½ cup	rice wine, such as sake	125 mL
2 oz	dried goji berries	60 g
2 oz	dried pitted red dates	60 g
2 oz	dried lotus seeds	60 g
1 tbsp	sea salt, or to taste	15 mL

1. Place shiitake mushrooms in a medium bowl. Pour in enough hot water to cover. Let stand for 10 minutes.

2. In a stockpot, combine 12 cups (3 L) water and kombu. Bring to a boil. Reduce heat and simmer for 15 minutes. Remove kombu.

3. Add shiitake mushrooms and soaking liquid, ginger, green onions, celery, onion, carrot and fennel. Cook over medium heat for 10 minutes.

4. Add rice wine, goji berries, red dates and lotus seeds. Reduce heat to low and simmer for 1 hour.

5. Stir in salt, adding more to taste if desired. Discard ginger. Let broth cool completely.

6. Strain broth through a fine-mesh sieve into a large bowl. Pour into airtight containers and refrigerate for 5 days or freeze for up to 3 months.

Pork Broth with Ginger

This long-cooked broth is very simple and exceptionally nourishing. It is an excellent option for sipping on its own or as a foundation for soup.

> **MAKES ABOUT
> 5 CUPS (1.25 L)**

2 lbs	pork, including some bones	1 kg
16	slices (quarter-size) gingerroot	16
1 tbsp	salt, or to taste	15 mL

Tip

Meaty pork neck bones or Chinese-cut spareribs are ideal choices for the pork, since they are about half meat and half bones.

Variation

Chicken Broth: To make chicken broth, substitute the same weight of chicken legs or thighs for the pork. Reduce simmering time to 3 hours.

1. Cut pork into pieces no thicker than $\frac{1}{2}$ inch (1 cm).

2. In a large saucepan, combine 8 cups (2 L) water, pork and ginger. Bring to a simmer over medium heat, skimming off any foam. Reduce heat to low and simmer for 4 hours.

3. Strain broth through a fine-mesh sieve into a large bowl. Stir in salt, adding more to taste if desired.

4. Pour into airtight containers and refrigerate for up to 5 days, already strained.

> ### Health Tips
>
> Pork is used medicinally to nourish the yin, enrich the blood and moisten dryness. It is useful during the postpartum period (especially for treating constipation), or if you have dry skin or a dry cough.
>
> The warming fresh ginger adds pungency and enhances the natural sweet and salty flavor of the pork.

Ginger-Braised Pork for New Moms

Pork braised in vinegar and ginger is a traditional postpartum dish served to women in China. The long cooking time makes the pork very tender and easier to digest, and it mellows the sharpness of the ginger. To get all the nutritional value from the soup, make sure to eat not only the pork and broth, but also the ginger.

> **MAKES**
> **3 TO 4 SERVINGS**

Tips

Black sugar is a minimally processed sugarcane product that comes in flat bars. It is available in Asian grocery stores and online.

Ask your butcher to cut the pork hocks into 1-inch (2.5 cm) slices for you.

This soup takes a long time to cook and reheats well, so you might as well make a larger batch. If you're doubling or quadrupling the recipe, it is not necessary to increase the cooking times. After cooking, it may be frozen for up to 3 weeks.

Caution

Supplementing foods, like this dish, are beneficial. However, if you have a cold or fever, they can strengthen pathogens or, as one of Ellen's Chinese medicine teachers, Dr. Heiner Fruehauf, says, "Lock the thief in the house." Do not eat this supplementing dish if you have a cold or fever; instead, try a simple congee or vegetable broth.

1 tbsp	avocado oil	15 mL
1 lb	skin-on pork hocks, preferably cut into 1-inch (2.5 cm) thick slices	500 g
4 oz	gingerroot, peeled and cut into quarter-size rounds	125 g
1 cup	unseasoned rice vinegar	250 mL
2 oz	black sugar (see tips, at left)	60 g
1 tsp	salt	5 mL

1. In a medium saucepan, heat oil over medium-high heat. Add pork and cook, turning often, for 3 to 5 minutes or until lightly browned all over.

2. Pour in enough water to cover and bring to a simmer. Skim off any foam. Add ginger and vinegar. Reduce heat to low and simmer, turning pork once or twice, for 2 hours.

3. Stir in sugar and salt. Simmer for 1 hour or until pork is very tender. Let cool slightly.

4. Using tongs, transfer pork to a cutting board. Remove and discard bones; cut pork and skin into bite-size pieces and return to broth. Let cool. Cover and refrigerate for at least 4 hours before serving, or for up to 3 days.

5. To serve, skim off and discard fat from surface. Reheat soup over medium heat until steaming. Serve immediately.

Health Tip

Pork has long been cooked for medicinal purposes — mainly to nourish yin and enrich the blood. This makes it a good ingredient to add to dishes for postpartum women. The long cooking time and the vinegar in this dish extract vital minerals from the bones in the pork hocks, which activate blood circulation and promote milk production.

Ginger supports breast milk flow, helps the body clear out excess fluids and supports digestion.

Sautéed Prawns in Rice Wine, Garlic, Ginger and Leeks

It is critically important to build vitality after childbirth or surgery. This warming and yang-building dish is a delicious way to do that. Aromatic leeks and garlic really complement the sweet-salty taste of prawns (a.k.a. shrimp). This combination, plus mellow rice wine and zippy ginger juice, produce a very flavorful dish. Have it with a side of cooked dark leafy greens.

MAKES 4 SERVINGS

Tips

Shrimp are sold by size, so the package will give a count, or a number per pound (500 g). There are about 25 jumbo shrimp in 1 lb (500 g).

To make ginger juice, grate gingerroot finely and press it through a fine-mesh sieve. Discard solids.

Variation

If you are sensitive to shrimp, substitute the same weight of boneless skinless trout fillets. Cut them into 2-inch (5 cm) pieces and cook as directed or until fish is just opaque. Trout is warming, like shrimp, and has a slightly sweet flavor.

Caution

If you have a cold or rash, do not eat this dish. It is warming, and can exacerbate these conditions.

2	large leeks	2
2 tbsp	avocado oil	30 mL
1 tsp	salt	5 mL
1 lb	jumbo shrimp (25 count), peeled and deveined	500 g
4	cloves garlic, thinly sliced	4
¼ cup	ginger juice (see tips, at left)	60 mL
¼ cup	rice wine, such as sake	60 mL

1. Trim roots and all but 1 inch (2.5 cm) of the dark green leaves off leeks and discard. Cut leeks in half lengthwise, then cut crosswise into ½-inch (1 cm) wide pieces. Rinse very well in 2 changes of water to remove grit.

2. In a large skillet, heat oil over high heat, swirling to coat bottom of pan. Add leeks and salt and cook, stirring often, for 1 to 2 minutes or until leeks are slightly wilted.

3. Add shrimp and garlic and cook, stirring often, for 2 to 3 minutes or until shrimp is almost opaque.

4. Stir in ginger juice and wine and cook, stirring often, for 1 to 2 minutes or until almost no liquid remains. Remove from heat. Spoon into serving dishes and serve immediately.

Health Tip

This sauté is especially beneficial for women who are *qi*-deficient after childbirth and aren't making enough breast milk. Shrimp are warming and build yang; so do the leeks, ginger and garlic. If you use freshwater shrimp, the dish will boost your breast milk production.

Dang Gui and Astragalus Tea with Ginger

This tea recipe is based on a classic Chinese herbal formula called dang gui bu xue tang, *which is a traditional blood tonic. The 5:1 ratio of qi-building astragalus to blood-building dang gui emphasizes building the* qi *to improve blood circulation. Since breast milk production is directly related to a woman's blood (essence), this tea can be beneficial for increasing milk supply as well as for women who need to build their vitality.*

	MAKES 1 SERVING	

5 tsp	dried astragalus root	25 mL
1 tsp	dried dang gui	5 mL
1	slice (quarter-size) gingerroot	1

Tip

If you can, it is always best to cook Chinese herbs in an enameled, stainless-steel or glass pot — never aluminum.

Variation

To sweeten the tea, add either 1 tsp (5 mL) goji berries or 1 dried red date in Step 1.

Health Tip

Childbirth and surgery are both traumatic physical events — they both exhaust *qi* (yang) and the blood (yin), which are interdependent. In childbirth and surgery, their interdependence is "interrupted" and can cause fatigue, slow healing or excessive bleeding. The astragalus in this tea takes the lead in restoring and replenishing *qi*, while the dang gui helps builds the blood. The ginger moderates the other herbs and balances the tea's flavor.

1. In a saucepan, combine 2 cups (500 mL) water, astragalus root, dang gui and ginger. Bring to a boil.
2. Reduce heat, cover and simmer for 15 minutes.
3. Strain into a teacup. Serve immediately or let cool slightly.

Other Recommended Postpartum and Post-Surgery Recipes

- Any of our Essential Seed and Nut Porridges (pages 213, 247, 290, 327, 328 and 370)
- Spring Nettle and Fragrant Flowers Tea (page 237)
- Ginger and Tangerine Peel Tea (page 238)
- Borscht (page 253)
- Arame Salad with Lemon and Chives (page 265)
- Steamed Egg Custard with Chopped Greens (page 294)
- Chunky Vegetable Bean Stew (page 299)
- Wakame Salad (page 307)
- Nourish the Qi and Blood Tea (page 313)
- Boost-the-Qi Chicken Soup (page 332)
- Braised Beef Brisket with Shiitakes (page 340)
- Black Soybeans and Kabocha with Walnuts (page 346)
- Brothy Salmon and Ginger Soup (page 377)
- Nourishing Lamb Stew with Butternut Squash and Dang Gui (page 382)
- Hijiki and Carrot Sauté with Ginger (page 392)
- Red Bean Soup with Tangerine Rind and Lotus Seeds (page 403)

Condiment Recipes

Why Condiments?

As you have learned in previous chapters, eating meals that include all of the five flavors — sweet, salty, sour, pungent and bitter — can be immensely satisfying as well as balancing. What better way to enhance a meal to each person's satisfaction than to have varied condiments on the table that are not only tasty but provide health benefits, too? Chinese nutritional therapy identifies condiments as a separate group unto themselves — these foods, herbs and spices enhance the flavor, palatability and digestibility of a meal. Throughout this book, we have included some condiments, such as salt, sweeteners, herbs, spices, wines, teas, fragrant flowers and vinegars, in the recipe ingredient lists.

However, we wanted to devote an entire chapter to homemade condiments that are flavor-dense and varied in texture. You can use these additions to round out or enhance a simple dish. By putting them on your table, everyone gets to customize his or her meal to meet particular flavor preferences or needs.

Each condiment was thoughtfully created to bring out unique and distinctive flavors that will activate your palate and balance your body. Please stretch your preferences and try them — we think you will enjoy the delight they bring to the table.

In order to make this chapter easier to use, we have divided the recipes into four sections:

1. **Pickles and Lightly Fermented Condiments:** Pickles are brined in a mix of salt and vinegar, while fermented condiments are fermented with salt — and both are cooling. None of the recipes in this book require long fermentation. In many cases, we're kick-starting a very light fermentation with an ingredient that has benefited from longer fermentation, such as kimchi or sauerkraut. It's the longer fermentation that gives you the health benefits, so those are the items you really want to get into your diet. Use our pickles and lightly fermented condiments when you want something a bit acidic or sour in your meal. The bonus is that these condiments support and invigorate digestion.

2. Savory, Pungent, Bitter and Aromatic Dry Condiments: This group contains a wide variety of seasonings that bring savory, pungent or aromatic flavors to foods. Use them whenever you want a bit of distinctive yet subtle flavor atop soups, salads, greens or grains. These dry condiments include "sprinkles," which are generally light in weight and texture, and furikake, a typical Japanese condiment that is used to complement and complete very simple dishes. Furikake is based on toasted sesame or other seeds, sea salt and nori; a variety of herbs, spices and ingredients are added to create variations on the theme. The dry seasonings in this section add minerals to the diet, as well as nourish *qi* and blood, yin and yang. They activate and balance the digestive system and can help with detoxification.

3. Vinegars: Vinegar is a common cooking and pickling ingredient. When infused with herbs or other ingredients, a simple vinegar adds flavor and brightness to dressings. It is also delicious drizzled over vegetables or even mixed with water to drink. It is always best to use unfiltered cider vinegar, wine vinegar or organic unseasoned rice vinegar. The infused vinegars in this chapter offer a variety of flavors and actions in the body, depending on which food or herb has been added.

4. Chutneys: Chutney is a condiment that comes in paste, sauce, relish or (sometimes) dry powdered form. It is usually served with meats and fish, but is delightful with other elements of a meal. Research tells us that chutney dates back to India in 500 BC and was developed as a method of preserving foods. Chutney has most been associated with Indian cuisine, but this condiment shows up across the world on many tables in the form of a cooked, concentrated combinations of fruit, vinegar and sweetener. Most chutneys are richly flavored and can be made from fresh, cooked or fermented ingredients. Adding a spoonful or two to your meal will add extra dimension and offer inviting new textures. Each chutney recipe has a different flavor and effect, so take a look at the ingredients to determine how it will enhance and balance your meal and your body.

Pungent Sichuan Turnip Pickles

Small amounts of pickles can enhance any meal and bring life to simple dishes, such as steamed vegetables or congee. The roasted Sichuan peppercorns and ginger add an earthy taste and enhance the natural pungency of the turnips. If you find them strong at first, don't worry — the pickles mellow out after a few days.

**MAKES
1 CUP (250 ML)**

Tips

Make sure to remove and discard the hard, shiny black seeds from the Sichuan peppercorns or they will give the finished pickles a gritty texture.

To toast sesame seeds, place them in a medium dry skillet. Toast over low heat, stirring or shaking pan often, for about 3 minutes or until fragrant.

- **2-cup (500 mL) canning jar**

1 cup	diced turnip	250 mL
1 tbsp	kosher or non-iodized sea salt	15 mL
2 tbsp	avocado oil	30 mL
1 tbsp	toasted sesame oil	15 mL
1 tbsp	Sichuan peppercorns, shiny black seeds removed (see tips, at left)	15 mL
1 tbsp	finely chopped gingerroot	15 mL
2 tbsp	black sesame seeds, toasted	30 mL

1. In a small bowl, toss turnip with salt. Let stand for 1 hour. Drain well and transfer to jar.

2. In a small saucepan or skillet, heat avocado oil and sesame oil over medium-high heat. Add Sichuan peppercorns and ginger and sauté for 2 to 3 minutes or until sizzling. Pour seasoned oil over turnip and sprinkle with sesame seeds.

3. Seal jar and refrigerate for at least 3 hours to allow flavors to meld before serving. Refrigerate in sealed jar for up to 2 weeks.

Health Tip

Sichuan peppercorns are warming and add a hot pungency to this turnip pickle, which soothes indigestion and boosts *qi*. If you eat a lot of raw food or foods straight from the refrigerator, adding this pickle to your meal will help warm your stomach and can actually relieve pain. Powdered Sichuan peppercorns can be rubbed onto the skin to relieve pain — just steer clear of mucous membranes and the eyes.

Pickled Mushrooms

These aromatic, tangy, brined mushrooms are nice on an appetizer tray, as a partner to green vegetables, or as a complement to roasted or grilled meat. We've used easy-to-find button mushrooms, but feel free to try other tasty varieties, such as shiitake, oyster, maitake or cremini, following the instructions below.

<table>
<tr><td colspan="4">MAKES GENEROUS 1 CUP (250 ML)</td></tr>
</table>

Tip

Always choose organic mushrooms. Commercially grown mushrooms usually contain high levels of pesticide residue.

- **2-cup (500 mL) canning jar**

¼ cup	unfiltered cider vinegar	60 mL
1 tsp	coriander seeds	5 mL
1 tsp	kosher or non-iodized sea salt	5 mL
½ tsp	black peppercorns	2 mL
1	bay leaf, broken in half	1
8 oz	button mushrooms, trimmed	250 g
1	clove garlic	1

1. In jar, combine vinegar, coriander seeds, salt, peppercorns and bay leaf.

2. In a medium saucepan, bring 2 cups (500 mL) water to a boil over medium-high heat. Add mushrooms and garlic. Return to a boil. Remove from heat, drain and stir into jar.

3. Seal jar with lid and refrigerate for 1 day to allow flavors to meld before serving. Refrigerate in sealed jar, shaking occasionally, for up to 1 week.

Health Tip

Common button mushrooms promote vitality, detoxify, support the immune system and clear out phlegm. Try this pickle if you have a wet cough. Button mushrooms moisten dry conditions and also benefit the stomach *qi*.

Kombu Vinegar Pickle

Kombu seaweed is filled with umami, that magical earthy and savory sixth flavor that can add depth to dishes. It is used as the foundation for dashi broth and is packed with minerals. This very traditional pickle is rich in its umami notes. Include it in simple meals served with plain rice, or serve it as a partner to a delicately flavored savory congee.

MAKES
½ CUP (125 ML)

Tip

If you have drained cooked kombu from a batch of Traditional or Vegetarian Dashi (page 297), you can use it in this recipe. Rinse it well and skip Step 1.

- **1-cup (250 mL) canning jar**

2	pieces (each 4 inches/10 cm square) dried kombu	2
¼ cup	tamari or soy sauce	60 mL
¼ cup	unseasoned rice vinegar	60 mL

1. In a medium saucepan, combine 4 cups (1 L) water and kombu. Bring to a boil. Turn off heat and let stand on burner for 10 minutes. Drain well.

2. Cut kombu into 1-inch (2.5 cm) squares. In jar, combine kombu, tamari and vinegar. Seal with lid and refrigerate for 1 day to allow flavors to meld before serving. Refrigerate in sealed jar for up to 2 weeks.

> ### Health Tip
>
> Pickles are generally cooling. This one adds a delicious savory note to a simple meal, is rich in minerals and is a good counterpoint to a rich seafood dish.

Fragrant Pickled Peaches

Aromatic, flavorful peaches come and go quickly in the summer. Pickling them in this delicious mixture lets you delight in them later on. After you've eaten all the peaches, save the leftover brine to use as a drinking vinegar (see tips, at left).

MAKES 4 CUPS (1 L)

Tips

If you don't have a canning jar handy, pour the vinegar mixture over the peaches in a stainless-steel bowl and let cool. Transfer to a glass or plastic container, cover and refrigerate as directed.

You can enjoy the leftover brine as a drinking vinegar. For a mocktail, mix equal parts vinegar and sparkling or still water. For a cocktail, mix equal parts vinegar and sake.

- **4-cup (1 L) canning jar**

1 cup	unfiltered cider vinegar	250 mL
1 cup	unsweetened apple juice	250 mL
5	whole cloves	5
1	piece (2 inches/5 cm long) cinnamon stick	1
1 lb	firm ripe peaches (about 2 large or 3 medium)	500 g

1. In a small nonreactive saucepan, combine vinegar, apple juice, cloves and cinnamon stick. Bring to a simmer over low heat.

2. Meanwhile, pit and cut peaches into $\frac{1}{2}$-inch (1 cm) thick wedges. Place in jar. Pour simmering vinegar mixture over top. Seal jar with lid and let cool completely.

3. Serve immediately or refrigerate in sealed jar for up to 4 weeks. Pickles will have the best flavor within the first week.

Health Tip
These tangy spiced peach pickles are beneficial for people who suffer from constipation. They stimulate digestion and satisfy cravings for sweet-and-sour foods.

Quince and Cinnamon Pickle

Ripe quinces are fragrant enough to scent a room, but their flesh is hard and dry and needs to be cooked before eating. This tender spiced pickle is especially delicious paired with simply prepared salmon.

**MAKES
5 CUPS (1.25 L)**

Tip

Quinces are ripe when they are yellow and fragrant, but they are still too hard and astringent to eat raw. If they are fuzzy (like peaches), gently rub off the fuzz before washing. The season for quinces is fall; sometimes you will find them coming out of cold storage in other times of the year. Specialty grocers and Asian markets are most likely to carry them.

2 cups	unsweetened apple juice	500 mL
½ cup	unfiltered cider vinegar	125 mL
¼ cup	liquid honey	60 mL
1	piece (2 inches/5 cm long) cinnamon stick	1
2	slices (quarter-size) gingerroot	2
1 lb	ripe quinces (about 1 large or 2 medium)	500 g

1. In a medium nonreactive saucepan, combine apple juice, vinegar, honey, cinnamon stick and ginger. Heat over low heat.

2. Meanwhile, quarter and core quinces. Cut into ¼-inch (0.5 cm) thick wedges. Add to pan and bring to a simmer. Cover and simmer for 45 minutes or until quince is tender and translucent.

3. Remove from heat. Let cool, covered, in pan. Transfer to glass or plastic container and serve immediately. Or refrigerate in sealed jar for up to 2 weeks. Pickles will have the best flavor within the first week.

Health Tips

Sweet, astringent quince is beneficial in cases of diarrhea, but not for people who suffer from chronic constipation. Its high pectin content makes it good for treating people who have elevated cholesterol.

As is the case with any condiment (or food), consuming it will not improve a health condition unless it's accompanied by a change in overall diet and lifestyle.

Digestive Shiso and Citrus Condiment

Shiso (also called perilla) is a member of the mint family. The leaves are used in Japanese and Chinese cuisine, and in herbal medicines. Its fragrance and pungency brightens, enlivens and adds balance to a variety of dishes. It is a fine accompaniment to rice, simply cooked greens, and steamed or grilled fish or poultry.

> **MAKES ABOUT
> ½ CUP (125 ML)**

Tip

To make ginger juice, grate gingerroot and press it through a fine-mesh sieve into a small bowl. Discard fibers.

- **1-cup (250 mL) canning jar**

8	fresh shiso leaves	8
1	lemon	1
1	small orange	1
1 tbsp	ginger juice (see tip, at left)	15 mL
1 tsp	liquid honey	5 mL
¼ tsp	kosher or non-iodized sea salt	1 mL

1. In a medium saucepan, bring 2 cups (500 mL) water to a boil. Add shiso leaves and stir once. Drain and transfer to a small plate. Let cool completely.

2. Grate ½ tsp (2 mL) zest each from lemon and orange. Using a sharp knife, peel lemon and orange. Cut fruit into segments.

3. Stack shiso leaves and roll up into a cylinder. Cut crosswise into thin shreds. Place in jar.

4. Add lemon and orange zests, lemon and orange segments, ginger juice, honey and salt.

5. Serve immediately or seal jar and refrigerate for up to 2 days. Bring to room temperature before serving.

> ### Health Tip
>
> Perilla is a powerful, delicious herb. It can settle the stomach, soothe nausea or morning sickness, and regulate *qi*. The leaves have potent anti-inflammatory powers and can counter mild allergic reactions. They are also high in iron.

Vegetable Top Green Sauce

If you are eating a simple meal and have a craving for some spiciness — but don't want to overheat — try these pungent and cooling vegetable tops. This relish-like sauce is a great way to use up the deliciously spicy tops (leaves and stems) of radishes and turnips, which are often discarded.

MAKES ABOUT 1 CUP (250 ML)

Tip

Omit the hot pepper flakes if your body tends to run hot.

Variations

Trimmed arugula or watercress makes a delicious substitute for the vegetable tops.

- **Blender or small food processor**
- **2-cup (500 mL) canning jar**

1 cup	packed chopped pungent vegetable tops, such as radish or turnip	250 mL
½ cup	packed chopped green onions	125 mL
6 tbsp	freshly squeezed lemon juice	90 mL
2 tbsp	avocado oil	30 mL
2 tsp	kosher or non-iodized sea salt, or to taste	10 mL
1 tsp	hot pepper flakes (optional)	5 mL

1. In blender, combine vegetable tops, green onions, lemon juice, oil, 2 tsp (10 mL) salt and hot pepper flakes (if using). Purée until almost smooth. Season to taste with additional salt, if desired.

2. Pour into jar. Serve immediately for best flavor. Or seal with lid and refrigerate for up to 3 days.

Health Tip

Spicy radish and turnip tops clear heat and dampness out of the body. They are marvelous in spring or summer and if you have been experiencing sluggish digestion or a cough with phlegm.

Pickled Lotus Root with Miso and Red Dates

This crunchy and refreshing condiment is both cooling and nourishing. The bland lotus root makes a terrific background for the sweet-and-earthy miso mixture.

MAKES SCANT 1 CUP (250 ML)

Tips

This pickle is mild enough to enjoy as a side dish.

Turning the jar ensures that the juices will be drawn out of all of the lotus root slices.

- **2-cup (500 mL) canning jar**

4 oz	lotus root	125 g
¼ cup	minced dried pitted red dates	60 mL
2 tbsp	white miso	30 mL
1 tsp	kosher or non-iodized sea salt	5 mL

1. Pour enough water into a medium saucepan to come 2 inches (5 cm) up side. Bring to a simmer. Trim ends off lotus root and peel. Immediately immerse in simmering water and cook for 25 to 30 minutes or until tender.

2. Drain and let cool to room temperature. Cut into ⅛-inch (3 mm) thick slices.

3. In a small bowl, stir together dates, miso, 2 tbsp (30 mL) water and salt to form a paste.

4. Spread a small amount of the red date paste on 1 lotus root slice and place in jar. Repeat with remaining paste and lotus root slices.

5. Seal jar with lid and refrigerate, upside down, for 24 hours to allow flavors to meld before serving. Refrigerate, right side up, in sealed jar for up 1 week.

Health Tip

Lotus root is cooling and sweet. On its own, it is beneficial to the stomach, and that action is enhanced by the miso, which adds healthy probiotic bacteria to the gut. Its nourishing component is enhanced by the sweet, *qi*-building red dates.

Pickled Umeboshi Radishes

This is a wonderfully satisfying pickle that is extremely good for your digestion. Small red globe radishes make a pretty pickle, but you can also use daikon radish — though the umeboshi plums will give them a light pink hue. Whenever spring comes around and the radishes are fresh and spicy, Ellen's family really enjoys having these on hand.

> **MAKES**
> **2 CUPS (500 ML)**

Tip

Be sure to purchase natural umeboshi, which don't contain added coloring or preservatives. See page 182 for more on this ingredient, and Resources (page 466) for sources.

- **2-cup (500 mL) canning jar**

2 cups	thinly sliced radishes	500 mL
1 tbsp	mashed pitted umeboshi	15 mL
1 tsp	kosher or non-iodized sea salt	5 mL

1. In a medium bowl, gently toss together radishes, mashed umeboshi and salt. Spoon into jar.

2. Seal with lid and refrigerate for at least 24 hours to allow flavors to meld before serving. Refrigerate in sealed jar for up to 1 week.

Health Tips

Umeboshi, the pickled fruit of the *Prunus mume* tree (a type of plum), is used as a home remedy in Japan and as a component in herbal medicines in China. The umeboshi's strong astringent and antiparasitic powers make it a go-to ingredient for treating digestive disturbances caused by viruses and bacteria, including cases of mild food poisoning (please note: any serious case of food poisoning requires immediate medical attention), diarrhea or even dysentery.

Have an upset stomach? Steep an umeboshi in a cup of hot water and drink as a tea. Drink it sparingly, though, as umeboshi plums are very salty.

Umeboshi with Jasmine Tea Leaves

Fermented tea leaf salad is a traditional dish eaten and enjoyed in Myanmar (formerly known as Burma). Fermented tea leaves are revered there and are served on special occasions and used in ceremonies. This variation is flavored with umeboshi, which kick-starts the very mild fermentation. A unique and delicious condiment, it lends a lovely fragrance and sour flavor to simple meals and adds balance to fish dishes.

> **MAKES SCANT
> 1 CUP (250 ML)**

Tip

To pit and mash the umeboshi, squeeze the fruit gently to extract the pit, and then chop finely or mash with a fork.

If you only have umeboshi paste on hand, you can use the same amount of that. However, be sure to buy only those brands that are free of preservatives. See Resources (page 466) for sources.

- **1-cup (250 mL) canning jar**

¼ cup	loose jasmine tea	60 mL
¼ cup	unsweetened white grape juice	60 mL
2 tbsp	mashed pitted umeboshi	30 mL

1. In a small saucepan, bring 2 cups (500 mL) water to a boil. Remove from heat and stir in tea leaves. Cover and let stand for 5 minutes.

2. Drain tea leaves well and let cool to room temperature. (Reserve tea and drink, or discard, as desired).

3. In jar, combine tea leaves, grape juice and mashed umeboshi. Seal with lid and shake vigorously to combine. Tap jar gently on work surface and let contents settle on bottom. Unseal lid but leave loosely on top of jar. Let stand at room temperature for 24 hours to allow flavors to meld before serving. Refrigerate sealed jar for up to 2 weeks.

> ## Health Tip
>
> Jasmine tea leaves are cooling and fragrant. They activate liver *qi*, clear up stagnation and balance digestion. Try small amounts of this condiment if you are transitioning from a meat-heavy diet, have a tendency toward slow digestion and run hot.

Parsley and Radish Top Sauerkraut

In many countries, fermented foods are made using a little bit of the leftovers from a previous batch. Here, sauerkraut juice acts as the starter. You may think this is a ton of greens, but fermentation greatly decreases their volume. Serve this condiment with any meal to increase your digestive juices.

**MAKES
½ CUP (125 ML)**

Tip

You can use different pungent greens in place of the parsley and radish tops: try arugula, mustard greens and stemmed tender kale leaves. Chop the leaves finely to make 2 cups (500 mL) total.

- **2-cup (500 mL) canning jar**

1 cup	packed coarsely chopped fresh parsley	250 g
1 cup	packed thinly sliced radish tops (leaves and stems)	250 g
1 tbsp	sauerkraut juice (from unpasteurized sauerkraut; store-bought or homemade)	15 mL
1 tsp	kosher or non-iodized sea salt	5 mL

1. In jar, combine parsley and radish tops. Sprinkle with sauerkraut juice and salt. Cover loosely with lid and let stand at room temperature for 24 hours before serving.

2. To store, using the back of a spoon, press parsley mixture down until submerged in liquid. Refrigerate in sealed jar for up to 2 weeks.

> ## Health Tip
>
> These strongly flavored greens activate digestion and break up stagnation in the body. They make a great spring and summer condiment.

Sauerkraut with Fennel and Caraway Seeds

Making your own fermented vegetables can be so satisfying — and somewhat magical. The combination of salt and a bit of starter juice makes this homemade sauerkraut an easy-to-prep introduction to fermentation.

> **MAKES**
> **2 CUPS (500 ML)**

Tips

This recipe creates a very mild fermentation; for a stronger one, you'll need to let the mixture stand at cool room temperature for 3 days before refrigerating it. Makes sure there's enough liquid to keep the cabbage submerged (see more info below).

After the cabbage mixture stands for 24 hours, there should be enough liquid to cover it. If there is not, dissolve 1/2 tsp (2 mL) salt in 7 tbsp (100 mL) water and pour it over the cabbage. Make sure you use this exact proportion of salt and water to ensure that the salt concentration is correct — it will prevent spoilage.

Once you refrigerate the cabbage mixture, the fermentation process slows down. That's why sauerkraut needs to stand at room temperature for a day.

Variations

Omit the seeds or substitute dill seeds or minced gingerroot for fennel or caraway seeds.

- **4-cup (1 L) canning jar**

2 cups	thinly sliced cabbage or mustard greens	500 mL
1 tbsp	sauerkraut juice (from unpasteurized sauerkraut; store-bought or homemade)	15 mL
1 tsp	kosher or non-iodized sea salt	5 mL
1/2 tsp	fennel seeds	2 mL
1/2 tsp	caraway seeds	2 mL

1. Place cabbage in jar and sprinkle with sauerkraut juice, salt, fennel seeds and caraway seeds. Seal lid and gently shake jar to make sure cabbage is evenly coated with juice mixture. Open jar. Using the back of a spoon, pack mixture down, making sure liquid covers cabbage. Cover loosely with lid and let stand at room temperature for 24 hours.

2. To store, using the back of a spoon, press cabbage down until submerged in liquid. Refrigerate in sealed jar for up to 2 weeks.

> ## Health Tip
>
> Fennel and caraway seeds enhance this condiment's positive effects on digestion. Their fragrance in the finished pickle will be subtle and enjoyable.
>
> Both seeds are very beneficial to digestion, warm the center of the body, dispel flatulence and ease abdominal cramping.

Dandelion Kimchi

This simple dandelion pickle is intensely bitter and palate-cleansing, making it the perfect spring condiment. If you have a lawn that is not sprayed with chemicals of any kind, get out there with your trowel and pick your own dandelion greens! Add this recipe to your spring menus to stimulate internal renewal.

**MAKES
1 CUP (250 ML)**

Tip

You can easily double or triple this recipe if you use the correct proportions. For every 1 cup (250 mL) tightly packed coarsely chopped dandelion greens, use ½ tsp (3 mL) salt. For example, if you use 2 cups (500 mL) greens, use 1 tsp (6 mL) salt.

- **2-cup (500 mL) canning jar**

1 cup	tightly packed coarsely chopped dandelion greens	250 mL
2 tbsp	finely chopped unpasteurized kimchi (store-bought or homemade)	30 mL
1 tbsp	kimchi juice (from kimchi jar)	15 mL
½ tsp	kosher or non-iodized sea salt	3 mL

1. In jar, combine dandelion greens, chopped kimchi, kimchi juice and salt. Using the back of a spoon, press down on greens to pack tightly. Cover jar with a paper towel and let stand at room temperature, pressing greens down every few hours with a spoon and re-covering with towel, for 24 hours. (Do not leave the spoon in the jar.)

2. Seal jar with lid and refrigerate for 3 days before serving. To store, refrigerate for up to 2 weeks. (This kimchi tastes best after about a week in the refrigerator.)

> ## Health Tips
>
> The word *dandelion* comes from the French *dent de lion,* which means "lion's tooth," for the toothed edges of the leaves. The French name for dandelion, *pissenlit,* literally means "wet the bed," for the plant's strong diuretic effects, which are due to its high potassium content.
>
> Dandelion greens are bitter and cooling and very beneficial to the liver; they stimulate liver metabolism and detoxification processes. The greens can help improve digestion and reduce swelling through their diuretic effect, while clearing heat and dampness from the body. Dandelion greens have traditionally been used to treat people suffering from water retention caused by high blood pressure.

Miso Daikon Pickles

In a Japanese household, it's practically a crisis when there aren't any pickles on hand! To the rescue: these quick Japanese-style pickles. Their earthy, very salty flavor makes them taste like they took much longer to make.

> **MAKES**
> **¾ CUP (175 ML)**

Tips

The pickles will keep for up to 1 week in the refrigerator, but they have the best flavor during the first 2 days.

Always buy the best-quality miso you can find (see page 173 for more on this ingredient). See Resources (page 466) for some good sources.

- **2-cup (500 mL) canning jar**

1	piece (6 oz/175 g) daikon radish	1
½ cup	white or red miso	125 mL
¼ cup	tamari	60 mL

1. Scrub or peel daikon and cut lengthwise into quarters. Cut quarters crosswise into ⅛-inch (3 mm) thick slices.

2. In a medium bowl, stir miso with tamari until smooth. Add daikon and stir to coat. Spoon into jar. Seal with lid and refrigerate for at least 6 hours before serving. Refrigerate in sealed jar for up to 1 week.

3. Rinse pickles and drain well before serving.

Health Tips

Daikon pickles enhance digestion and fat metabolism when you're eating an oily or rich meal. The addition of miso makes this version especially helpful for treating indigestion. They're also good for supporting detoxification if you're transitioning away from a diet high in processed foods.

If you eat a meat-heavy diet, eat these salty pickles in moderation.

Aromatic Nori Basil Sprinkle

This seasoning is subtly fragrant and a little bit pungent, built on a foundation of ingredients that are rich in minerals. Dust it over a quick salad or some cooled steam-sautéed vegetables.

MAKES
¾ CUP (175 ML)

Tips

Drying the blender ensures the nori will stay crisp and dry. Moisture causes nori to clump.

To toast black sesame seeds, place them in a medium dry skillet. Toast over low heat, stirring or shaking pan often, for about 3 minutes or until fragrant.

- **Preheat oven to 300°F (150°C)**
- **Rimmed baking sheet, lined with parchment paper**
- **8-inch (20 cm) square metal baking pan**
- **Blender**

½ tsp	Sichuan peppercorns, shiny black seeds removed (see tip, page 219)	2 mL
1	sheet nori	1
2 tbsp	hulled hemp seeds	30 mL
2 tbsp	black sesame seeds, toasted	30 mL
1 tsp	dried basil	5 mL
1 tsp	coconut sugar	5 mL
1 tsp	salt	5 mL

1. Spread Sichuan peppercorns and nori on prepared baking sheet. Bake in preheated oven for 5 to 7 minutes or until nori is crisp. Let cool completely on pan on a wire rack.

2. Spread hemp seeds in baking pan and bake in preheated oven for 5 to 7 minutes or until golden. Let cool completely in pan on a wire rack.

3. Dry blender completely with a towel (see tips, at left). Break nori into several pieces. In blender, combine nori and Sichuan peppercorns and grind until a coarse powder forms.

4. Pour nori mixture into an airtight container. Stir in hemp seeds, sesame seeds, basil, coconut sugar and salt. Seal tightly and store in a cool dry place for up to 2 weeks.

Health Tip

This aromatic and balanced sprinkle is mildly warming. It complements all sorts of simple meals and is especially delightful in the spring and summer.

Nettle and Chive Seaweed Sprinkle

Nettles and chives are some of the first greens that appear in spring in temperate climates. They are both wonderful spring tonic herbs. This springtime condiment has a mild onion flavor, thanks to the dried chives.

> **MAKES**
> **¾ CUP (175 ML)**

Tip

Drying the blender ensures the nori will stay crisp and dry. Moisture causes nori to clump.

- **Preheat oven to 300°F (150°C)**
- **Rimmed baking sheet, lined with parchment paper**
- **8-inch (20 cm) square metal baking pan**
- **Blender**

2	sheets nori	2
½ cup	hulled hemp seeds	125 mL
1 tbsp	dried nettles	15 mL
1 tbsp	dried chives	15 mL
¼ tsp	salt	1 mL

1. Place nori on prepared baking sheet. Bake in preheated oven for 5 to 7 minutes or until crisp. Let cool completely on pan on a wire rack.

2. Spread hemp seeds in baking pan and bake in preheated oven for 5 to 7 minutes or until golden. Let cool completely in pan on a wire rack.

3. Dry blender completely with a towel (see tip, at left). Break nori into several pieces. In blender, grind nori until a coarse powder forms.

4. Pour nori into an airtight container. Stir in hemp seeds, nettles, chives and salt. Seal tightly and store in a cool dry place for up to 2 weeks.

Health Tips

Nettles are cooling. They act as a natural diuretic and antihistamine and are very helpful for people who have allergies. Nettles are also nourishing to the blood and yin.

Chives give this condiment a warming action, which is excellent in the spring, when the weather is changeable. Hemp seeds and nori add important essential fatty acids and minerals.

Cooling Savory Nori Sprinkle

Here, tea leaves, nori and kale work together to create a lively "green" flavor. This condiment is especially nice sprinkled over sliced fresh tomatoes.

<table>
<tr><td>MAKES
¾ CUP (175 ML)</td></tr>
</table>

Tip

Use green tea that is made of only leaves, not a blend of leaves and twigs. If you don't have loose tea on hand, it's perfectly fine to open up a couple of tea bags and use the contents.

- **Preheat oven to 300°F (150°C)**
- **2 rimmed baking sheets, lined with parchment paper**
- **8-inch (20 cm) square metal baking pan**
- **Blender**

1 cup	coarsely chopped stemmed kale	250 mL
1 tbsp	loose green tea (see tip, at left)	15 mL
2	sheets nori	2
¼ cup	hulled hemp seeds	60 mL
1 tsp	salt	5 mL

1. Spread kale on 1 of the prepared baking sheets. Bake in preheated oven, stirring once or twice, for 20 to 25 minutes or until very crisp. Let cool completely on pan on a wire rack.

2. Meanwhile, spread green tea and nori on remaining prepared baking sheet. Bake in preheated oven for 5 to 7 minutes or until crisp. Let cool completely on pan on a wire rack.

3. Spread hemp seeds in baking pan and bake in preheated oven for 5 to 7 minutes or until golden. Let cool completely in pan on a wire rack.

4. Dry blender completely with a towel (see tips, page 440). In blender, grind tea leaves with kale until a coarse powder forms. Break nori into several pieces and add to blend and grind until a coarse powder forms.

5. Pour tea mixture into an airtight container. Stir in hemp seeds and salt. Seal tightly and store in a cool dry place for up to 2 weeks.

> ## Health Tip
>
> Enjoy this condiment in the spring and summer, when the cooling tea leaves and mildly bitter flavor will counter the heat of the season and clear out excess heat buildup in the body.

Walnut and Chive Condiment

This warming, rich and mildly spiced condiment is delicious with grilled fish and rice. The inclusion of fresh chives make it a little moister than other dry condiments, but the mixture is textured and crunchy, with a surprising, complex flavor.

	MAKES
	½ CUP (125 ML)

Tip

Letting the cooked mixture cool completely in the pan helps dry out the chives.

½ cup	coarsely chopped walnuts	125 mL
2 tbsp	minced fresh chives	30 mL
1 tsp	dill seeds	5 mL
1 tsp	avocado oil	5 mL
¼ tsp	salt	1 mL

1. In a medium dry skillet, toast walnuts over medium-low heat for 5 minutes or until slightly fragrant.

2. Stir in chives, dill seeds, oil and salt. Heat, stirring constantly, for 1 to 2 minutes or until chives are wilted. Remove from heat and let cool completely.

3. Refrigerate in airtight container for up to 3 days.

Health Tip

Walnuts and chives are both yang and warming foods that benefit the kidneys. They are a perfect choice if you often feel cold and run-down. Use this condiment in the colder months if you tend to run cold, or to warm up a vegan or vegetarian meal.

Bonito and Seed Furikake

Furikake is a Japanese seasoning used to add flavor and nutrients to plain rice. Its rich mineral content comes from the nori and katsuobushi (fish flakes). It adds savory notes and is delicious on steamed greens, roasted sweet vegetables, noodles or any other food that needs a boost of seasoning and protein.

MAKES
⅔ CUP (150 ML)

Tip

To toast hemp, sesame and chia seeds, place them in a medium dry skillet. Toast over low heat, stirring or shaking pan often, for about 3 minutes or until fragrant.

- **Preheat oven to 200°F (100°C)**
- **Rimmed baking sheet, lined with parchment paper**

2	sheets nori	2
2 tbsp	hulled hemp seeds, toasted	30 mL
2 tbsp	white sesame seeds, toasted	30 mL
2 tbsp	chia seeds, toasted	30 mL
2 tbsp	finely crumbled katsuobushi (see page 171)	30 mL
1 tsp	date or coconut sugar	5 mL
1 tsp	salt	5 mL

1. Tear nori into large strips and place on prepared baking sheet, without overlapping. Bake in preheated oven for 20 minutes or until nori is crisp and dry. Let cool completely on pan on a wire rack.

2. Using kitchen shears and working over paper on pan, cut nori into strips about ½ inch (1 cm) wide. Stacking 5 or 6 strips at a time, cut strips crosswise into very thin shreds.

3. Gather up edges of paper and pour nori into a medium bowl. Gently stir in hemp seeds, sesame seeds, chia seeds, katsuobushi, date sugar and salt.

4. Pour nori mixture into an airtight container. Seal tightly and store in a cool dry place for up to 2 months.

Health Tip

The foundation of nori, sesame, salt and katsuobushi makes this topping not only delicious but also nourishing for the kidney yin and *jing* (essence). The katsuobushi adds protein and an umami, or savory, dimension.

Black and White Sesame Furikake

This furikake is a little bit of a mash-up between the usual Japanese rice topper and another Japanese seasoning called shichimi togarashi *(seven-flavor chili pepper). It stimulates digestion with a bit of spice and is a tasty complement to almost any simple food, including soups, steamed rice, noodles or sweet, earthy vegetables.*

MAKES
½ CUP (125 ML)

Tip

To toast sesame seeds, place them in a medium dry skillet. Toast over low heat, stirring or shaking pan often, for about 3 minutes or until fragrant.

- **Preheat oven to 200°F (100°C)**
- **Rimmed baking sheet, lined with parchment paper**

2	sheets nori	2
½ tsp	grated tangerine zest	2 mL
2 tbsp	white sesame seeds, toasted	30 mL
2 tbsp	black sesame seeds, toasted	30 mL
1 tsp	date or coconut sugar	5 mL
1 tsp	salt	5 mL
½ tsp	coarsely ground cayenne pepper or hot pepper flakes	2 mL

1. Tear nori into large strips and place on prepared baking sheet, without overlapping. Bake in preheated oven for 20 minutes or until nori is crisp and dry. Let cool completely on pan on a wire rack.

2. Slide paper with nori onto work surface. Line baking sheet with another piece of parchment paper. Spread tangerine zest in center. Bake for 6 to 8 minutes or until fragrant and dry. Let cool completely on pan on a wire rack.

3. Meanwhile, using kitchen shears and working over paper, cut nori into strips about ½ inch (1 cm) wide. Stacking 5 or 6 strips at a time, cut strips crosswise into very thin shreds. Gather up edges of paper and pour nori into a medium bowl. Set aside.

4. Add tangerine zest to nori. Gently stir in white and black sesame seeds, date sugar, salt and cayenne.

5. Pour nori mixture into an airtight container. Seal tightly and store in a cool dry place for up to 2 months.

Health Tip

This sprinkle is sweet and aromatic, with a bit of spice from the cayenne. If you are looking for a condiment that offers mild heat, this is a well-balanced, flavorful choice.

Dried Lime Furikake

This tasty sprinkle is sour and zesty at the same time. Enjoy it over steamed rice, or grilled fish or chicken. It makes a lovely addition to summer and autumn meals, thanks to its mild tartness.

MAKES
½ CUP (125 ML)

Tips

Once you've stripped the fresh parsley leaves from the stems, be sure to pat them with a towel until they are completely dry. This will ensure they crisp up well in the oven.

To toast hemp seeds, place them in a medium dry skillet. Toast over low heat, stirring or shaking pan often, for about 3 minutes or until fragrant.

- **Preheat oven to 200°F (100°C)**
- **Rimmed baking sheet, lined with parchment paper**

2	sheets nori	2
1 tsp	freshly squeezed lime juice	5 mL
½ tsp	grated lime zest	2 mL
2 tbsp	fresh parsley leaves (see tips, at left)	30 mL
¼ cup	hulled hemp seeds, toasted	60 mL
1 tsp	salt	5 mL

1. Tear nori into large strips and place on prepared baking sheet, without overlapping. Drizzle with lime juice (nori will wrinkle). Bake in preheated oven for 20 minutes or until nori is crisp and dry. Let cool completely on pan on a wire rack.

2. Slide paper with nori onto work surface. Line baking sheet with another piece of parchment paper. Spread lime zest in center and arrange parsley near edges of pan. Bake for 6 to 8 minutes or until dry and crisp. Let cool completely on pan on a wire rack.

3. Meanwhile, using kitchen shears and working over paper, cut nori into strips about ½ inch (1 cm) wide. Stacking 5 or 6 strips at a time, cut strips crosswise into very thin shreds.

4. Gather up edges of paper and pour nori into a medium bowl. Gently stir in lime zest, parsley, hemp seeds and salt.

5. Pour nori mixture into an airtight container. Seal tightly and store in a cool dry place for up to 2 months.

Health Tip

The cooling lime adds a sour undertone to this condiment that is beneficial in summer and autumn. If you crave a bit of acidity in your meal, this furikake makes a perfect topping. The tart flavor astringes and contains, so if you are feeling a bit scattered, try this condiment to calm and soothe your energy. The warming parsley also serves as a blood tonic; this herb, like the nori, also acts as a mild diuretic.

Gomashio

The name of this Japanese savory condiment is a combination of goma, meaning "sesame," and shio, meaning "salt." Sesame seeds give this blend a nutty taste and help you cut down on the amount of salt you might add at the table. The combination of black and white seeds brings yin-yang balance to the condiment and is very pretty atop greens, noodles or grains during any season.

> **MAKES**
> **1/3 CUP (75 ML)**

Tips

There's a quick test you can do to ensure that your sesame seeds are perfectly toasted. When the oil begins to release and the white sesame seeds turn a slightly darker color, remove one and crush it between your pinky and thumb. If it crushes easily, the seeds are done.

In Japan, gomashio is traditionally ground using a mortar (*suribachi*) and pestle (*surikogi*). See page 160 for more information on suribachis and other mortars and pestles.

Variation

Feel free to substitute hemp seeds for half of the sesame seeds. For a more aromatic result, add a pinch of fennel seeds (which also aid digestion), cumin seeds or caraway seeds. Or add a pinch of dried herbs such as basil, thyme or oregano for their warming powers.

- **Mortar and pestle (see tips, at left)**

1/3 cup	mixed black and white sesame seeds	75 mL
1 tsp	sea, Himalayan pink or Celtic salt	5 mL

1. Toast sesame seeds in a medium dry skillet over low heat, stirring or shaking pan often, for 5 to 7 minutes or until fragrant and seeds can be crushed easily (see tips, at left). Immediately transfer to mortar. Set aside.

2. Add salt to skillet and cook, stirring, for 2 minutes or until slightly gray. Immediately transfer to mortar. Using pestle, grind sesame seeds with salt until coarse powder forms. Let cool completely.

3. Spoon sesame mixture into an airtight container. Seal tightly and store in a cool dry place for up to 3 weeks.

> ## Health Tip
>
> Sesame seeds are a blood and yin tonic that benefits the kidneys. They also lubricate the intestines and relieve constipation. Gomashio is a beneficial condiment for nursing mothers because it supports breast milk production. It is also a delicious alternative for anyone who likes the taste of salt but is wary of consuming too much sodium.

Ras el Hanout Dukkah

Dukkah (also spelled duqqa) is an Egyptian condiment made from a variety of nuts, herbs and spices. Our recipe uses fragrant homemade Ras el Hanout as the seasoning. Mix dukkah with a little olive oil and use it as a dip for bread or vegetables, or sprinkle the dry mixture over a delicate soup.

| **MAKES** |
| **1 CUP (250 ML)** |

Tips

To toast hazelnuts, place them in a medium dry skillet. Toast over low heat, stirring or shaking pan often, for about 7 minutes or until fragrant.

- **Blender or small food processor**

½ cup	hazelnuts, toasted	125 mL
¼ cup	sesame seeds, toasted (see tip, page 445)	60 mL
¼ cup	Ras el Hanout (page 227)	60 mL
1 tsp	salt	5 mL

1. In blender, combine hazelnuts and sesame seeds. Grind until the texture is slightly coarser than brown sugar.

2. Spoon into an airtight container. Stir in ras el hanout and salt. Seal tightly and store in a cool dry place for up to 2 weeks.

Health Tip

Nuts and spices make this fragrant mixture a nourishing condiment. It is warming and energizing, with the subtle fragrance of rose to lift your spirits.

Four-Flavor Savory Sprinkle

This vegan condiment is dense and rich in umami ingredients. It adds a nice, deep, savory hit of flavor to dishes.

MAKES
1½ CUPS (375 ML)

Tip

If the finished condiment seems like it isn't completely dry, store it in the refrigerator and use it up within 1 week.

Health Tip

This condiment contains all four flavors, which work in harmony to give it salty, sour, sweet and bitter overtones. If you are craving a more substantial condiment, look no further — this one rounds out the simplest of meals and has a satisfying taste.

- **Preheat oven to 250°F (120°C)**
- **1 piece (16 by 12 inches/40 by 30 cm) parchment paper**
- **2 large rimmed baking sheets**
- **Blender or food processor**

¼ cup	white miso	60 mL
¼ cup	tomato paste	60 mL
1 tbsp	unsweetened cocoa powder	15 mL
4	dried shiitake mushrooms	4
½ cup	walnut halves	125 mL

1. In a small bowl, stir together miso, tomato paste and cocoa powder. Using a long, flexible spatula, spread mixture as thinly as possible on parchment paper, making sure edges are slightly thicker than center. Slide paper onto 1 of the baking sheets.

2. Bake in preheated oven for about 20 minutes or until surface looks dry. (Watch carefully so that mixture doesn't overbrown.) Let cool completely on pan on a wire rack.

3. Meanwhile, break or cut stems off mushrooms and discard. Place mushrooms and walnuts on remaining baking sheet. Bake in preheated oven for 5 to 10 minutes or until walnuts are lightly browned. Let cool completely on pan on a wire rack.

4. Peel miso mixture off paper and break into pieces. If any pieces remain moist, return to paper, place on baking sheet and bake for 5 minutes or until dry.

5. Dry blender completely with a towel (see tips, page 440). In blender, grind mushrooms until a coarse powder forms.

6. Add miso mixture pieces and walnuts. Grind until a coarse powder forms.

7. Pour into an airtight container. Seal tightly and store in a cool dry place for up to 2 weeks.

Salty Juniper Berry and Tangerine Sprinkle

This pleasingly sharp, salty condiment gets its resinous flavor from dried juniper berries. If you are looking to add a delicious aroma and hearty flavor, serve it with braised meat or sweet vegetables.

> **MAKES ABOUT ½ CUP (125 ML)**

Tip

To toast hemp seeds, place them in a medium dry skillet. Toast over low heat, stirring or shaking pan often, for about 3 minutes or until fragrant.

Caution

Juniper berries are contraindicated if you are pregnant, have kidney inflammation or nephritis. Avoid this dish in those cases.

- **Mortar and pestle, or spice grinder**

½ tsp	dried juniper berries	2 mL
½ tsp	dried tangerine peel	2 mL
½ cup	hulled hemp seeds, toasted	125 mL
1½ tsp	salt	7 mL
½ tsp	minced dried rosemary	2 mL

1. In mortar, combine juniper berries and tangerine peel. Using pestle, grind until coarse powder forms.

2. Pour into an airtight container. Stir in hemp seeds, salt and rosemary. Seal tightly and store in a cool dry place for up to 2 weeks.

Health Tip

Juniper berries are bitter, sweet and drying. They can dispel cold, warm the body, relieve flatulence and support digestion. Juniper berries are also used medicinally for mild urinary tract infections. Their powers are enhanced by dried tangerine peel, which moves *qi*. When paired with dried rosemary, their warming and yang-fortifying actions are heightened. This condiment is great for people who live in chilly, damp climates.

Walnut and Black Sesame Sprinkle

Be careful when you make this — we promise it's so good you might eat it all in one sitting! Walnuts and black sesame both nourish the kidney yin and yang from a Chinese medicinal point of view. The Chinese say that eating 1 tbsp (15 mL) of this blend each morning will ensure longevity and youthful vigor. It is delicious on top of congee or your favorite fruit compote.

**MAKES
½ CUP (125 ML)**

Tips

We like to rub the walnuts to remove the skins, because they are unpleasantly bitter.

There's a quick test you can do to ensure that your sesame seeds are perfectly toasted. When the oil begins to release, remove one and crush it between your pinky and thumb. If it crushes easily, the seeds are done.

- **Mortar and pestle (see tips, page 447)**

¼ cup	walnut halves	60 mL
¼ cup	black sesame seeds	60 mL
1 tbsp	coconut sugar or date sugar	15 mL

1. Toast walnuts in a medium dry skillet over low heat, stirring or shaking pan often, for 6 to 8 minutes or until fragrant. Immediately transfer to a tea towel and let cool enough to handle. Rub briskly to remove skins (see tips, at left). Pick nuts off towel and place in mortar. Let cool.

2. Meanwhile, add sesame seeds to skillet. Toast over low heat, stirring or shaking pan often, for 3 minutes or until fragrant (see tips, at left). Immediately transfer to mortar and let cool completely.

3. Using pestle, grind walnuts and sesame seeds until a medium-fine powder forms. Stir in sugar.

4. Spoon walnut mixture into an airtight container. Seal tightly and store in a cool dry place for up to 3 weeks.

Health Tips

Walnuts nourish the kidney *qi* and yang, while the black sesame seeds nourish the kidney yin. This is a condiment that gets to the root of all *qi*: the kidney yin and yang.

If you experience insomnia, take 1 tbsp (15 mL) of this condiment 2 hours prior to bedtime.

This recipe can also be used to nourish the hair and skin and to prevent premature grays. In this case, take 1 tbsp (15 mL) every morning on an empty stomach.

Crataegus, Dried Cherry, Walnut and Nutmeg Sprinkle

This topping is fragrant, with a sweet flavor and bold texture. It is delicious with water-sautéed or puréed cooked Asian sweet potatoes and ghee. The dried Chinese hawthorn fruit is different from the Western hawthorn berry; it is often known by its Latin name, crataegus, and retains a slightly hard texture even when ground.

> **MAKES**
> **1 CUP (250 ML)**

Tips

To toast walnuts, place them in a medium skillet. Toast over low heat, stirring or shaking pan often, for 5 to 7 minutes or until fragrant.

Be sure you purchase the Chinese variety of crataegus, also known in Mandarin as *shan zha*. This herb is not the same as Western hawthorn berries, which have a different effect on the body. You can purchase Chinese crataegus at Asian grocery stores and from Chinese herb suppliers. See Resources (page 466) for our recommendations.

- **Blender or small food processor**

2 tbsp	dried crataegus	30 mL
2 tbsp	dried pitted cherries	30 mL
2 tbsp	finely chopped dried apricots	30 mL
Pinch	salt	Pinch
½ cup	walnuts, toasted and cooled	125 mL
¼ tsp	ground nutmeg	1 mL

1. In blender, combine crataegus, cherries, apricots and salt. Grind until finely chopped. Add walnuts and grind just until finely chopped.

2. Spoon crataegus mixture into an airtight container. Stir in nutmeg. Seal tightly and store in a cool dry place for up to 2 weeks.

> ### Health Tips
>
> Dried hawthorn fruit (crataegus) is often used in Chinese herbal formulas to invigorate blood circulation, improve digestion and eliminate food stagnation. This condiment helps speed up sluggish digestion. Dried hawthorn fruit is often sold in candied or fruit-leather form and eaten as a snack in China.
>
> The fruits and nuts are warming and nourishing, and benefit the kidney yang.

Five-Seed Crunchy Condiment

If you are looking for your daily dose of essential fatty acids, this is your condiment. Enjoy its nourishing crunch atop plain vegetables, salads or fish.

> **MAKES**
> **⅔ CUP (150 ML)**

Tip

The seeds toast at slightly different rates. Remove them from the pan as soon as the mixture is fragrant so the smaller seeds don't get scorched.

- **Blender, or large mortar and pestle**

2 tbsp	chia seeds	30 mL
2 tbsp	flax seeds	30 mL
2 tbsp	hulled hemp seeds	30 mL
2 tbsp	sunflower seeds	30 mL
2 tbsp	sesame seeds	30 mL
1 tsp	coconut sugar	5 mL
1 tsp	salt	5 mL

1. In a large skillet, combine chia, flax, hemp, sunflower and sesame seeds. Toast over medium heat, stirring or shaking pan often, for about 5 minutes or until fragrant. Transfer to a small bowl and let cool completely.

2. In blender, grind seed mixture until the texture of brown sugar.

3. Pour seed mixture into an airtight container. Stir in coconut sugar and salt. Seal tightly and store in a cool dry place for up to 2 weeks.

Health Tip

In Chinese medicine, seeds are used to nourish the yin, jing and brain. This condiment is an excellent choice for seniors, and others who are yin deficient, such as women who are going through perimenopause and menopause. It is also good for women who are trying to boost their fertility. For everyone else, a sprinkle of this condiment will up your intake of essential fatty acids, which have anti-inflammatory and lubricating effects in the body.

Ginger Vinegar

This warming and spicy vinegar is excellent for digestion. You can take it a couple of different ways: add a splash to your favorite simple vegetable dish, or stir 1 tbsp (15 mL) into a glass of water or tea. Feel free to add a bit of honey to sweeten up your beverage.

> **MAKES**
> **2 CUPS (500 ML)**

Tips

When you make flavored vinegar, wash your canning jars well with soap and rinse them in very hot water before using.

Placing a piece of waxed paper between mouth of the jar and the lid will keep the vinegar from corroding the metal.

Health Tip

The combination of raw ginger and vinegar has a strong warming effect on the digestive system. Take 1 tbsp (15 mL) with a meal, once or twice a day.

Use this vinegar, or eat a piece of the steeped ginger, to soothe indigestion. These can also help you feel better if you consume large amounts of fish or cold-natured foods, such as salads, juices, and raw fruits and vegetables, which can irritate the stomach.

- **4-cup (1 L) canning jar (see tips, at left)**

½ cup	julienned gingerroot	125 mL
1¾ cups	unseasoned rice vinegar or unfiltered cider vinegar (approx.)	425 mL

1. Place ginger in jar and pour vinegar over top, adding a little more vinegar if necessary to fill jar. Place a piece of waxed paper over jar mouth and seal with lid (see tips, at left). Let stand in a cool dry place for 1 week.

2. Taste vinegar; if the ginger flavor is strong enough, strain through a fine-mesh sieve into a clean jar and store in a cool, dark, dry place for up to 6 months or in the refrigerator for up to 1 year. If you would like a stronger flavor, do not strain; refrigerate sealed jar for up to 1 year.

What Vinegars Do

All of our vinegars are made using the same basic method. Their therapeutic effects and flavors, are, of course, distinctly different depending on the herb or food that is being infused. Feel free to extend your repertoire of herbal and therapeutic vinegars by experimenting with other ingredients, such as mint, rosemary, oregano, thyme, nettles, green onions, garlic, black, white or red (pink) peppercorns and so on.

Vinegar has an alkalinizing effect on the body. It is beneficial for digestion, and aids in the breakdown of animal fats. When added to vegetables and fruits, it can help extract essential minerals and make them more absorbable.

Rosemary and Thyme Vinegar

This herbaceous vinegar is warming and good for the lungs and digestive system. Drizzle it over cooked greens or meat dishes. Or use it if you have a cold or need extra warming yang in your meal.

> **MAKES**
> **2 CUPS (500 ML)**

Tips

When you make flavored vinegar, wash your canning jars well with soap and rinse them in very hot water before using.

Placing a piece of waxed paper between mouth of the jar and the lid will keep the vinegar from corroding the metal.

- **4-cup (1 L) canning jar (see tips, at left)**

½ cup	fresh rosemary leaves (6 to 8 sprigs)	125 mL
½ cup	fresh thyme leaves (6 to 8 sprigs)	125 mL
1¾ cups	unseasoned rice vinegar or unfiltered cider vinegar (approx.)	425 mL

1. Place rosemary and thyme in jar and pour vinegar over top, adding a little more vinegar if necessary to fill jar. Place a piece of waxed paper over jar mouth and seal with lid (see tips, at left). Let stand in a cool dry place for 1 week.

2. Taste vinegar; if the herbal flavor is strong enough, strain through a fine-mesh sieve into a clean jar and store in a cool, dark, dry place for up to 6 months or in the refrigerator for up to 1 year. If you would like a stronger flavor, do not strain; refrigerate sealed jar for up to 1 year.

> ### Health Tip
>
> Rosemary and thyme are both warming herbs that stimulate digestion and soothe indigestion. Thyme moves *qi* and benefits the lungs; rosemary stimulates and improves circulation, stimulates the mind and memory, and is rich in antioxidants.

Rose Vinegar

The fragrant, qi-moving rose adds a light floral flavor to foods. It eases stress, lifts the spirits and benefits the liver. To make a delicious spring or summer beverage, mix a little of this vinegar into a glass of still or sparkling water and add a little honey to taste.

**MAKES
2 CUPS (500 ML)**

Tips

When you make flavored vinegar, wash your canning jars well with soap and rinse them in very hot water before using.

Placing a piece of waxed paper between mouth of the jar and the lid will keep the vinegar from corroding the metal.

It's important to buy food-grade petals or dried buds from organically grown roses that have not been sprayed with pesticides or herbicides.

- **4-cup (1 L) canning jar (see tips, at left)**

1 cup	food-grade fresh red rose petals (or ¾ cup/175 mL food-grade dried red rose buds)	250 mL
1¾ cups	unseasoned rice vinegar or unfiltered cider vinegar (approx.)	425 mL

1. Place rose petals in jar and pour vinegar over top, adding a little more vinegar if necessary to fill jar. Place a piece of waxed paper over jar mouth and seal with lid (see tips, at left). Let stand in a cool dry place for 1 week.

2. Taste vinegar; if the rose flavor is strong enough, strain through a fine-mesh sieve into a clean jar and store in a cool, dark, dry place for up to 6 months or in the refrigerator for up to 1 year. If you would like a stronger flavor, do not strain; refrigerate sealed jar for up to 3 weeks. (Do not refrigerate unstrained vinegar for longer, as the flavor becomes bitter.)

> ## Health Tips
>
> This vinegar works as a stress reliever and nervine, or calming agent; take 1 tbsp (15 mL) before eating or mix it into a glass of water. It can also ease menstrual cramps and mild premenstrual symptoms, and it relieves hot flashes without sweating.
>
> Rose vinegar is also good for topical use. Spray it over your face to reduce redness, or dab it onto bug bites or sunburned skin to get some relief. It makes a soothing addition to warm bathwater, too.

Lemon Zest Vinegar

This cooling, ultra-tangy vinegar helps disperse superficial body heat. Use it as a seasoning on simple vegetable dishes, or as a tea or a spring-into-summer beverage (see health tip, below).

MAKES
2 CUPS (500 ML)

Tips

When you make flavored vinegar, wash your canning jars well with soap and rinse them in very hot water before using.

Placing a piece of waxed paper between mouth of the jar and the lid will keep the vinegar from corroding the metal.

- **4-cup (1 L) canning jar (see tips, at left)**

1	lemon	1
2 cups	unseasoned rice vinegar or unfiltered cider vinegar	500 mL

1. Using a sharp paring knife or vegetable peeler, cut zest off lemon, avoiding any of the bitter white pith.

2. Place lemon zest in jar and pour vinegar over top. Place a piece of waxed paper over jar mouth and seal with lid (see tips, at left). Let stand in a cool dry place for 1 week.

3. Taste vinegar; if the lemon flavor is strong enough, strain through a fine-mesh sieve into a clean jar and store in a cool, dark, dry place for up to 6 months or in the refrigerator for up to 1 year. If you would like a stronger flavor, do not strain; refrigerate sealed jar for up to 3 months.

Health Tip

This cooling vinegar is just right for late spring and summer. Add it to either still or sparkling water for a refreshing cool beverage. If you feel a sore throat coming on, stir a bit into a cup of hot tea along with a few fresh mint leaves and a spoonful of honey.

Endive, Raisin and Pine Nut Chutney

This chutney makes a delicious complement to a warming dish of curry or meat. The bitterness of the endive is tempered by the sweetness of the raisins.

> **MAKES**
> **1½ CUPS (375 ML)**

Tip

To toast pine nuts, place them in a medium dry skillet. Toast over low heat, stirring or shaking pan often, for 3 to 5 minutes or until fragrant.

- **2-cup (500 mL) canning jar**

1 cup	minced curly endive leaves	250 mL
¼ cup	raisins	60 mL
2 tbsp	unfiltered cider vinegar	30 mL
½ tsp	salt	2 mL
½ cup	pine nuts, toasted	125 mL

1. In jar, combine endive, raisins, vinegar and salt. Seal with lid and refrigerate for at least 2 hours or up to 3 days.

2. Stir in pine nuts just before serving.

> ### Health Tip
>
> Endive, a member of the bitter chicory family, is cooling and helps cleanse the blood. It can counter any heat buildup in the body and makes a perfect spring tonic. Members of the chicory family contain inulin, a soluble plant fiber that promotes good digestion, helps keep blood sugar levels steady and has been shown to reduce low-density lipoprotein (LDL), or cholesterol, levels in people with diabetes and those who are obese.

Mulberry and Goji Berry Chutney

Mulberries and goji berries — two essence-building fruits — make this chutney a unique qi, yin and blood tonic. Try a spoonful of it with congee, simple braised dishes or fried eggs.

MAKES
½ CUP (125 ML)

Tip

If the mixture is too thick, you can stir in a little more juice to thin it out.

¼ cup	dried mulberries	60 mL
¼ cup	dried goji berries	60 mL
2 tbsp	unseasoned rice vinegar	30 mL
2 tbsp	pomegranate juice	30 mL
1 tbsp	liquid honey	15 mL
¼ tsp	ground cinnamon	1 mL
¼ tsp	ground nutmeg	1 mL
Pinch	salt	Pinch

1. In a small nonreactive saucepan, combine mulberries, goji berries, vinegar, pomegranate juice, honey, cinnamon, nutmeg and salt. Bring to a boil.

2. Remove from heat, cover and let stand for 20 minutes.

3. Spoon into an airtight container and refrigerate for up to 1 week.

Health Tip

This is a beneficial blood-tonic condiment for people who are blood deficient; these people experience dry hair and skin, dry or brittle nails and insomnia. Women who are blood deficient may also experience irregular periods. This condiment is also terrific for seniors, because it is warming and eases constipation.

Sweet Cherry, Date and Walnut Warming Chutney

There is something so wonderfully tempting about cherries and dates paired together. Try this chutney if you are looking for a concentrated, sweet-tart flavor addition to your meal. It is balanced, with a sweet-and-spicy taste that goes well with curry dishes, sweet vegetables, braised meats and fish.

MAKES
¾ CUP (175 ML)

Tips

Don't spend a ton on balsamic vinegar or use your best bottle for this chutney. Regular, inexpensive varieties from the supermarket will work just fine.

To toast walnuts, place them in a medium dry skillet. Toast over low heat, stirring or shaking pan often, for 5 to 7 minutes or until fragrant.

¼ cup	minced toasted walnuts	60 mL
¼ cup	minced pitted fresh or thawed frozen dark cherries	60 mL
¼ cup	minced pitted dates	60 mL
1 tbsp	balsamic vinegar	15 mL
¼ tsp	salt	1 mL
¼ tsp	black pepper	1 mL

1. In a medium bowl, stir together walnuts, cherries, dates, vinegar, salt and pepper.

2. Spoon into an airtight container and refrigerate for up to 1 week.

Health Tip

This warming *qi* and yang chutney is great for anyone who runs cold, has poor energy or sluggish digestion. Use this condiment to add warmth to cooling dishes.

Fig and Cardamom Charoset

Charoset is a sweet condiment eaten during the Passover Seder to symbolize the mortar used by enslaved Jews in Egypt during the time of the Pharaohs. The ingredients vary from country to country. This tasty, warming and aromatic version is typical of the Sephardic communities of Northern Africa, Greece, Turkey and southern Spain. Add it to your meals when you want a touch of rich and filling sweetness.

MAKES SCANT 2 CUPS (500 ML)

Tips

To toast walnuts, place them in a medium skillet. Toast over low heat, stirring or shaking pan often, for 5 to 7 minutes or until fragrant.

Other dried fruits, such as cherries or plums, may be substituted for the figs, dates and apricots.

Caution

Cinnamon is one of the most common spices used in the kitchen. However, in high doses it can cause uterine contractions, so be moderate in your consumption if you are pregnant. Typical amounts used in recipes are just fine.

- **2-cup (500 mL) canning jar**

½ cup	chopped walnuts, toasted	125 mL
½ cup	minced stemmed dried figs	125 mL
¼ cup	minced pitted dates	60 mL
¼ cup	minced dried apricots	60 mL
¼ cup	red wine (kosher for Passover, if desired) or unsweetened grape juice	60 mL
½ tsp	ground cinnamon	2 mL
¼ tsp	ground cardamom	1 mL

1. In jar, combine walnuts, figs, dates, apricots, wine, cinnamon and cardamom. Shake or stir to combine.

2. Seal with lid and refrigerate for up to 2 weeks.

Health Tips

Warming, aromatic cinnamon and cardamom enhance digestion and counter the effects of eating a diet of cooling raw foods. These two spices are beneficial if your digestion is sluggish.

If you suffer from night sweat or hot flashes, often feel warm or are significantly overweight, do not eat large amounts of this warming condiment.

Ginger, Turmeric and Tamarind Chutney

Enticing, pungent aromas and tangy flavors are delightfully balanced in this chutney. Mildly sweet and bracingly acidic at the same time, it is scrumptious drizzled over greens, or served with simple congee or eggs.

MAKES
MAKES **1½ CUPS (375 ML)**

Tip

Tamarind paste is often labeled "seedless" but it usually still contains seeds. Pressing the soaked paste through a fine-mesh sieve fixes that.

- **Blender or food processor**

¼ cup	tamarind paste	60 mL
2 cups	hot water	500 mL
¼ cup	finely chopped gingerroot	60 mL
¼ cup	coarsely chopped pitted dates	60 mL
2 tbsp	finely chopped peeled fresh turmeric	30 mL
1 tbsp	coconut sugar	15 mL
¼ tsp	salt	1 mL

1. Break tamarind paste into almond-size lumps. In a small bowl, stir tamarind paste with hot water. Let stand for 1 hour.

2. Transfer tamarind mixture to blender. Purée until thickened. Using a spatula, press through a fine-mesh sieve into a small bowl. Discard seeds and fibers.

3. In a medium nonreactive skillet, combine tamarind purée, ginger, dates, turmeric, coconut sugar and salt. Bring to a simmer over medium heat. Simmer, stirring often, for 20 minutes or until thickened and glossy. Let cool completely.

4. Spoon into an airtight container and refrigerate for up to 2 weeks.

Health Tip

Paired together in this chutney, ginger and turmeric are potent anti-inflammatories. Their powers are further enhanced by the addition of tamarind, an excellent nausea fighter. This chutney is best for people who suffer from inflammatory pain, nausea or blood sugar imbalances.

Pungent Ginger and Mustard Seed Spread

This intensely delightful spread is packed with pungency from the radishes, ginger and mustard. The small addition of honey, lemon and salt only enhances the vibrancy of this spread. You must try it! Eat it on the side with congee or roasted squash, or anytime you want to liven up a plain meal.

> **MAKES SCANT
> 1 CUP (250 ML)**

Tip

Any kind of radish works well in this recipe. Red radishes make a pretty orange spread, but pale daikon radishes are just as tasty.

½ cup	chopped radish (see tip, at left)	125 mL
¼ cup	chopped gingerroot	60 mL
2 tbsp	brown or yellow mustard seeds	30 mL
2 tbsp	liquid honey	30 mL
2 tbsp	freshly squeezed lemon juice	30 mL
½ tsp	salt	2 mL

1. In a small nonreactive skillet, combine radish, ginger, mustard seeds and honey. Cook over medium-low heat, stirring often, for 5 minutes or until thickened.

2. Stir in lemon juice and salt. Let cool completely. Spoon into an airtight container and refrigerate for up to 1 week.

> ## Health Tips
>
> Mustard seeds have a long medicinal history. They have traditionally been used topically in plasters to increase blood circulation to the surface of the skin. These plasters break up congestion and reduce inflammation in cases of sprains, respiratory congestion and arthritis. Internally, mustard seeds are warming; they stimulate *qi* and promote circulation.
>
> Ginger is warming and beneficial to the stomach and digestion, while radish clears out excessive heat and has a pungent flavor.
>
> Packed with healing ingredients, this condiment is terrific if you're suffering from a cold or cough, have a poor appetite, eat too many cooling foods, feel fatigued, generally feel cold or experience digestive distress.

Fresh Turmeric and Umeboshi Relish

This engaging condiment is hard to resist. Enjoy good digestion by serving it with salmon, tofu or well-cooked warm vegetables.

MAKES
²⁄₃ CUP (150 ML)

Tip

This relish is especially strong when it's first mixed up, but it mellows as it ferments.

- **Mortar and pestle, or spice grinder**
- **1-cup (250 mL) canning jar**

¼ tsp	cumin seeds	1 mL
¼ tsp	coriander seeds	1 mL
¼ tsp	fennel seeds	1 mL
¼ cup	grated peeled fresh turmeric	60 mL
2 tbsp	mashed pitted umeboshi	30 mL
¼ tsp	salt	1 mL

1. In a small skillet, combine cumin, coriander and fennel seeds. Toast over low heat, stirring or shaking pan often, for 2 to 3 minutes or until fragrant. Transfer to mortar and let cool completely.

2. Using pestle, grind seed mixture until a coarse powder forms. Pour into jar. Stir in turmeric, mashed umeboshi and salt. Cover loosely with lid and let stand at room temperature for 24 hours.

3. Seal jar with lid and refrigerate for at least 1 week before serving. Refrigerate sealed jar for up to 1 month.

Health Tips

Turmeric is an herb that has been well researched for its health-promoting effects. It is a powerful anti-inflammatory and has been shown to help reduce arthritis pain. It is high in beta-carotene, acts as a powerful antioxidant and can be used to help regulate blood sugar.

Umeboshi are a beneficial digestive and are also used in Chinese herbal medicine to relieve coughs.

If you are looking for a slightly warming, aromatic, digestive condiment with a savory and sour flavor, this is it! It prevents and soothes mild indigestion.

Chunky Bitter Melon Relish with Miso and Tomato

If you have not tried the inimitable and distinctively bitter vegetable known as bitter melon, this condiment might be a good introduction. This relish is a powerful detoxifier — and a tasty condiment. The strong umami flavors in the sauce temper the sharp flavor of the bitter melon.

**MAKES
1 CUP (250 ML)**

Tip

There are two varieties of bitter melon. One is shiny and light green, with smooth, elongated bumps. The other is darker green with sharp, pointy bumps. We prefer the latter for its firmer texture.

Caution

If you are pregnant, nursing or trying to conceive, be moderate in your bitter melon intake. Eating too much can cause digestive issues, such as bloating, diarrhea or abdominal cramping. In pregnancy, the medicinal element, *Momordica charantia*, can cause toxicity in some people. It also can disturb the fetus and cause premature labor.

8 oz	bitter melons (2 or 3 small)	250 g
1 tsp	salt	5 mL
1 tbsp	avocado oil	15 mL
1 tbsp	hulled hemp seeds	15 mL
1 tsp	yellow or brown mustard seeds	5 mL
1 tbsp	tomato paste	15 mL
1 tbsp	white or red miso	15 mL
1 tsp	freshly squeezed lime juice	5 mL

1. Cut bitter melons in half lengthwise and scrape out seeds and white pulp. Cut crosswise into $1/8$-inch (3 mm) thick slices. In a medium bowl, toss bitter melon slices with salt. Let stand for 30 minutes.

2. In a medium saucepan, bring 4 cups (1 L) water to a boil. Drain bitter melon and add to pan. Return to a boil. Remove from heat and drain well.

3. In a large skillet, heat oil over medium-high heat, swirling to coat bottom of pan. Add hemp and mustard seeds. Cook, stirring, for 30 seconds. Add bitter melon, tomato paste, miso and lime juice.

4. Reduce heat to low and cook, stirring often and adding a little water if necessary to prevent sticking, for 5 to 7 minutes or until bitter melon is tender. Serve immediately or refrigerate in sealed jar for up to 1 week.

Health Tip

If you have a tendency toward high blood sugar or suffer from diabetes, eat this condiment once or twice a week.

Resources and Recommended Reading

The books below served as sources of learning, understanding and inspiration in the writing of this book.

Chinese Medicine

Flaws, Bob. *Chinese Medicinal Wines and Elixirs*. Boulder, CO: Blue Poppy Press, 1994.

Flaws, Bob. *The Book of Jook: Chinese Medicinal Porridges — A Healthy Alternative to the Typical Western Breakfast*. Boulder, CO: Blue Poppy Press, 1995.

Flaws, Bob, and Honora Lee Wolfe. *Prince Wen Hui's Cook: Chinese Dietary Therapy*. Brookline, MA: Paradigm, 1983.

Fruehauf, Heiner. *The Five Organ Networks of Chinese Medicine*. Portland, OR: National University of Natural Medicine, 1997.

Kaptchuk, Ted. *The Web That Has No Weaver: Understanding Chinese Medicine*. New York: Congdon and Weed, 1983.

Larre, Claude, and Elisabeth Rocha de la Vallée. *Spleen and Stomach*. London: Monkey Press, 2004.

Maciocia, Giovanni. *The Foundations of Chinese Medicine*. New York: Churchill Livingstone, 1998.

Maciocia, Giovanni. *Obstetrics and Gynecology in Chinese Medicine*. New York: Churchill Livingstone, 1998.

Ni, Maoshing. *The Yellow Emperor's Classic of Medicine: A New Translation of the Neijing Suwen with Commentary*. Boulder, CO: Shambala Press, 1995.

O'Neill, Molly. *Using Chinese Medicine During the Postpartum Period: Zuo Yue Zi for All Women and Common Postpartum Conditions*. Masters thesis. Portland OR: National University of Natural Medicine, Spring 2006.

Unschuld, Paul U. *Forgotten Traditions of Ancient Chinese Medicine: A Chinese View from the 18th Century*. Brookline, MA: Paradigm, 1990.

Wilms, Sabine. "Nurturing Life in Classical Chinese Medicine: Sun Simiao on Healing without Drugs, Transforming Bodies and Cultivating Life." *Journal of Chinese Medicine* 93 (June 2010): 5–13. Online at https://www.happygoatproductions.com

Wilms, Sabine. "Eating for Long Life: Sun Simiao on Dietetics." *Register of Chinese Herbal Medicine Journal* 10 (Autumn 2013): 28–34. Online at https://www.happygoatproductions.com

Yang, Shou-zhong. *The Divine Farmer's Materia Medica: A Translation of the Shen Ning Ben Cao Jing*. Boulder, CO: Blue Poppy Press, 1997.

Yang, Shou-zhong, and Jian-yong Li. *Li Dong Yuan's Treatise on the Spleen and Stomach: A Translation of the Li Wei Lun*. Boulder, CO: Blue Poppy Press, 1993.

Zhang, Zhongjing. *Jin Gui Yao Lue: Essential Prescriptions of the Golden Cabinet: Translation and Commentaries, translated by Nigel Wiseman and Sabine Wilms*. Brookline, MA: Paradigm, 2000.

Chinese Nutritional Therapy

Buell, Paul D., and Eugene N. Anderson. *A Soup for the Qan: Chinese Dietary Medicine of the Mongol Era as seen in Hu Sihui's Yinshan Zhengyao*. New York: Columbia University Press, 2000.

Clogstoun-Willmott, Jonathan. "Food in Traditional Chinese Medicine." *Journal of Chinese Medicine* 24/25 (1987): 25–30.

Jilin, Liu, and Gordon Peack. *Chinese Dietary Therapy*. New York: Churchill Livingstone, 1995.

Kastner, Joerg. *Chinese Nutrition Therapy: Dietetics in Traditional Chinese Medicine*. New York: Thieme, 2009.

Leggett, Daverick, *Helping Ourselves: A Guide to Traditional Chinese Food Energetics*. Dartington, UK: Meridian Press, 2014.

Losso, Jack N., Fereidoon Shahidi and Debasis Baghchi, Eds. *Anti-Angiogenic Functional and Medicinal Foods*. Boca Raton, FL: CRC Press, 2007.

Lu, Henry. *Chinese System of Food Cures: Prevention and Remedies*. New York: Sterling Press, 1986.

Pieroni, Andrea, and Lisa Leimar Price, Eds. *Eating and Healing: Traditional Food as Medicine.* Boca Raton, FL: CRC Press, 2006.

Pitchford, Paul. *Healing with Whole Foods: Asian Traditions and Modern Nutrition.* Berkley, CA: North Atlantic Books, 2002.

Yifang, Zhang. *Your Guide to Health with Foods and Herbs: Using the Wisdom of Traditional Chinese Medicine.* Shanghai: Shanghai Press, 2012.

Weng, Wei Jiang, and Junshi Chen. "The Eastern Perspective on Functional Foods Based in Chinese Medicine." *Nutrition Reviews* 54, no. 11 (November 1996): S11–S16.

Zhang, Enqin, Ed. *Chinese Medicated Diet.* Shanghai: Shanghai College of Traditional Chinese Medicine, 1988.

Zhang, Haosheng. "The Energetics of Food from a Classical Chinese Medicine Perspective." *Qi: The Journal of Traditional Eastern Health and Fitness* 14, no. 5 (Winter 2004–05): 32–36.

Cookbooks

Andoh, Elizabeth. *Washoku: Recipes from the Japanese Home Kitchen.* Emeryville, CA: Ten Speed Press, 2005.

Andoh, Elizabeth. *Kansha: Celebrating Japan's Vegan and Vegetarian Traditions.* Emeryville, CA: Ten Speed Press, 2010.

Bradford, Peter, and Montse Bradford. *Cooking with Sea Vegetables.* Rochester, VT: Healing Arts Press, 1988.

Dunlop, Fuchsia. *Revolutionary Chinese Cookbook: Recipes from Hunan Province.* New York: W. W. Norton, 2007.

Dunlop, Fuchsia. *The Land of Fish and Rice: Recipes from the Culinary Heart of China.* New York: W. W. Norton, 2016.

Hachisu, Nancy Singleton. *Japanese Farm Food.* Kansas City, MO: Andrews McMeel, 2012.

Hachisu, Nancy Singleton. *Preserving the Japanese Way: Traditions of Salting, Fermenting and Pickling for the Modern Kitchen.* Kansas City, MO: Andrews McMeel, 2015.

Hutton, Wendy. *The Food of China: Authentic Recipes from the Middle Kingdom.* New York: Periplus, 1999.

Magariños-Rey. Hélène. *Cuisine-santé aux algues marines*, Condé-sur-Poireau, France: Charles Corlet, 1997.

McEachern, Leslie. *The Angelica Home Kitchen: Recipes and Rabble Rousing from an Organic Vegan Restaurant.* Emeryville, CA: Ten Speed Press, 2003.

Simonds, Nina. *A Spoonful of Ginger: Irresistible, Health-Giving Recipes from Asian Kitchens.* New York: Knopf, 1999.

Trang, Corinne. *Essentials of Asian Cuisine: Fundamentals and Favorite Recipes.* New York: Simon and Schuster, 2003.

Wang, Yuan, Warren Sheir and Mika Ono. *Ancient Wisdom, Modern Kitchen: Recipes from the East for Health, Healing, and Long Life.* Boston, MA: Da Capo Lifelong Books, 2010.

Yin-Fei Lo, Eileen. *Mastering the Art of Chinese Cooking.* San Francisco, CA: Chronicle Books, 2009.

Young, Grace. *The Wisdom of the Chinese Kitchen: Classic Family Recipes for Celebration and Healing.* New York: Simon and Schuster, 1999.

Zhao, Zhuo, and George Ellis. *The Healing Cuisine of China: 300 Recipes for Vibrant Health and Longevity.* Rochester, VT: Healing Arts Press, 1998.

Information on Herbs

Bensky, Dan, Steven Clavey and Erich Stöger. *Chinese Herbal Medicine: Materia Medica.* Seattle, WA: Eastland Press, 2004.

Dharmananda, Subhuti. Perilla *Leaf.* Online at www.itmonline.org/articles/perilla/perilla.htm

Dharmananda, Subhuti. *Turmeric: What's in an Herb Name? How Turmeric (Jiang Huang) and Curcuma (Yu Jin) Became Confused.* Portland, OR: Institute for Traditional Medicine, 1999.

Foster, Steven, and Yue Congxi. *Herbal Emissaries: Bringing Chinese Herbs to the West.* Rochester, VT: Healing Arts Press, 1992.

Holmes, Peter. *The Energetics of Western Herbs: A Materia Medica Integrating Western and Chinese Herbal Therapeutics, Volumes 1 and 2.* Santa Rosa, CA: Snow Lotus Press, 1997.

Tierra, Michael. *The Way of Herbs: Revised Edition — Updated with the Latest Developments in Herbal Science.* New York: Pocket Books: 1980.

Zong, Xiao-fan, and Gary Liscum. *Chinese Medicinal Teas: Simple, Proven, Folk Formulas for Common Diseases and Promoting Health*. Boulder, CO: Blue Poppy Press, 1996.

General Writings on Food, Food and Health, Food and Culture

Ang, Audra. *To the People, Food is Heaven: Stories of Food and Life in a Changing China*. Guilford, CT: Lyons Press, 2012.

Briley, Julie, and Courtney Jackson. *Food as Medicine Everyday: Reclaim Your Health with Whole Foods*. Portland, OR: NUNM Press, 2016.

Brillat-Savarin, Jean Anthelme. *The Physiology of Taste: or Meditations on Transcendental Gastronomy*. New York: Heritage Press, 1949.

Clissold, Lorraine. *Why the Chinese Don't Count Calories: 15 Secrets of a 3,000-Year-Old culture*. New York: Skyhorse, 2008.

Colbin, Annemarie. *Food and Healing: How What You Eat Determines Your Health, Your Well-Being, and the Quality of Your Life*. New York: Ballantine, 1986.

Katz, Sandor Ellix. *Wild Fermentation: The Flavor, Nutrition and Craft of Live-Culture Foods*. White River Junction, VT: Chelsea Green, 2003.

Katz, Sandor Ellix. *The Art of Fermentation: An In-Depth Exploration of Essential Concepts and Processes from around the World*. White River Junction, VT: Chelsea Green, 2012.

Kurlansky, Mark. *Salt: A World History*. New York: Penguin, 2002.

McGee, Harold. *On Food and Cooking: The Science and Lore of the Kitchen — Completely Revised and Updated*. New York: Scribner, 2004.

Nordstrom, Karin, Christian Coff, Hakan Jonsson, Lennart Nordenfelt and Ulf Gorman. "Food and Health: Individual, Cultural, or Scientific Matters." *Genes and Nutrition* 8, no. 4 (July 2013): 357–63. Online at doi 10.1007/s12263-013-0336-8

Pollan, Michael. *In Defense of Food: An Eater's Manifesto*. New York: Penguin, 2009.

Pollan, Michael. *Food Rules: An Eater's Manual*. New York: Penguin, 2009.

Pollan, Michael. *Cooked: A Natural History of Transformation*. New York: Penguin, 2013.

Valera, Stephanie. Food in Chinese Culture. *Asia Society Blog*, September 2, 2008. Online at http://asiasociety.org/blog/asia/food-chinese-culture

Zhao, Rongguang. *A History of Food Culture in China*, translated by Gangliu Wang and Aimee Yiran Wang. New York: SCPG, 2015.

Books about Foods

Creasy, Rosalind. *The Edible Asian Garden*. Clarendon, VT: Tuttle, 2000.

Larkcom, Joy. *Oriental Vegetables: The Complete Guide for the Gardening Cook*. London: Frances Lincoln, 2007.

Page, Karen, and Andrew Dornenburg. *The Flavor Bible: The Essential Guide to Culinary Creativity, Based on the Wisdom of America's Most Imaginative Chefs*. Boston, MA: Little, Brown, 2008.

Page, Karen, and Andrew Dornenburg. *The Vegetarian Flavor Bible: The Essential Guide to Culinary Creativity with Vegetables, Fruits, Grains, Legumes, Nuts, Seeds, and More, Based on the Wisdom of Leading American Chefs*. Boston, MA: Little, Brown, 2014.

Wood, Rebecca. *The New Whole Foods Encyclopedia*. New York: Penguin, 1988.

Food Resources

Many of the foods mentioned in this book may not be readily available at your local grocery store. Use the resources below to source ingredients such as herbs, spices and other foods.

CHINESE HERBS
Root and Spring
rootandspring.com
Ready-made Chinese herbal soup mixes.

Spring Wind Herbs
springwind.com
Food-grade Chinese herbs. The company's herbs are tested for pesticides and many of them are also organic.

GRAINS, BEANS/LEGUMES, NUTS, SPICES/HERBS AND INTERNATIONAL FOODS
Asian Food Grocer
asianfoodgrocer.com
Most East Asian ingredients. Read ingredient lists to make sure that what you purchase does not include added sulfites, coloring, MSG or preservatives.

Bob's Red Mill
bobsredmill.com
Grains, legumes, seeds, whole-grain flours, nuts.

Eden Foods

edenfoods.com

Grains, legumes, seeds, whole-grain flours, seaweed, dried fruits, herbs, spices, teas, oils, vinegars, many East Asian ingredients. All products are non-GMO, organic or locally sourced. All cans are BPA-free.

Gold Mine Natural Food Co.

shop.goldminenaturalfoods.com

Purveyor of organic, heirloom, kosher and high-quality grains, beans, legumes, miso, seaweeds, dried foods and fruits, umeboshi, teas, fermented foods.

Kalustyan's

kalustyans.com

Grains, legumes, seeds, whole-grain flours, coconut milk, seaweeds, dried fruits, nuts, ghee, herbs, spices, teas, oils, vinegars and many Middle Eastern ingredients.

Lundberg Family Farms

lundberg.com

Fine-quality rice and rice products.

Sadaf

sadaf.com

Grains, legumes, seeds, whole-grain flours, seaweeds, dried fruits, nuts, oils, ghee, herbs, spices, teas, vinegars, many Middle Eastern ingredients.

Sahadi's

sahadis.com

Grains, legumes, seeds, whole-grain flours, dried fruits, nuts, oils, herbs, spices, teas, vinegars, many Middle Eastern ingredients.

South River Miso

southrivermiso.com

A wide variety of delicious artisan and organic miso, including these varieties: rice, adzuki, chickpea, barley, dandelion leek, sweet white and garlic red pepper miso.

ORGANIC PRODUCE AND FOODS

Community Supported Agriculture Resources throughout North America

localharvest.org/csa

A resource to find and join a Community Supported Agriculture (CSA), where consumers buy local, seasonal food directly from a farmer.

Local Farmers Market Directory

(U.S., Canada and International)

localfarmmarkets.org

Organic Consumers Association

Organicconsumers.org

Online source for all issues that promote interests of organic and socially responsible consumers.

SEAWEEDS

Maine Coast Sea Vegetables

seaveg.com

Offers eight organically certified North Atlantic varieties of sea vegetables: alaria, dulse, kelp, laver, sea lettuce, Irish moss, rockweed and bladderwrack. It also imports well-tested organic nori sheets from China.

Maine Seaweed

theseaweedman.com

Hand-harvested dry Atlantic seaweeds and sea vegetables.

SUSTAINABLE SEAFOOD

The Monterey Bay Aquarium's Seafood Watch program (North America)

Seafoodwatch.org

Information on how to choose and buy seafood from sustainable sources.

WESTERN HERBS AND SPICES

Frontier Co-op

Frontiercoop.com

Organic herbs and spices, teas, dried fruits and vegetables.

Mountain Rose Herbs

mountainroseherbs.com

Seeds, seaweeds, oils, herbs, bulk spices, teas.

Real Salt

Realsalt.com

High-quality, mineral-rich, unrefined fine, coarse, kosher or powder sea salt.

WILD FOODS

Ryan Drum

ryandrum.com

Seaweeds and sea vegetables, herbs, wild foods and wild food seeds.

"Wildman" Steve Brill

wildmanstevebrill.com

Wild plants and mushrooms.

COOKING INSTRUCTIONS/ FOOD INFORMATION

Food & Water Watch (U.S.)

Foodandwaterwatch.org

Public-interest group that champions healthy food and clean water for all.

Rouxbe

Rouxbe.com

Online cooking school with a variety of cooking instruction for non-professionals.

United States Department of Agriculture

Food Safety and Inspection Service

fsis.usda.gov

References

CHAPTER 1

Buksh, Jacqueline. "Curing Ailments the Chinese Way." *China Eye Magazine* 23 (Autumn 2009). Online at www.sacu.org/chinesefood.html

Economic Research Service, United States Department of Agriculture. "Frequency of Food Insecurity." Updated September 6, 2017. Online at https://www.ers.usda.gov/topics/food-nutrition-assistance/food-security-in-the-us/frequency-of-food-insecurity

Feeding America. "Child Food-Insecurity Reports, 2011–17." Online at www.feedingamerica.org/hunger-in-america/our-research/map-the-meal-gap/child-food-insecurity-executive-summary.html

Wilms, Sabine. "Eating for Long Life: Sun Simiao on Dietetics." *Register of Chinese Herbal Medicine Journal* 10 (Autumn 2013): 28–34. Online at https://www.happygoatproductions.com

CHAPTER 2

Einstein, Albert. Letter to Margot Einstein, after his sister's Maja's death, 1951. Memorable Albert Einstein Quotes. Online at www.asl-associates.com/einsteinquotes.htm

Littlejohn, Ronnie. "Wuxing (Wu-hsing)." Internet Encyclopedia of Philosophy. Online at www.iep.utm.edu/wuxing

Ni, Maoshing. *Huang Di Nei Jing Suwen: The Yellow Emperor's Classic of Medicine: A New Translation of the Neijing Suwen with Commentary*. Boston, MA: Shambala, 1995: 1.

Sagan, Carl. *Cosmos*. New York: Ballantine, 1985: 59.

Violatti, Cristian. "Science." Ancient History Encyclopedia. Online at www.ancient.eu /science

Xichun, Zhang. "On the Relationship between Medicine and Philosophy." Translated and introduced by Heiner Fruehauf. *Online at https://classicalchinesemedicine.org/gpa/on-the-relationship-between-medicine-and-philosophy*

CHAPTER 3

Dharmananda, Subhuti. "Taste and Action of Chinese Herbs: Traditional and Modern Viewpoints." Institute for Traditional Medicine, 2010: 1–8. Online at www.itmonline.org/articles/taste_action/taste_action_herbs.htm

Lansky E., S. Shubert and I. Neeman. "Pharmacological and Therapeutic Properties of Pomegranate." In Melgarejo P., J.J. Martínez-Nicolás and J. Martínez-Tomé, Eds. *Production, Processing and Marketing of Pomegranate in the Mediterranean Region: Advances in Research and Technology*. Zaragoza, Israel: CIHEAM, *Options Méditerranéennes* 42 (2000): 231–35.

New Hampshire Department of Health and Social Services. *How Much Sugar Do You Eat? You May Be Surprised*. Online at https://www.dhhs.nh.gov/dphs/nhp/documents/sugar.pdf

CHAPTER 4

Dharmananda, Subhuti. *Turmeric: What's in an Herb Name? How Turmeric (Jiang Huang) and Curcuma (Yu Jin) Became Confused*. Portland, OR: Institute for Traditional Medicine, 1999. Online at www.itmonline.org/arts/turmeri3.htm

Jiang, Yong Ping. "Vinegar, the 'Bitter' Herb." *Acupuncture Today* 5, no. 7 (July 2004). Online at www.acupuncturetoday.com/mpacms/at/article.php?id=28488

CHAPTER 5

Fruehauf, Heiner. *The Five Organ Networks of Chinese Medicine*. Portland, OR: National University of Natural Medicine, 1997: 63.

Fruehauf, Heiner. *The Five Organ Networks of Chinese Medicine*: 119.

Yang, Joy. "The Human Microbiome Project: Extending the Definition of What Constitutes a Human." National Human Genome Research Institute, July 16, 2012. Online at www.genome.gov/27549400/the-human-microbiome-project-extending-the-definition-of-what-constitutes-a-human/

CHAPTER 6

Ephron, Nora. *I Feel Bad About My Neck: And Other Thoughts on Being a Woman*. New York: Vintage, 2008: 25.

Katz, Sandor Ellix. *The Art of Fermentation: An In-Depth Exploration of Essential Concepts and Processes from around the World*. White River Junction, VT: Chelsea Green, 2012: 24.

Katz, Sandor Ellix. Workshop on Fermentation at the National University of Natural Medicine. Portland, OR, February 10, 2017.

National Cancer Institute, National Institutes of Health. "Chemicals in Meat Cooked at High Temperatures and Cancer Risk." Reviewed October 19, 2015. Online at https://www.cancer.gov/about-cancer/causes-prevention/risk/diet/cooked-meats-fact-sheet

Wang, Hwa L., and S. F. Fang. *History of Chinese Fermented Foods*. Chapter 2 in C.W. Hesseltine and Hwa L. Wang, Eds., *Mycologia Memoir No. 11, Indigenous Fermented Food of Non-Western Origin*: 34. Online at https://naldc.nal.usda.gov/download/23848/PDF

CHAPTER 7

Fruehauf, Heiner. *The Five Organ Networks of Chinese Medicine*. Portland, OR, 1998: 67–68.

Maciocia, Giovanni. *The Foundations of Chinese Medicine*. New York: Churchill Livingstone, 1989: 111.

Sun, Jing, et al. "To Unveil the Molecular Mechanisms of Qi and Blood through Systems Biology-Based Investigation into Si-Jun-Zi-Tang and Si-Wu-Tang Formulae." *Scientific Reports* 6 (2016): 34328. Online at doi: 10.1038/srep34328

CHAPTER 8

Baldwa, V. S., C. M. Bhandari, A. Pangaria and R. K. Goyal. "Clinical Trial in Patients with Diabetes Mellitus of an Insulin-Like Compound Obtained from Plant Source." *Upsala Journal of Medical Sciences* 82 (1977): 39–41.

CHAPTER 9

Fruehauf, Heiner. "Alcohol Use in Traditional Chinese Formulas," 2006. Online at https://classical chinesemedicine.org/?s=alcohol+use +in+traditional+chinese+formulas

Kirkpatrick, Kristin. "Avoid These 10 Foods Full of Trans Fats." Cleveland Clinic. Online at https://health.clevelandclinic. org/2015/07/avoid-these-10-foods-full-of-trans-fats

Mayo Clinic Staff. "Artificial Sweeteners and Other Sugar Substitutes." Mayo Clinic. Online at www.mayoclinic.org/ healthy-lifestyle/nutrition-and-healthy-eating/in-depth/artificial-sweeteners/art-20046936

Mercola, Joseph. "Top 10 Food Additives to Avoid." Food Matters. Online at www.foodmatters.com/ article/top-10-food-additives-to-avoid

Ni, Maoshing. *The Yellow Emperor's Classic of Internal Medicine: A New Translation of the Neijing Suwen with Commentary.* Boulder, CO: Shambhala Press, 1995: 59.

Non-GMO Project. "High-Risk Crops and Inputs." Online at https:// www.nongmoproject.org/gmo-facts/high-risk/

Potera Carol. "Diet and Nutrition: The Artificial Food Dye Blues." *Environmental Health Perspective* 118, no. 10 (October 2010): A428. Online at https://www.ncbi.nlm. nih.gov/pmc/articles/PMC2957945

Sugar Science, University of California-San Francisco. "Hidden in Plain Sight." Online at http://sugarscience.ucsf. edu/hidden-in-plain-sight/#. WduTJsZrzm4

Young, Grace. "How to Care for Your Carbon-Steel Wok." *Fine Cooking* 117: 66. Online at https://www.finecooking.com/ item/42905/how-to-care-for-your-carbon-steel-wok

Wilson, Brian, and Sami Bahna. "Adverse Reactions to Food Additives." *Annals of Allergy, Asthma and Immunology* 95, no. 6 (December 2005): 499–507. Review PMID. Online (limited) at *https://www.ncbi.nlm.nih.gov/ pubmed/16400887.*

Food and Nutrition Labeling

United States Food and Drug Administration. "How To Understand and Use the Nutrition Facts Label." Updated October 2, 2017. Online at https://www.fda.gov/food/ ingredientspackaginglabeling/ labelingnutrition/ucm274593.htm

Wolfram, Taylor. "The Basics of the Nutrition Facts Label." Academy of Nutrition and Dietetics. Reviewed August 2017. Online at www.eatright.org/resource/food/ nutrition/nutrition-facts-and-food-labels/the-basics-of-the-nutrition-facts-panel

CHAPTER 10

Chinese Herbs Healing. "Schizandra Berry (Wu Wei Zi)." Chinese Herbs Healing. Online at www.chineseherbshealing.com/ schizandra-berry

Dharmananda, Subhuti. *Perilla Leaf.* Online at www.itmonline.org/ articles/perilla/perilla.htm

Foster, Steven, and Yue Congxi. *Herbal Emissaries: Bringing Chinese Herbs to the West.* Rochester, VT: Healing Arts Press, 1992: 93, 194.

Ji, Liu. *Chinese Dietary Therapy.* New York: Churchill Livingstone, 1995: 58.

Katz, Sandor Ellix. *Wild Fermentation: The Flavor, Nutrition and Craft of Live-Culture Foods.* White River Junction, VT: Chelsea Green, 2003: 139, 185.

Mountain Rose Herbs. "White Peony Root." Online at www.mountain roseherbs.com/products/peony-root/profile

Ried, Karin, Thomas R. Sullivan, Peter Fakler, Oliver R. Frank and Nigel P. Stocks. "Effect of Cocoa on Blood Pressure." *Cochrane Database of Systematic Reviews* 8 (August 15, 2012): CD008893. Online (limited) at doi: 10.1002/14651858. CD008893.pub2

Suttie, Emma. "The Healing Power of Turmeric." Chinese Medicine Living. March 27, 2017. Online at https://www. chinesemedicineliving.com/ health-2/healing-power-of-turmeric/

Tang, Weici, and Eisenbrand, Gerhard. "*Cinnamomum cassia* Presl." *In Chinese Drugs of Plant Origin: Chemistry, Pharmacology and Use in Traditional and Modern Medicine.* Berlin: Springer-Verlag, 1992: 319–30. Online (limited) at *https://link.springer.com/chapter/10.1 007%2F978-3-642-73739-8_42*

Vogl, S., et al. "Ethnopharmacological in Vitro Studies on Austria's Folk Medicine — An Unexplored Lore in Vitro Anti-inflammatory Activities of 71 Austrian Traditional Herbal Drugs." *Journal of Ethnopharmacology* 149, no. 3 (October 2013): 750–51. PMID 23770053. Online (limited) at doi:10.1016/j.jep2013.06.007

Yamamoto, Seiichiro, Tomataka Sobue, Minatsu Kobayashi, Satoshi Sasaki and Shoichiro Tsugane. "Soy, Isoflavones, and Breast Cancer Risk in Japan." *Journal of the National Cancer Institute* 95, no. 12 (June 18, 2003): 906–13. Online at https://academic.oup.com/jnci/ article/95/12/906/2520284/Soy-Isoflavones-and-Breast-Cancer-Risk-in-Japan

Acknowledgments

The writing of this book would not have been possible without several serendipitous connections and many people who have contributed directly and indirectly to its writing.

First, I'd like to thank Dr. Denise Dallman, former associate dean of undergraduate studies and distance learning at the National University of Natural Medicine in Portland, Oregon, who introduced me to Bob Dees of Robert Rose Inc. — without whom this book might still be in my head and whose patience and curiosity fueled many conversations to bring this book to light. Thank you Marlene Zichlinsky for introducing me to Maya Klein, PhD. I could not have conceived more than 175 recipes without Maya's sensitive, conceptual and clear-eyed brilliance. She started out as the recipe developer for this book but became so much more and, ultimately, an invaluable collaborator. Maya, thank you for creating delicious recipes that deliver vitality with such pleasure and sensory delight.

To all my teachers, who have influenced how I perceived the world, nature, health and food, I honor you: Shizuko Yamamoto, Keichi Murata, Jeffrey Yuen, Heiner Fruehauf, PhD, Rihui Long, LAc, Mengke Kou, LAc, Huosheng Zhang, LAc, Yafei Liu, Hélène Magariños-Rey, Roger Leggett and Angelika Haring. To all the patients who have entrusted me with their care over three decades. Thank you to the National University of Natural Medicine (NUNM) and the College of Classical Chinese Medicine, my educational and professional home where I immersed myself in the spirit of medicine, to my Chinese medicine and nutrition students who teach me through their questions and to all my colleagues at NUNM. A special thank you to David Schleich, PhD, president of NUNM, who was always on my case to "write that book." Thanks to Sabine Wilms, PhD, for her input on women's health and the importance of tending to women post-partum.

Thank you Leslie McEachern, author and owner of the groundbreaking Angelica Kitchen in New York City, for preparing my first taste of organic steamed winter squash and collard greens, whose pure and vibrant flavors I can conjure in my taste memory to this day, and to her ever-steady cheering. Acknowledgments also go to: Ann Gentry, who continually encouraged me during the journey of writing; William Spear, with whom I shared years of teaching, using food as a main tool in supporting people's transformation; and David Gould, food scientist and friend who was my go-to person about everything organic and GMO. To Mary Elliott, whose discerning designer's eye and friendship is constant. A shout-out to Tara Gentile and Robin Mesch, who helped me distill big ideas down into something that could be useful in a book. Thank you to Nikol Wells, my student, who diligently entered the data for the food property tables and saved me days of work.

I want to also thank my editor, Fina Scroppo, who waded into the task of polishing my writing with great positivity and expertise. This book would not be possible without her clear editing, tenacity, patience and creativity. Thank you to the team at Robert Rose Inc. — Martine Quibell and Kelly Glover — and to the book designers at PageWave Graphics Inc., in particular Daniella Zanchetta, for making this book lovely to read.

To my mother and father, without whom I would not be who I am today. To Amy, David and Jonah, my siblings and their families, with whom I share a love for good food. My village family in Brooklyn: Sarah Safford, Gary Singer, Thai Singer, my dear departed Sylvia Harris (how I miss all the possible conversations we would have had about this book, how to make it accessible and of value to readers), Fo Wilson, Juliette Harris, Susan Siegel, Saundra Thomas and Karen McMullen — your heartfelt love is manna. To my "girl pile," Carole Warner, Lori Soule and Tami Staudt, you sustain me.

My boundless gratitude goes to my husband, Gary Weiner, who gladly tasted our recipes, worked hard to carry the burden and to support me in the writing of this book, helped bring clarity to complex thoughts, shared his medical expertise on all matters digestive, and was always brimming with ideas throughout the process. Your love and support are my foundation. And finally to our daughter, You Lian, who brings us joy, made us a family and reminds me each and every day how powerful love is.

— *Ellen*

From Maya:

Thank you to everyone who has helped me to understand what people like to consume and how to prepare it: To Mom, for imparting a joy of eating. To Ellen Goldsmith, for teaching me about a whole different world of ingredients. To Alice, for teaching me how to communicate about food. To Fina Scroppo and everyone at Robert Rose for always making it better. To Nate for field-testing the Velvety Pears. And especially to Wade and Steve for their patience through the whirlwind of recipe testing.

This book is dedicated to all those seeking health.

Index

Note: Recipes are listed under the following entries: autumn recipes; blood tonic recipes; condiment recipes; spring recipes; summer recipes; seasonal transition recipes and winter recipes.

Page references containing "t" refer to content in tables; references containing "f" refer to content in illustrations.

Library and Archives Canada Cataloguing in Publication

Goldsmith, Ellen, 1954-, author
  Nutritional healing with Chinese medicine : +175 recipes for optimal health / Ellen Goldsmith, MSOM, LAc, DipCH with Maya Klein, PhD.

Includes index.
ISBN 978-0-7788-0584-7 (softcover)

  1. Diet therapy — Popular works. 2. Medicine, Chinese — Popular works. 3. Nutrition — Popular works.
4. Cookbooks. I. Klein, Maya, author II. Title.

RM217.G65 2017   615.8'54   C2017-905975-0